BILE ACIDS
IN HEALTH
AND DISEASE

BILE ACIDS
IN HEALTH
AND DISEASE

Update on Cholesterol Gallstones and Bile Acid Diarrhoea

Editors

**Tim Northfield, Riadh Jazrawi and
Patrick Zentler-Munro**

*Department of Medicine, St. George's Hospital Medical School
London, UK*

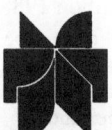

KLUWER ACADEMIC PUBLISHERS
DORDRECHT / BOSTON / LONDON

Distributors

---

for the United States and Canada: Kluwer Academic Publishers, PO Box 358, Accord Station, Hingham, MA 02018-0358, USA
for all other countries: Kluwer Academic Publishers Group, Distribution Center, PO Box 322, 3300 AH Dordrecht, The Netherlands

British Library Cataloguing in Publication Data

Bile acids in health and disease.
  1. Man. Bile acids
  I. Northfield, Tim II. Jazrawi, Riadh
  III. Zentler-Munro, Patrick
  612'.35

ISBN-13: 978-94-010-7054-6   e-ISBN-13: 978-94-009-1249-6
DOI: 10.1007/978-94-009-1249-6

Copyright

Published in the United Kingdom by Kluwer Academic Publishers,
PO Box 55, Lancaster, UK

Kluwer Academic Publishers BV incorporates the publishing programmes of
D. Reidel, Martinus Nijhoff, Dr W. Junk and MTP Press

Contents

SECTION G   DIAGNOSIS OF BILE ACID MALABSORPTION – ROLE OF ^{75}SeHCAT

Preface

Bile acids occupy a central position in in the absorption, excretion and metabolism of lipids within the body. Our understanding of their unique properties has illuminated many biochemical and biophysical processes. Animals have evolved a unique system of preserving these important detergent-like molecules within the body and reusing them many times – the enterohepatic circulation.

Disorders of the enterohepatic circulation contribute to a correspondingly wide range of diseases, and recent developments have centred in particular on cholesterol gallstone disease and bile acid diarrhoea. Successful management of these diseases is increasingly based on an understanding of the physicochemical and biochemical properties of bile acids, and of their pathophysiological role in disease.

Professor Alan Hofmann starts this book with an overview of the enterohepatic circulation of bile acids. The first section then discusses biliary lipid synthesis, transport and secretion by the liver and the solubilisation of cholesterol in the bile. The next section applies this knowledge to the pathogenesis of cholesterol gallstones. Separate chapters focus on defects in biliary lipid secretion, in cholesterol solubilisation and in gallbladder motility. The succeeding sections then review posssible approaches to gallstone prevention, and assess recent developments in non-surgical forms of treatment. Two exciting new therapies that receive particular attention are contact dissolution therapy with methyl tert-butyl ether and extracorporeal shock wave lithotripsy. Further sections turn to the absorptive functions of bile acids in health. These relate to the absorption of fat and electrolytes, and to the subsequent reabsorption of the bile acids themselves. There follows a discussion of the contribution of bile acids to the pathogenesis of diarrhoea and steatorrhoea. The most noteworthy clinical advance has been in the diagnosis of bile acid malabsorption and bile acid diarrhoea using the gamma emitting ^{75}Se radiolabelled bile acid SeHCAT, which has provided a diagnostic tool available for the first time in any hospital with a gamma camera.

This book is addressed primarily to gastrointestinal physicians and physiologists. However, anyone who shares our interest in these fascinating molecules will glean new insights fom this compendium. The invited authors are drawn from those international centres which have contributed most to our understanding. Their contributions have been heavily edited to achieve a cohesive volume of uniform style and format. As editors, we accept responsibility for any deficiencies in the final result.

Department of Medicine   *Tim Northfield*
St. George's Hospital Medical School   *Riadh Jazrawi*
London   *Patrick Zentler-Munro*

Acknowledgements

The preparation of this book was stimulated by the enthusiasm of the contributors at a meeting entitled "Bile Acids in Health and Disease" held at the Royal Society of Medicine, London in September, 1987. This meeting was generously sponsored by Dr. Herbert Falk through the Falk Foundation, and by his UK collaborators, Thames Laboratories. We would also like to thank Miss Marion Amos and Mr. Martin Lister for their valuable assistance in the production of the book.

List of Invited Contributors

Professor Helmut Ammon, Henry Ford Hospital, Detroit, USA

Professor Luigi Barbara, Università di Bologna, Italy

Professor Bengt Borgström, University of Lund, Sweden

Professor Martin Carey, Harvard Medical School, Boston, USA

Dr. Roger Coleman, University of Birmingham, UK

Dr. Martin Eastwood, Western General Hospital, Edinburgh, UK

Dr. Kurt Einarsson, Huddinge University Hospital, Sweden

Professor Serge Erlinger, Hopital Beaujon, Clichy, France

Dr. Roberto Ferraris, Ospedale Mauriziano, Turin, Italy

Dr. Ian Forgacs, King's College Hospital, London, UK

Dr. John Graham, St. George's Hospital Medical School, London, UK

Dr. Ken Heaton, Bristol Royal Infirmary, UK

Professor Alan Hofmann, University of California, San Diego, USA

Dr. Thomas Holzbach, Cleveland Clinic, USA

Dr. Kathryn Hood, Guy's Hospital Medical School, London, UK

Dr. Riadh Jazrawi, St. George's Hospital Medical School, London, UK

Dr. Alberto Lanzini, Ospedale Civili, Brescia, Italy

Dr. Patrick Zentler-Munro, Raigmore Hospital, UK

Dr. Tim Northfield, St. George's Hospital Medical School, London, UK

Professor Gustav Paumgartner, Klinikum Grosshadern, Munich, FRG

Professor Mauro Podda, Istituto di Medicina Interna, Milan, Italy

Dr. Giuseppe Sciarretta, Ospedale Maggiore, Bologna, Italy

Professor Adolf Steihl, University of Heidelberg, FRG

Professor John Thistle, Mayo Medical School, USA

1

Overview: Enterohepatic Circulation of Bile Acids – a Topic in Molecular Physiology

A.F. Hofmann
Division of Gastroenterology, University of California, San Diego
La Jolla, California 92093, USA

INTRODUCTION

In principle, the scope of physiology should begin where cell biology ends. Physiology deals with the orchestration of functions of multiple cells in different organs, the end results of which are co-ordinated physiological processes such as digestion and absorption or glucose homoeostasis. A triumph of cell biology has been the elucidation of cellular regulatory circuits, and the limiting case is that in which cells regulate their own activities so reliably that there is no need for regulatory circuits involving many organs. In a sense, by analogy, the governance of a university faculty usually uses a tiny proportion of total energy expenditure at the university because most facilities govern themselves effectively, at least most of the time.

For the enterohepatic circulation of bile acids, the major regulatory circuits are at a molecular and cell biological level, rather than at a higher level of integration. The one obvious exception to this generalisation is gastrointestinal motility, which is co-ordinated both enterally and centrally. In this brief essay, I wish to summarise my own views of the four subcirculations of bile acids encompassed in the inclusive term 'enterohepatic circulation'. It is probably useful to include the cholehepatic or biliohepatic circulation within the term enterohepatic, since the Greek word 'entero' is not very specific and could well include the biliary tract. Indeed, the tradition has been for gastroenterology to include considerations of hepatic and biliary function, physiology, and pathology, so this view has ample precedent.

In this article, four subcirculations of the enterohepatic circulation will be distinguished – by their location, mechanism of transport, and consequence of transport. Since these enterohepatic circulations involve many organs, the appropriate discipline is physiology. Yet any consideration of the

1

enterohepatic circulation must consider the relationship between chemical structure, physico-chemical properties, and cell transport. Thus, the term 'molecular physiology' seems appropriate.

BIOLOGICAL OVERVIEW

Where digestive surfactants arise in animal evolution is unclear. Digestive surfactants have been identified in invertebrates such as the crab[1], but as yet our knowledge of structure and function of digestive surfactants in invertebrates is meagre. In vertebrates, cholesterol is converted to water-soluble derivatives, termed bile salts. In primitive vertebrates, these are bile alcohol sulphates; and in higher vertebrates, bile acids are formed[2]. There are two striking physico-chemical properties of these molecules. The first is that they are large and hydrophilic, so that passive entry across the lipid domains of cell membranes is extremely limited. The second is that bile acids, and presumably some bile alcohols (as their sulphates) are amphipathic. They self-associate to form micelles which are capable of solubilising digestive lipids and also binding counterions, such as calcium[3].

A paradigm of pharmacology is the division of drug biotransformations into two general classes[4]. Type I biotransformation involves hydroxylation, oxidation/reduction of existing hydroxyl groups, but does not in general involve the addition of carbon atoms. Thus, the biotransformation of cholesterol to a C_{27} bile acid may be considered a Type I biotransformation. Type II biotransformations involve the addition of solubilising groups such as amino acids, sugars or peptides. As a result of such addition, the molecules become water-soluble, actively transported by anion carriers, and non-absorbable after secretion into bile or urine. The remarkable exception to this is bile acid amidation, in that the glycine and taurine amidates are actively reabsorbed by the terminal ileum. In contrast, bile acid glucuronides and sulphates do not undergo efficient active reabsorption[5]. Thus, amidation with glycine or taurine, in addition to all of its other physico-chemical results, leads to active bile acid reabsorption by ileal enterocytes.

Whether bile alcohol sulphates function as digestive surfactants, or whether they are actively reabsorbed by a distal intestinal transport system, is not known. If they were not actively absorbed, they would be deconjugated by the intestinal flora, or conceivably even by pancreatic or intestinal surface enzymes, and the resultant bile alcohol reabsorbed. For this to occur, a bile alcohol would have to have no more than three hydroxy groups, based on the rules of passive reabsorption of bile acids. Most of the common bile alcohols in lower vertebrates are tetrols or pentols, and consequently should not undergo passive absorption[2].

2

Cholehepatic Circulation

It has been traditional teaching, largely based on analysis of hepatic or gallbladder bile, that the bile acid molecules secreted into canalicular bile are fully conjugated. It is now clear that traces of unconjugated bile acids are present in human bile and indeed in one species (the Australian opossum) the unusual trihydroxy bile acids occurring in this species are secreted into bile completely in unconjugated form[6]. Recent work from our laboratory has suggested that C_{23} nor-bile acids are secreted into canalicular bile in part in unconjugated form, and that dihydroxy C_{23} nor-bile acids are reabsorbed passively in the biliary tree as bile flows toward the hepatic ducts[7-9]. Reabsorption is thought to occur in the protonated form, and the source of the proton is thought to be luminal carbonic acid. The absorbed bile acid molecule is resecreted into bile, and each molecule generates a manyfold increase in osmotic bile flow many times. As a consequence of this 'cholehepatic shunt' pathway, a bicarbonate-rich hypercholeresis is generated. (The term 'hypercholeresis' refers to the finding that bile acid dependent bile flow is greater than can be accounted for by the recovery of bile acids in bile.) The cholehepatic shunt pathway hypothesis predicts that one bicarbonate anion will be generated each time a bile acid molecule is absorbed passively in the biliary tree. Thus, each bile acid molecule is used at least twice for the generation of bile acid dependent bile flow; and each cycle in the cholehepatic circulation induces osmotic secretion at the canalicular level. Biliary osmolarity is maintained by the generation of bicarbonate anions, as the bile acid molecule is absorbed in its protonated form. The current view of the cholehepatic circulation is shown in Figure 1.

Cholehepatic shunting is observed when C_{23} nor-dihydroxy bile acids are administered to rodents and man, and is likely to occur when C_{24} dihydroxy bile acids are administered under conditions where they are secreted in unconjugated form into bile[10].

Whether cholehepatic shunting occurs naturally in vertebrates is not known. To demonstrate it would require (1) the presence in bile of an unconjugated lipophilic bile acid, (2) bicarbonate enrichment of bile above plasma bicarbonate concentrations, and (3) evidence that ductular bicarbonate secretion is not responsible for the bicarbonate enrichment – using a marker for canalicular bile flow such as mannitol or erythritol. In animals whose bile contains only conjugated bile acids, but in whom bile flow is high and bicarbonate rich (rabbit and guinea pig), it remains possible that there is active reabsorption of *conjugated* bile acid anions by the biliary tract epithelium – that is, that the bile ductules function in the same manner as the terminal ileum.

The surface area of the biliary tract must be many times greater than

3

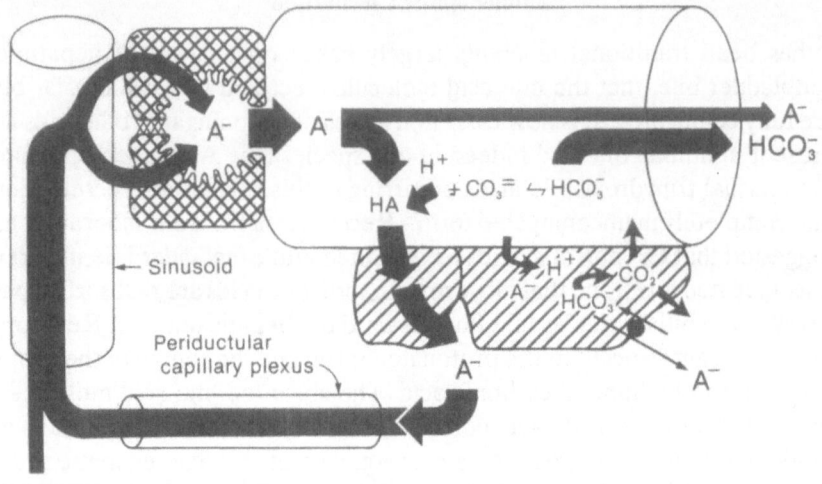

Figure 1 Schematic depiction of the cholehepatic circulation of unconjugated lipophilic dihydroxy bile acids, for example nor-ursodeoxycholic acid. The bile acid is secreted actively into the canaliculus, but is reabsorbed passively in protonated form by the biliary ductular cell, thereby generating a luminal bicarbonate ion, which maintains luminal osmolarity. The bile acid molecule crosses the luminal membrane of the cholangiocyte passively, but ionises in the cytosol. The bile acid molecule exits the cell across the basolateral membrane using a proposed bicarbonate/bile acid exchange mechanism, which results in a bicarbonate anion entering the cell. The bicarbonate anion and proton combine to form CO_2 and water, catalysed by cytosolic carbonic anhydrase. The molecule returns to the sinusoid via the periductular capillary plexus and is resecreted into bile. With each cycle through the cholehepatic shunt, bile acid dependent flow is generated by the bile acid anion, and maintained in the lumen by generation of a bicarbonate anion as the bile acid molecule is absorbed in the protonated form (modified from reference 8). Many details of this scheme remain to be proved experimentally, and it should be viewed as a working hypothesis.

that of the gallbladder and, in my judgement, it is unlikely that there is an appreciable flux of conjugated bile acids through the gallbladder epithelial cell. Ostrow showed many years ago that the rodent gallbladder is impermeable to conjugated bile acids unless it is injured[11].

Jejuno-hepatic Circulation

The discovery of active transport of bile acids by the terminal ileum[12] solved a longstanding paradox in physiology: how could bile acids undergo such efficient enterohepatic cycling, yet be so poorly absorbed from the jejunum? Evidence that the jejunum could absorb some bile acid was provided by the first perfusion studies with micellar bile acid solutions. These showed some absorption of the glycine conjugate of chenodeoxycholic (chenodeoxycholyl-

4

glycine) from the jejunum in man[13]. Later experiments supported this[14]. The development of a successful radioimmunoassay for chenodeoxycholylglycine allowed the demonstration of an early postprandial elevation in chenodeoxy-cholyl conjugates, before that of cholyl conjugates[15]. This again suggested absorption of dihydroxy glycine conjugated bile acids proximal to the terminal ileum. Angelin and Einarsson provided additional evidence for this by showing that mainly dihydroxy bile acids disappeared from small intestinal contents collected from the proximal ileum[16], and by using mass spectrometry on serum to show an early peak in dihydroxy bile acids[17]. Finally, studies in patients ingesting chenodeoxycholic acid again confirmed more rapid enterohepatic cycling of chenodeoxycholic acid conjugates than of cholic acid conjugates[18].

Several lines of evidence have thus suggested that the most hydrophobic bile acid conjugates could be absorbed from the proximal small intestine. Presumably, such absorption is passive. Unconjugated dihydroxy bile acids are absorbed extremely rapidly and passively, the rate being limited by diffusion[19,20]. The glycine conjugates of dihydroxy bile acids have a pK_a of about 3.8^{21}, and when protonated, therefore, have a hydrophilicity not very different from that of trihydroxy bile acids which are absorbed slowly but detectably at alkaline pH by the small intestine[14].

The enterohepatic circulation has been simulated using a linear physiological pharmacokinetic model. This technique shows that for chenodeoxycholic acid conjugates about 15% of the total bile acids are absorbed passively from the proximal small intestine[22]. The site of this absorption has not been determined precisely in man. Recent work suggests that the duodenum actively secretes bicarbonate anions[23], and it is quite possible that the duodenum has an alkaline microenvironment close to the enterocytes. If so, the absorption of protonated glycine conjugated dihydroxy bile acids would be inhibited in the duodenum compared to the jejunum, where there is believed to be an acid microclimate in the diffusion layer coating the enterocyte[24].

The jejuno-hepatic circulation of bile acids can be considered to be useful for bile acid reclamation, but disadvantageous for lipid digestion. All in all, it does not seem to be very important, at least in man, because its magnitude is small. The arguments against its importance are:

(1)   Maximal jejuno-hepatic reclamation of bile acids should occur when the bile acid pool is changed to predominantly decxycholic acid or chenodeoxycholic acid (assuming that most bile acid is amidated with glycine). Even then, there appears to be little increase in overall bile acid secretion, which means that there is little increase in overall intestinal absorption[25-28].

(2)   The passive absorption of bile acids from the jejunum should be diminished by taurine feeding, as taurine conjugated bile acids, irrespective of the degree of nuclear hydroxylation, presumably cannot be absorbed passively from the proximal intestine. In fact, taurine feeding does cause a small diminution in the size of the bile acid pool, but the effect is not marked[29].

Recent experimental evidence suggests that, in the neonatal rat, the jejunal mucosal permeability is greatly increased: the increase in permeability to polar molecules is so great that conjugated bile acids are absorbed passively[30]. If this occurs in humans, it could contribute to the low intrajejunal concentration of bile acids reported in infants. In fish, the jejunum also appears to be permeable to taurocholate[31]. Whether this is passive paracellular permeability, or whether the enterocyte actively or passively transports taurocholate, is not clear.

Ileo-hepatic Circulation

The ileo-hepatic circulation is the key transport system in the intestinal part of the enterohepatic loop (Figure 2). Lack and Weiner deserve credit for establishing its existence[12], although important experimental observations were made previously by Baker and Searle[32], and by Tappeiner nearly a century ago[33]. Verzar indicated in his monograph[34] his 'puzzlement' that conjugated bile acids were not well absorbed from the proximal small intestine, but sodium coupled active transport was not envisioned at that time. Lack and his colleagues subsequently extended their pioneering studies and showed that the transport system transported monovalent bile acids most efficiently and that the system was a sodium-coupled secondary active transport system[35]. Presumably, the carrier protein responsible for uptake will be isolated in the next few years, and photoaffinity labelling experiments have already begun[36]. Whether it will be identical to the canalicular transport protein remains to be established.

The efficiency of ileal transport is high. In man, it appears to be close to 90% per meal, or 70 to 80% per day, depending on the bile acid. In general dihydroxy bile acids have a lower K_m and V_{max} than trihydroxy bile acids[37].

Molecules other than bile acids which are transported by the ileal uptake system have not yet been identified. Presumably, conjugated bile acids are not biotransformed during transport by the ileocyte. It is not known whether they are protein bound and, if so, to which cytoplasmic proteins.

Exit from the ileocyte via the basolateral membrane is considered to involve an anion exchange protein, and presumably is not 'uphill' in contrast to uptake from the brush border[38]. The unbound concentration of bile acids in plasma is likely to be in the nanomolar range, so that it is very easy to im-

6

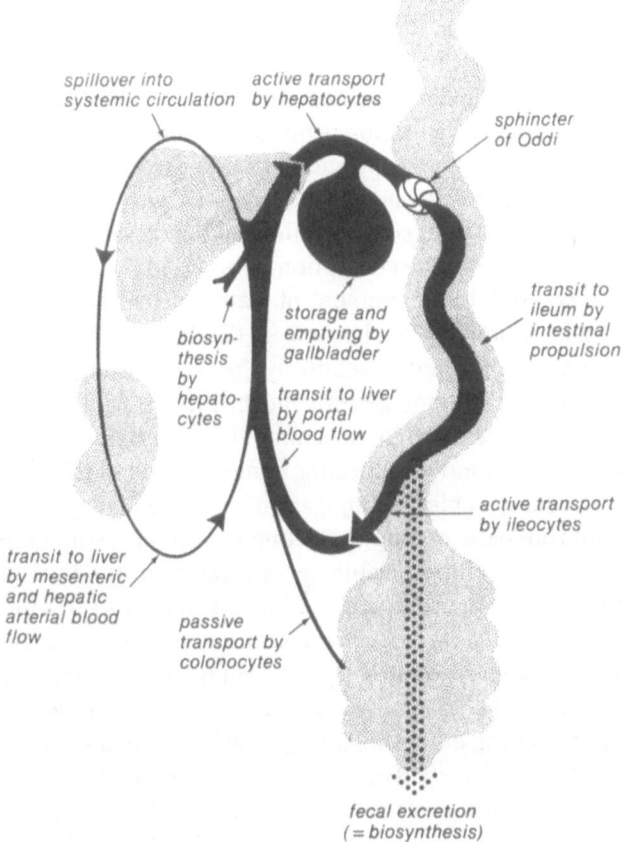

spillover into
systemic circulation

active transport
by hepatocytes

sphincter
of Oddi

transit to
ileum by
intestinal
propulsion

storage and
emptying by
gallbladder

biosyn-
thesis
by
hepato-
cytes

transit to liver
by portal
blood flow

active transport
by ileocytes

transit to liver
by mesenteric
and hepatic
arterial blood
flow

passive
transport by
colonocytes

fecal excretion
(= biosynthesis)

Figure 2 A schematic view of the enterohepatic circulation of bile acids in man. The two primary bile acids (cholic acid and chenodeoxycholic acid) are biosynthesised in the liver from cholesterol and after conjugation with glycine or taurine, are secreted into bile. The two most common secondary bile acids (deoxycholic acid and lithocholic acid) are formed in the colon by bacterial 7-hydroxylation of their corresponding primary bile acid precursor; they are then absorbed passively from the colon to enter the portal blood and join other cycling bile acids. Other components of the enterohepatic circulation include storage in, and subsequent discharge from, the gallbladder, propulsion along the small intestine to the distal ileum where efficient, active absorption occurs, and transit to the liver where efficient active uptake is followed by active resecretion into bile. The small fraction of bile acids which spills past the liver into the systemic circulation is shown. In the steady state, biosynthesis is balanced by fecal excretion.

agine that bile acid transport from the ileocyte into plasma is downhill.

The most remarkable aspect of the ileo-hepatic circulation, in addition to its capacity, specificity and efficiency, is that it is apparently 'saturated'[39]. The evidence for this is the failure of biliary bile acid secretion to increase during chronic bile acid feeding. In the new steady state that obtains, the loss of conjugates must equal the input of administered unconjugated bile acids, suggesting that the terminal ileum transport system is saturated even before bile acids are administered[40].

The mechanism of saturation is not understood. One would normally assume that the bile acid concentration in a bolus would decline exponentially as it moved caudad in the terminal ileum. More distal cells would therefore be exposed to lower concentrations of bile acids and would not be saturated. It is possible that the absorption of bile acid by the ileocytes is associated with a comparable movement of water so that the bile acid concentration remains relatively unchanged in the lumen. Were this so, the monomer concentration would be relatively the same throughout the ileum; the total concentration (the monomer concentration plus the micellar concentration) might decline through the ileum. The critical micellar concentration thus functions as a kind of saturating concentration in this theory.

There is considerable deconjugation – and reconjugation – of bile acids during enterohepatic cycling[41]. Deconjugation is presumed to occur in the terminal ileum, since appreciable deconjugation in the liver is unlikely (although a little occurs in the rodent)[42]. The magnitude of this ileal deconjugation is considerable – about 20%/cycle for glycine amidated bile acids – resulting in the amino acid moiety of glycine conjugated bile acids undergoing complete turnover daily. In contrast, taurine-amidated bile acids undergo less deconjugation during enterohepatic cycling[43]. Much of the liberated unconjugated bile acid is absorbed and reconjugated in the liver.

The fate of the carbon atoms of the glycine has been traced using ^{14}C-glycine, and most found in the breath as ^{14}CO$_2$. The chemical form in which these atoms are absorbed is not known. The rate of recovery of CO_2 from the carboxyl carbon of glycine from a glycine-conjugated bile acid is correlated with the turnover of the glycine moiety of the bile acid[44,45]. The recovery of ^{14}CO$_2$ after the administration of cholyl-l-^{14}C-glycine can be used to detect increased bile acid deconjugation[46], and this principle forms the basis of the 'bile acid breath test' whose sensitivity, specificity and general utility have been extensively studied[47,48]. Although it is generally held that the bile acid breath test is not as sensitive as some other breath tests, this work appears to have stimulated the development of a number of non-invasive methods for detecting intestinal events[49,50].

Bile acid molecules which are not absorbed by the terminal ileum cross the ileo-cecal valve. The chemical and physical form of these molecules has not been defined. Two limiting situations can be envisioned. In one, since there is considerable deconjugation in the terminal ileum, both unconjugated and conjugated bile acids will be present: the unconjugated bile acids are rapidly absorbed by passive diffusion, so that most of the bile acids passing across the ileo-cecal valve would be conjugated. In the other, the bile acids, especially unconjugated bile acids, are bound to bacteria: what would pass across the ileo-cecal valve would be those largely unconjugated bound bile acids. Probably the truth is somewhere in between.

Colono-hepatic Circulation

The flux of bile acids through the colonic mucosa is far less than that through the ileal mucosa. It is passive, and involves only unconjugated bile acids. The current view is that it probably contributes to chenodeoxycholic acid reclamation, in that the colon should be equally permeable to chenodeoxycholic acid and deoxycholic acid, the latter obviously entering the enterohepatic circulation by absorption from the colon[39]. There is no way that measurements of systemic levels of unconjugated chenodeoxycholic acid can be used to infer colonic absorption, and all simulations indicate that the magnitude of absorption of unconjugated chenodeoxycholic acid from the ileum is likely to be greater than that from the colon[39]. Nonetheless, absorption from the colon could be important because it could greatly decrease the fractional turnover rate of chenodeoxycholic acid.

Cholic acid is assumed to undergo little absorption from the colon but, as with chenodeoxycholic acid, no data are available. The absence of appreciable colonic absorption is assumed because the colon has a much lower passive permeability to cholic acid, and because cholic acid probably binds rapidly to bacteria with subsequent 7-dehydroxylation to deoxycholic acid.

Clearly, the most significant flux of bile acids from the colon is that of deoxycholic acid, which, by isotope dilution techniques, achieves one-third to one half the rate of cholic acid synthesis[39]. The proportion of deoxycholic acid in bile may exceed that of cholic acid because the turnover of deoxycholic acid is much slower than that of cholic acid. If all cholic acid is converted to deoxycholic acid, and over 50% of the deoxycholic acid is absorbed, then the proportion of deoxycholic acid in the circulating bile acids will exceed that of cholic acid[51].

Relatively little is known about factors influencing deoxycholic acid formation or absorption in man. In the Western world, where colonic transit time is long, most cholic acid entering the colon is converted to deoxycholic acid by the time stools are evacuated. The administration of antibiotics decreases deoxycholic acid formation, and slowing of colonic transit increases deoxycholic acid absorption[52]. The administration of cholestyramine decreases colonic absorption from the colon, in all probability, although no experimental observations of deoxycholic acid absorption in patients ingesting cholestyramine have been reported.

Some fraction of deoxycholic acid formed in the colon is absorbed passively and returns to the liver. In man and rabbit, deoxycholic acid is not 7-hydroxylated ,and its only biotransformation is amidation with glycine or taurine. These deoxycholyl amidates circulate with the primary bile acids. When deoxycholic acid is fed, the biliary bile acid composition becomes enriched in deoxycholic acid in a manner similar to that when chenodeoxycholic acid is fed[25]. In each case, dihydroxy bile acid conjugates appear to be preferentially transported by the terminal ileum, but whether deoxycholyl conjugates are preferred to chenodeoxycholyl conjugates is not known. If this were so, then deoxycholic acid feed would enrich the bile acid pool to a greater extent than chenodeoxycholic acid feeding would enrich the pool in chenodeoxycholic acid.

We have speculated that, in the ageing population, endogenous primary bile acids are displaced from the enterohepatic circulation by deoxycholic acid[39], but our speculation remains untested.

Lithocholic acid is also absorbed from the colon in man, although there is only one study of lithocholic acid input measured by isotope dilution kinetics[53]. When lithocholic acid reaches the liver, it is fully amidated and in part sulphated[54]. The sulphated lithocholyl amidates appear to be poorly conserved by the small intestine, so that the net conservation of lithocholate conjugates by the enterohepatic circulation is much poorer than that of deoxycholyl conjugates[55]. The unsulphated lithocholyl amidates secreted into bile are presumably absorbed passively or actively in the small intestine and return to the liver where they are again partly sulfated. With two or three passes through the liver, most lithocholate molecules are sulfated, so that the proportion of lithocholate in the enterohepatic circulation remains extremely low.

We have recently examined the proportion of lithocholate species sulfated in biliary bile acids in man. The majority of lithocholyl conjugates were sulfated, but the fraction sulfated was extremely variable[56]. The reasons for this sulfation variability are not known. One possibility is that sulfation during hepatic transport varies widely within individuals.

COMPARTMENTAL MODELLING OF THE ENTEROHEPATIC CIRCULATION

Lindstedt, in his doctoral thesis, described his classical studies which indicated that the metabolism of cholic acid could be described by a one-pool linear model[57]. Subsequent work by Vlahcevic and Swell and their colleagues indicated that this was also true for chenodeoxycholic acid[58]. Deoxycholic acid metabolism is also described by a single linear compartment model. However, lithocholic acid metabolism is more complex, requiring at least two compartments (for a reviews, see 59,60).

10

These steady state descriptions of the metabolism of the steroid moiety of bile acids were extended by experiments which characterised the turnover of the amino acid moiety. These indicated that glycine turnover was

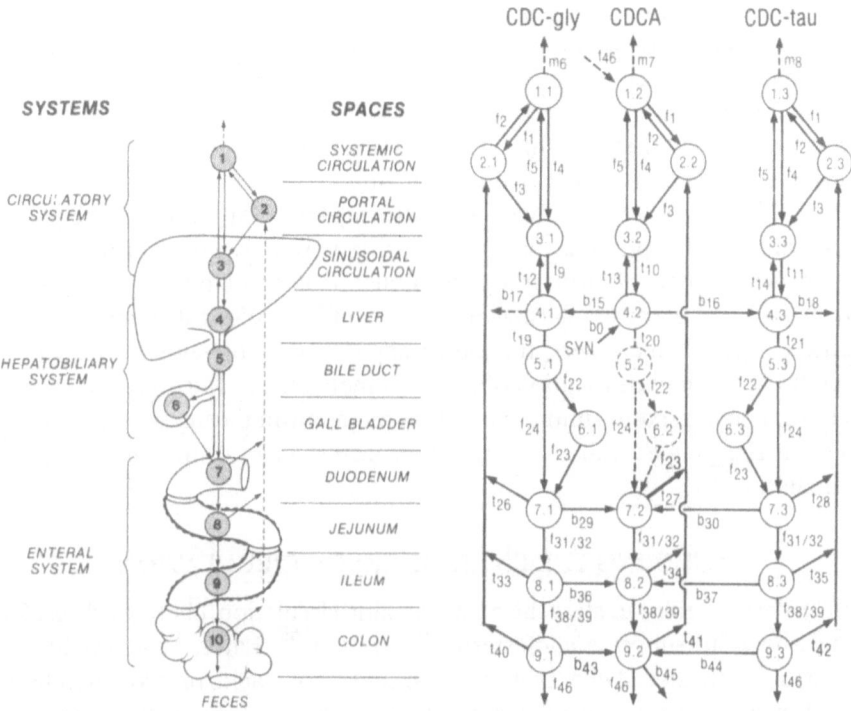

Figure 3 A physiological multicompartmental model of the enterohepatic circulation of chenodeoxycholic acid. Left, the general model with 'lumped' compartments. Right, the model with individual compartments; the three classes of compounds (glycine conjugates, taurine conjugates, and unconjugated bile acids) are shown as well as the transfer coefficients which denote movement from one compartment to another by flow (f), transport (t), or biotransformation (b). For details, see references 22, 39 and 66.

far more rapid than that of the associated steroid moiety[44,45]. Steady state models were thus developed which included both the steroid and amino acid moieties; such models were the result of the talented endeavours of Neville Hoffman[51,61]. These models were used to simulate the experimental data collected previously by Gershon Hepner[43-45], with excellent agreement.

Radioimmunoassays for conjugated bile acids were then developed, first by Wilfred Simmonds in consultation with VLW Go[62]. It was clearly desirable to describe a model which dealt with dynamic aspects of bile acid metabolism. During this time the general field of physiological pharmacokinetic modelling had been conceived by Bischoff and Brown[63] (for

11

review, see 64), but the development of a model for bile acid metabolism was the result of a collaboration with a group of colleagues in Torino, who had already performed elegant pharmacokinetic analyses of bromosulphthalein metabolism[65]. In collaboration with Gianpaolo Molino and with the encouragement of Mario Milanese, as well as the talented labours and insights of Gustavo Belforte and Basilio Bono, models for cholic acid metabolism[66] and subsequently chenodeoxycholic acid metabolism[22] were described and used for simulation. Last year the model was satisfactorily applied to deoxycholic acid metabolism[39]. Figure 3 illustrates the model, as applied to chenodeoxycholic acid metabolism in man.

This work seems to have had little impact so far on other disciplines including clinical pharmacology and gastroenterology. This is probably because bile acid metabolism differs from that of all common drugs (or so it is believed) and because pharmacokinetics is of little interest to most gastroenterologists. Nonetheless, the model appears to be of value for providing the first complete description of bile acid metabolism. Recently, the model has also been used to simulate bile acid metabolism during portal-systemic venous shunting as well as several other disturbances of the enterohepatic circulation[67].

ALTERING THE ENTEROHEPATIC CIRCULATION

In an early attempt to alter the enterohepatic circulation, cholic acid was fed and shown to suppress cholesterol biosynthesis[68]. Later, Schoenfield and Thistle administered chenodeoxycholic acid, cholic acid, or hyodeoxycholic acid in an attempt to expand the bile acid pool and diminish cholesterol saturation in bile[69]. Of these three bile acids, only chenodeoxycholic acid was found to induce bile desaturation and, with time, to induce cholesterol gallstone dissolution[70]. This started a world-wide campaign to define the safety, efficacy, and utility of bile acid administration for cholesterol gallstone dissolution[70]. Subsequently investigators have administered deoxycholic acid[25] or ursodeoxycholic acid[27]; in each instance, enrichment of the administered bile acid was observed.

Administered hyodeoxycholic acid, in contrast, does not accumulate in bile. This remarkable finding, first noted by Thistle and Schoenfield, was explained some 15 years later when Saquet, Parquet, and Infante and their colleagues showed that hyodeoxycholic acid was actively glucuronidated at the 6-position and excreted in urine as well as bile[71].

When a bile acid is administered in unconjugated form, it is likely to be absorbed from the small intestine: the more hydrophobic the bile acid, the greater the degree of passive absorption. Its conservation in the enterohepatic circulation requires amidation by the liver and subsequent efficient reclamation by the ileum. If a bile acid is glucuronidated or sulfated, it will not be efficiently conserved by the small intestine[15]. If a bile acid amidate is administered, its absorption depends on its affinity for the ileal transport system. The current strategy for promoting bile acid accumulation in the enterohepatic circulation is to identify bile acids which are rapidly (passively) absorbed and efficiently amidated in the liver, and whose amidates are well absorbed by the ileal transport system. The one remarkable exception is cholic acid, whose administration leads to accumulation of deoxycholyl conjugates in the enterohepatic circulation[26].

Bile acid administration has so far been used primarily for the induction of biliary cholesterol desaturation and cholesterol gallstone dissolution. Following the provocative report from Poupon *et al.*[72] experiments are planned to test whether ursodeoxycholic acid administration is of benefit in patients with primary biliary cirrhosis or other types of chronic inflammatory liver disease. The utility of 'enterohepatic drugs' has been discussed elsewhere[73]. The great advantage, at least in principle, is to deliver high drug concentrations to the epithelial cells lining the organs participating in the enterohepatic circulation. To the extent that such molecules increase the flux through the enterohepatic circulation, they will also induce bile acid dependent bile flow, and possibly modulate biliary lipid secretion as well as other hepatocyte or ileocyte events.

SUMMARY

The overall description of the enterohepatic circulation of bile acids in man is approaching completion. The enterohepatic circulation has not been characterised in any other vertebrate as completely as in man. So, much remains to be done in comparative pharmacology just from a descriptive standpoint.

Bile acids in plasma can now be measured with sensitivity and specificity, although methods remain rather difficult and not widely available[74]. A satisfactory gamma-emitting bile acid is now available to the clinical community[75,76]. Although its clinical utility remains unclear, it is an elegant radiochemical achievement, and it will certainly prove to be of value to the bile acid researcher.

The discovery that C_{23} nor-bile acids are metabolised by the liver as drugs and do not circulate in the enterohepatic circulation highlights the key role of the isopentanoic acid side-chain structure as a determinant of the hepatic biotransformation and subsequent intestinal reabsorption of bile acids. The essential role of the ileum in closing the loop of the enterohepatic circulation has become progressively clearer with each decade.

The challenge for the future is to develop bile acid derivatives which

13

can solve the problem of bile acid deficiency in cholestatic disease or conditions of bile acid malabsorption, and to find new bile acids which will achieve desired effects on bile flow and biliary lipid secretion. Another obvious deficiency in our knowledge is the structure of the enzymes that are responsible for bile acid biosynthesis and the transport proteins mediating transmembrane transport. The isolation, sequencing, and cloning of these key proteins is an exciting challenge to us.

Acknowledgement

The author's work is supported by NIH Grants DK 21506 and DK 32130, as well as a grant-in-aid from the Falk Foundation, e.V. of Freiburg, West Germany. This article was delivered as the Burroughs–Wellcome Lecture at a symposium sponsored by the Royal Society of Medicine

REFERENCES

1. Vonk, H.J. (1962). Emulgators in the digestive fluids of invertebrates. *Arch. Intern. Physiol.*, 70, 67–85
2. Hoshita, T. (1985). Bile alcohols and primitive bile acids. In: Danielsson, H. and Sjövall, J. (ed), *Sterols and Bile Acids*, pp. 279–302. (Amsterdam: Elsevier)
3. Hofmann, A.F. and Mysels, K.J. (1988). Bile salts as biological surfactants. *Colloids and Surfaces*, 30, 145–73
4. Williams, R.T. (1971). Introduction: pathways of drug metabolism. *Handb. Exp. Pharmacol.*, 28, 226
5. Cohen, B.I., Hofmann, A.F., Mosbach, E.H., Stenger, R.J., Rotschild, M.A., Hagey, L.R. and Yoon, Y.B. (1986). Differing effects of nor-ursodeoxycholic or ursodeoxycholic acid on hepatic histology and bile acid metabolism in the rabbit. *Gastroenterology*, 91, 189–97
6. Lee, S.P., Lester, R. and St. Pyrek, J. (1987). Vulpecholic acid (1α, 3α, 7α-trihydroxy-5β-cholan-24-oic acid): a novel bile acid of a marsupial, Trichosurus vulpecula lesson. *J. Lipid Res.*, 28, 19-31
7. Hofmann, A.F., Palmer, K.R., Yoon, Y.B., Hagey, L.R., Gurantz, D., Huijghebaert, S., Converse, J.L., Cecchetti, S. and Michelotti, E. (1985). The biological utility of bile acid conjugation with glycine or taurine. In: Matern, S, Bock, KW and Gerok, W (eds), *Advances in Glucuronide Conjugation*, pp. 245–64. (Lancaster: MTP Press)
8. Yoon, Y.B., Hagey, L.R., Hofmann, A.F., Gurantz, D., Michelotti, E.L. and Steinbach, J.H. (1986). Effect of side-chain shortening on the physiologic properties of bile acids: hepatic transport and effect on biliary secretion of 23-nor-ursodeoxycholate in rodents. *Gastroenterology*, 90, 837–52
9. Palmer, K.R., Gurantz, D., Hofmann, A.F., Clayton, L.M., Hagey, L.R. and Cecchetti, S. (1987). Hypercholeresis induced by nor-chenodeoxycholate in biliary fistula rodent. *Am. J. Physiol.*, 252, G219–28
10. Lake, J.R., Renner, E.L., Scharschmidt, B.F., Cragoe, E.J. Jr, Hagey, L.R., Lambert, K.J., Gurantz, D. and Hofmann, A.F. The relationship between ursodeoxycholate hypercholeresis and ursodeoxycholate biotransformation. *Gastroenteroly*, (In press)
11. Ostrow, J.D. (1971). Absorption of organic compounds by injured gallbladder. *J. Lab. Clin. Med.*, 78, 255–64
12. Lack, L. and Weiner, I.M. (1961). *In vitro* absorption of bile salts by small intestine of rats and guinea pigs. *Am. J. Physiol.*, 200, 313–17

13. Borgstrom, B., Lundh, G. and Hofmann, A.F. (1963). The site of absorption of conjugated bile salts in man. *Gastroenterology*, **45**, 229–38
14. Hislop, I.G., Hofmann, A.F. and Schoenfield, L.J. (1967). Determinants of the rate and site of bile acid absorption in man. *J. Clin. Invest.*, **46**, 1070, (abstract)
15. Schalm, S.W., LaRusso, N.F., Hofmann, A.F., Hoffman, N.E., van Berge Henegouwen, G.P. and Korman, M.G. (1978). Diurnal serum levels of primary conjugated bile acids. Assessment by specific radioimmunoassays for conjugates of cholic and chenodeoxycholic acid. *Gut*, **19**, 1006–14
16. Angelin, B., Einarsson, K. and Hellstrom, K. (1976). Evidence for the absorption of bile acids in the proximal small intestine of normo- and hyperlipidaemic subjects. *Gut*, **17**, 420–5
17. Angelin, B., Bjorkhem, I., Einarsson, K. and Ewerth, S. (1982). Hepatic uptake of bile acids in man. Fasting and postprandial concentrations of individual bile acids in portal venous and systemic blood serum. *J. Clin. Invest.*, **70**, 724–31
18. Einarsson, K. and Grundy, S. (1980). Effects of feeding cholic acid and chenodeoxycholic acid on cholesterol absorption and hepatic secretion of biliary lipids in man. *J. Lipid Res.*, **21**, 23–34
19. van Berge Henegouwen, G.P. and Hofmann, A.F. (1977). Pharmacology of chenodeoxycholic acid. II. Absorption and metabolism. *Gastroenterology*, **73**, 300–9
20. Dupas, J.L. and Hofmann, A.F. (1984). Passive jejunal absorption of bile acids *in vivo*: Structure–activity relationships and rate limiting steps. *Gastroenterology*, **86**, 1067 (Abstract)
21. Fini, A. and Roda, A. (1987). Chemical properties of bile acids. IV. Acidity constants of glycine-conjugated bile acids. *J. Lipid Res.*, **28**, 755–9
22. Molino, G., Hofmann, A.F., Cravetto, C., Belforte, G. and Bona, B. (1986). Simulation of the metabolism and enterohepatic circulation of endogenous chenodeoxycholic acid in man using a physiological pharmacokinetic model. *Europ. J. Clin. Invest.*, **16**, 397–414
23. Isenberg, J.I., Hogan, D.L., Koss, M.A. and Selling, J.A. (1986). Human duodenal mucosal bicarbonate secretion: evidence for basal secretion and stimulation by hydrochloric acid and a synthetic prostaglandin E_1 analogue. *Gastroenterology*, **91**, 370–8
24. Lucas, M. (1983). Determination of acid surface pH *in vivo* in rat proximal jejunum. *Gut*, **24**, 734–9
25. LaRusso, N.F., Szczepanik, P.A., Hofmann, A.F. and Coffin, S.B. (1977). Effect of deoxycholic acid ingestion on bile acid metabolism and biliary lipid secretion in normal subjects. *Gastroenterology*, **72**, 132–40
26. LaRusso, N.F., Hoffman, N.E., Hofmann, A.F., Northfield, T.C. and Thistle, J.L. (1975). Effect of primary bile acid ingestion on bile acid metabolism and biliary lipid secretion in gallstone patients. *Gastroenterology*, **69**, 1301–14
27. Nilsell, K., Angelin, B., Leijd, B. and Einarsson, K. (1983). Comparative effects of ursodeoxycholic and chenodeoxycholic acid on bile acid kinetics and biliary lipid secretion in humans. Evidence for different modes of action on bile acid synthesis. *Gastroenterology*, **85**, 1248–56
28. von Bergmann, K., Epple-Gutsfeld, M. and Leiss, O. (1984). Differences in the effects of chenodeoxycholic and ursodeoxycholic acids on biliary lipid secretion and bile acid synthesis in patients with gallstones. *Gastroenterology*, **87**, 136–43
29. Hardison, W.G.M. and Grundy, S.M. (1984). Effect of ursodeoxycholate and its taurine conjugate on bile acid synthesis and cholesterol absorption. *Gastroenterology*, **87**, 130–5
30. Stahl, G.E., Fayer, J.C. and Watkins, J.B. (1987). Rapid passive proximal bile salt (BS) absorption alters the enterohepatic circulation (EHC) in young rats. *Gastroenterology*, **92**, 1781 (Abstract)
31. Honkanen, R.E., Rigler, M.W. and Patton, J.S. (1985). Dietary fat assimilation and bile salt absorption in the killifish intestine. *Am. J. Physiol.*, **249**, G399–407

32. Baker, R.D. and Searle, G.W. (1960). Bile salt absorption at various levels of rat small intestine. *Proc. Soc. Exp. Biol. Med.*, **105**, 521–3
33. Tappeiner, A.J.F.H. (1878). Ueber die Aufsaugung der Gallsauren alkalien im Dunndarme. *Wien. Akad. Sitzber.*, **77**, 281–304
34. Verzar, F. (1936). *Absorption from the Intestine*, 294 pp. (London: Longmans, Green & Co)
35. Weiner, I.M. and Lack, L. (1968). Bile salt absorption. Enterohepatic circulation. In: Code, CF (ed), *Handbook of Physiology*, Section 6: Alimentary Canal, pp. 1439–55. (Washington DC: American Physiological Society)
36. Kramer, W., Burckhardt, G., Wilson, F.A. and Kurz, G. (1983). Bile salt-binding polypeptides in brush-border membrane vesicles from rat small intestine revealed by photoaffinity labeling. *J. Biol. Chem.*, **258**, 3623–7
37. Wilson, FA. The intestinal transport of bile acids. In: *Handbook of Physiology*. (In press)
38. Weinberg, S.L., Burckhardt, G. and Wilson, F.A. (1986). Taurocholate transport by rat intestinal basolateral membrane vesicles. Evidence for the presence of an anion exchange transport system. *J. Clin. Invest.*, **78**, 44–50
39. Hofmann, A.F., Cravetto, C., Molino, G., Belforte, G. and Bona, B. (1987). Simulation of the metabolism and enterohepatic circulation of endogenous deoxycholic acid in man using a physiological pharmacokinetic model for bile acid metabolism. *Gastroenterology*, **93**, 693–709
40. Hofmann, A.F. (1983). Pharmacology of chenodeoxycholic and ursodeoxycholic acid in man. In: Paumgartner, G., Stiehl, A. and Gerok, W. (eds), *Bile Acids and Cholesterol in Health and Disease*, pp. 301–36. (Lancaster: MTP Press)
41. Hofmann, A.F. (1977). The enterohepatic circulation of bile acids in man. *Clin. Gastroenterol.*, **6**, 3–24
42. Hagey, L.R., Neoptolemos, J.P., Rossi, S.S., Ton-Nu, H.-T., Hofmann, A.F. and Whitney, J.O. (1985). Deamidation and ester glucuronidation: New side chain biotransformations of bile acids occurring in mammals. *Hepatology*, **5**, 1023 (Abstract)
43. Hepner, G.W., Sturman, J.A., Hofmann, A.F. and Thomas, P.J. (1973). Metabolism of steroid and amino acid moieties of conjugated bile acids in man. III. Cholyltaurine (taurocholic acid). *J. Clin. Invest.*, **52**, 433–40
44. Hepner, G.W., Hofmann, A.F. and Thomas, P.J. (1972). Metabolism of steroid and amino acid moieties of conjugated bile acids in man. I. Cholylglycine. *J. Clin. Invest.*, **51**, 1889–97
45. Hepner, G.W., Hofmann, A.F. and Thomas, P.J. (1972). Metabolism of steroid and amino acid moieties of conjugated bile acids in man. II. Glycine-conjugated dihydroxy bile acids. *J. Clin. Invest.*, **51**, 1898–1905
46. Fromm, H., Thomas, P.J. and Hofmann, A.F. (1973). Sensitivity and specificity in tests of distal ileal function. Prospective comparison of bile acid and vitamin B12 absorption in ileal resection patients. *Gastroenterology*, **64**, 1077–90
47. Lauterberg, B.H., Newcomer, A.D. and Hofmann, A.F. (1978). Clinical value of the bile acid breath test: evaluation of the Mayo Clinic experience. *Mayo. Clin. Proc.*, **53**, 227–33
48. O'Connor, M.P., Healy, M., Kehely, A., Keane, C.T., O'Moore, R.R. and Weir, D.G. (1987). H2- or ^{14}C-breath tests in the diagnosis of small intestinal bacterial overgrowth. *Gut*, **10**, A1353 (Abstract)
49. Newcomer, A.D., Hofmann, A.F., DiMagno, E.P., Thomas, P.J. and Carlson, G.L. (1979). Triolein breath test: a sensitive and specific test for fat malabsorption. *Gastroenterology*, **76**, 6–13
50. Graham, D.Y., Klein, P.D., Evans, D.J., Alpert, L.C., Opekun, A. and Boutton, T.W. (1987). *Campylobacter pylori* detected noninvasively by the ^{13}C-urea breath test. *Lancet*, **1**, 1174–7
51. Hoffman, N.E. and Hofmann, A.F. (1977). Metabolism of steroid and amino acid moieties of conjugated bile acids in man. V. Equations for the perturbed enterohepatic

circulation and their application. *Gastroenterology*, 72, 141–8

52. Marcus, S.N. and Heaton, K.W. (1986). Intestinal transit, deoxycholic acid and the cholesterol saturation of bile – three inter-related factors. *Gut*, 27, 550–8

53. Allan, R.N., Thistle, J.L. and Hofmann, A.F. (1976). Lithocholate metabolism during chenotherapy for gallstone dissolution. II. Absorption and sulphation. *Gut*, 17, 413–9

54. Cowen, A.E., Korman, M.G., Hofmann, A.F. and Cass, O.W. (1975). Metabolism of lithocholate in healthy men. I. Biotransformation and biliary excretion of intravenously administered lithocholate, lithocholylglycine, and their sulfates. *Gastroenterology*, 69, 59–66

55. Cowen, A.E., Korman, M.G., Hofmann, A.F., Cass, O.W. and Coffin, S.B. (1975). Metabolism of lithocholate in healthy men. II. Enterohepatic circulation. *Gastroenterology*, 69, 67–76

56. Fisher, R.L., Hofmann, A.F., Rossi, S., Converse, J.L. and Lan, S.P. (1986). Pathogenesis of morphological damage and major serum amino-transferase (AT) elevation in NCGS patients: Enhanced liver cell sensitivity – not defective lithocholate metabolism. *Hepatology*, 6, 1169

57. Lindstedt, S. (1957). The turnover of cholic acid in man. *Acta Physiol. Scand.*, 40, 1–9

58. Vlahcevic, Z.R., Bell, C.C. Jr, Buhac, I., Farrar, J.T. and Swell, L. (1970). Diminished bile acid pool size in patients with gallstones. *Gastroenterology*, 59, 165–73

59. Hofmann, A.F. and Hoffman, N.E. (1974). Measurement of bile acid kinetics by isotope dilution in man. *Gastroenterology*, 67, 314–23

60. Hofmann, A.F. and Cummings, S.A. (1983). Measurement of bile acid and cholesterol kinetics in man by isotope dilution: principles and applications. In: Barbara, L., Dowling, R.H., Hofmann, A.F. and Roda, E. (eds), *Bile Acids in Gastroenterology*, pp. 75–117. (Lancaster: MTP Press)

61. Hoffman, N.E. and Hofmann, A.F. (1974). Metabolism of steroid and amino acid moieties of conjugated bile acids in man. IV. Description and validation of a multicompartmental model. *Gastroenterology*, 67, 887–97

62. Simmonds, W.J., Korman, M.G., Go, V.L.W. and Hofmann, A.F. (1973). Radioimmunoassay of conjugated cholyl bile acids in serum. *Gastroenterology*, 65, 705–11

63. Bischoff, K.B. and Brown, R.G. (1966). Drug distribution in mammals. *Chem. Eng. Progr. Symp. Ser.*, 62, 32–45

64. Lutz, R.J., Dedrick, R.L. and Zaharko, D.S. (1980). Physiological pharmacokinetics: an *in vivo* approach to membrane transport. *Pharmac. Ther.*, 11, 559–92

65. Molino, G., Milanese, M., Villa, A., Gaidano, G. and Cavanna, A. (1978). Discrimination of hepatobiliary diseases by the evaluation of bromosulphophthalein blood kinetics. *J. Lab. Clin. Med.*, 91, 396

66. Hofmann, A.F., Molino, G., Milanese, M. and Belforte, G. (1983). Description and simulation of a physiological pharmacokinetic model for the metabolism and enterohepatic circulation of bile acids in man. Cholic acid in healthy man. *J. Clin. Invest.*, 71, 1003–22

67. Cravetto, C., Molino, G., Hofmann, A.F., Belforte, G. and Bona, B. Computer simulation of portal venous shunting and other isolated hepatobiliary defects of the enterohepatic circulation of bile acids using a physiological pharmacokinetc model. *Hepatology*, (In press)

68. Grundy, S.M., Hofmann, A.F., Davignon, J. and Ahrens, E.H. Jr (1966). Human cholesterol synthesis is regulated by bile acids. *J. Clin. Invest.*, 45, 1018–19

69. Thistle, J.L. and Schoenfield, L.J. (1971). Induced alterations in composition of bile of persons having cholelithias. *Gastroenterology*, 61, 488–96

70. Danzinger, R.G., Hofmann, A.F., Schoenfield, L.J. and Thistle, J.L. (1972). Dissolution of cholesterol gallstones by chenodeoxycholic acid. *N. Engl. J. Med.*, 286, 1–8

71. Sacquet, E., Parquet, M., Riottot, M., Raizman, A., Jarrige, P., Huguet, C. and Infante, R. (1983). Intestinal absorption, excretion, and biotransformation of hyodeoxycholic acid in man. *J. Lipid Res.*, 24, 604–13

17

72. Poupon, R., Poupon, R.E., Calmus, Y., Chretein, Y., Ballet, F. and Darnis, F. (1987). Is ursodeoxycholic acid an effective treatment for primary biliary cirrhosis? *Lancet*, 1, 834–6

73. Hofmann, A.F. (1985). Targeting drugs to the enterohepatic circulation: Lessons from bile acids and other endobiotics. *J. Controlled Release*, 2, 2–11

74. Roda, A. (1983). Sensitive methods for serum bile acid analysis. In: Barbara, L., Dowling, R.H., Hofmann, A.F. and Roda, E. (eds), *Bile Acids in Gastroenterology*, pp. 57–68. (Lancaster: MTP Press)

75. Merrick, M.V., Eastwood, M.A., Anderson, J.R. and Ross, H.M. (1982). Enterohepatic circulation in man of a gamma-emitting bile-acid conjugate. 23-selena-25-homotaurocholic acid (SeHCAT). *J. Nucl. Med.*, 23, 126-30

76. Malaguti, P., Sciarretta, G., Abbati, A. and Furno, A. (1986). *New Radioisotope Tests in Gastroenterology*, 139 pp. (Milan: Masson Italia Editori)

SECTION A
BILIARY CHEMISTRY
AND PHYSIOLOGY

2

Hepatic Bile Acid Transport and Secretion

S. Erlinger
Unité de Recherches de Physiopathologie Hépatique
INSERM U-24 Hôpital Beaujon,
92118 Clichy Cedex France

INTRODUCTION

Bile acid transport and secretion by the liver is one of the important steps in the recirculation of bile acid within the body. After bile acids return from the intestine, they have first to be taken up by the parenchymal liver cell, then transported from the sinusoidal pole to the canalicular pole of the cell, and finally secreted into the bile canalicular lumen. In addition, unconjugated bile acids have to be conjugated, chiefly with taurine or glycine, before secretion. The purpose of this review is to examine the cellular mechanisms of bile acid transport by the liver, with particular emphasis on intracellular transport, the step which is at present least well understood.

METHODS OF STUDY

Until now, bile secretion has been generally studied by methods involving the collection of bile from the common bile duct : from a bile fistula *in vivo* in anaesthetised or non-anaesthetised animals, or from an isolated perfused liver. This has given only indirect information on events occurring at the hepatocellular level. Recently, more direct methods have been used which have provided information on the mechanisms involved : the use of isolated or cultured hepatocytes, isolated membrane vesicle preparations and isolated hepatocyte couplets. In order to study the fate of bile acids within the liver cell, autoradiography using labelled bile acids or bile acid analogues has also been employed.

UPTAKE

The liver has a high extraction efficiency for bile acids. The uptake of bile acids by the liver cells meets the criteria of a carrier-mediated process. It appears to be saturable, as shown by an indicator dilution technique in the intact dog[1,2], in the rat liver perfused *in situ* [3,4], and by studies with isolated and cultured liver cells[5-7]. Competitive inhibition may be shown when two bile acids are given simultaneously[2], but not with other organic anions, such as indocyanine green[8].

The marked dependence of bile acid uptake on extracellular sodium has been clearly demonstrated in the isolated perfused liver[4], in isolated[7] and cultured[6] hepatocytes, and in plasma membrane vesicles[9-12]. This strongly suggests that bile acid uptake involves a secondary active transport energised by the transmembrane sodium gradient. The carrier probably moves the bile acid and sodium simultaneously across the membrane (symport or cotransport). The sodium gradient is continuously maintained by sodium-potassium activated adenosine triphosphatase ($Na^+ - K^+$-ATPase), the enzymatic basis of the sodium pump.

The carrier, a 54 kDa protein, has been identified by photoaffinity labelling techniques[13,14] and reconstituted in artificial proteoliposomes[15].

The maximal capacity for uptake (about 4.5 μmol/s/100 g liver) is approximately 10 times greater than the maximal capacity for uptake of bromosulphophthalein (BSP), and greatly exceeds the maximal capacity for biliary excretion (see below).

INTRACELLULAR TRANSPORT

Less is known about intracellular transport from the sinusoidal to the canalicular pole of the hepatocyte. Bile acids appear to have little affinity for the Y (ligandin) or Z proteins that bind a variety of other organic anions, including BSP and iodinated contrast agents. Cytoplasmic bile acid-binding proteins which could play a role in transport have, however, been detected and partially purified[16,17]. One of these exhibits glutathione transferase activity and could be identical to ligandin[17]. Others differing from ligandin have also been identified[18,19]

During this phase of hepatic transport, unconjugated bile acids are conjugated to taurine and glycine. Conjugation could be a rate limiting step in overall hepatic transport for certain bile acids, as the maximal biliary transport capacity (transport maximum or T_m, maximal secretory rate or SRm) of some conjugated bile acids after intravenous administration is far greater than that of the unconjugated compounds[20,21,22]. Recently, we have used an immunoperoxidase technique to localise bile acids in liver cells, employing antibodies against cholic acid conjugates and against ursodeoxycholic acid[23]. An indirect immunoperoxidase technique was used on rat liver sections fixed either with paraformaldehyde and saponin (a membrane-permeabilising agent which allows penetration of antibodies into the cell) or with paraformaldehyde alone. When sections fixed with paraformaldehyde and saponin were incubated with the antibody against conjugated cholic acid, a granular cytoplasmic staining was observed by light microscopy in all hepatocytes. Strong electron-dense deposits were observed by electron microscopy, mostly on vesicles of the Golgi apparatus and sometimes on the smooth endoplasmic reticulum. After infusing taurocholate, the intensity of the reaction increased. When sections were fixed with paraformaldehyde alone, almost no reaction was visible on light microscopy but on electron microscopy the label was localised to the hepatocyte plasma membrane - mainly on the bile canalicular domain and to a lesser extent on the sinusoidal domain. With the antibody against ursodeoxycholic acid, no staining was observed in three of four livers, and a slight staining in one. After infusing ursodeoxycholic acid, the Golgi apparatus and smooth endoplasmic reticulum vesicles were stained when the liver was fixed with paraformaldehyde and saponin, whilst with paraformaldehyde alone intense staining was seen on the canalicular membrane. These results support the view that, after uptake by the sinusoidal plasma membrane, vesicles from the Golgi apparatus and possibly from the smooth endoplasmic reticulum are involved in the intracellular transport of bile acids before canalicular secretion.

Results using autoradiography with cholyl-glycine histamine, cholyl-glycine tyrosine and ^{3}H-taurocholate are also consistent with this possibility[24,25,26]. A specific transport system has been isolated on the Golgi apparatus, which is able to translocate bile acids from the cytosol (outside the Golgi) into the Golgi apparatus lumen[27]. Vesicular transport in the cell is well known to be inhibited by colchicine and it is interesting that colchicine inhibits bile acid transport after a bile acid load in the rat[28].

CANALICULAR SECRETION

The secretion of bile acids into bile probably takes place through another carrier-mediated mechanism. The process is saturable, with a maximal capacity (T_m) of 8–8.5 μmol/min/kg in dogs, 14 μmol/min/kg in sheep, and 10–12 μmol/min/kg in rats. Three lines of evidence suggest that the hepatic secretory mechanism for bile acids is not the same as that for other organic anions excreted in bile such as bilirubin, BSP, and iodinated contrast agents. Firstly, the T_m for bile acids is 5–10 times higher than that of BSP. Secondly, bile acids and BSP do not compete for biliary excretion. On the contrary, administration of bile acids increases the apparent T_m for BSP. Thirdly, in mutant Corriedale sheep (which have an inherited defect in biliary excretion of organic anions closely related to the Dubin-Johnson syndrome in humans) maximal biliary excretion of BSP is low, whereas that of bile acids is normal.

23

The canalicular carrier system appears to be independent of sodium, as has been demonstrated in canalicular membrane vesicles[29], and there is no evidence that it requires a source of energy. It could therefore be a carrier-mediated system (facilitated diffusion) driven perhaps by the membrane potential[30]. The carrier, a 100 kDa protein, has been identified by photoaffinity labelling[31], and transport has recently been reconstituted in artificial liposomes[32]. If one accepts that a vesicular mechanism is important in the transport of bile acids from the sinusoidal to the canalicular membrane, exocytosis could contribute to secretion into the canalicular lumen.

The active step in overall transport from blood to bile is probably uptake, which allows concentration within the hepatocyte. This step is probably responsible, in part, for the concentration gradient between blood and bile: the biliary concentration (10–100 mmol/l) is approximately 100–1,000 times higher than the plasma concentration in systemic or portal blood. Part of this concentration gradient, however, is probably best explained by micelle formation, which prevents reabsorption from bile.

Because of their efficient transhepatic transport and their enterohepatic circulation, bile acids are secreted into bile in considerable amounts: with a synthetic rate of approximately 600 mg per day, the liver is able to maintain a bile acid pool of 2–3 g and to secrete 20–30 g of bile acids into the bile each day.

SUMMARY

Hepatic bile acid secretion is a key determinant of the secretion of bile and biliary lipids. It involves uptake at the sinusoidal pole of the hepatocyte, intracellular transport to the canalicular pole and secretion into the canalicular lumen. Uptake of conjugated bile acids is sodium-dependent and is thought to be mediated by a sodium-bile acid co-transport (or symport) system, energised by the transmembrane sodium gradient maintained by the Na^+,K^+-ATPase. The mechanisms of intracellular transport are largely unknown. Bile acid binding proteins have been identified but their role in transport has not been established. Studies with autoradiography and recent studies from this laboratory using anti-bile acid antibodies and immunoperoxidase techniques suggest that a vesicular system including the Golgi apparatus may be involved. Observations with inhibitors of vesicular transport, such as colchicine, also support this hypothesis. There is a lobular gradient in bile acid transport, periportal hepatocytes removing most of the bile acid load at physiological concentrations. For some unconjugated bile acids, conjugation may be the limiting factor in overall transport from blood to bile. Canalicular secretion occurs via carrier-mediated diffusion sensitive to the membrane potential.

References

1. Glasinovic, J.C., Dumont, M., Duval, M. and Erlinger, S. (1975). Hepatocellular uptake of taurocholate in the dog. *J. Clin. Invest.*, **55**, 419-26
2. Glasinovic, J.C., Dumont, M., Duval, M. and Erlinger, S. (1975). Hepatocellular uptake of bile acids in the dog : Evidence for a common carrier-mediated transport system. An indicator dilution study. *Gastroenterology*, **69**, 973-81
3. Reichen, J. and Paumgartner, G. (1975). Kinetics of taurocholate uptake by the perfused rat liver. *Gastroenterology*, **68**, 132-6
4. Reichen, J. and Paumgartner, G. (1976). Uptake of bile acids by the perfused rat liver. *Am. J. Physiol.*, **231**, 734-42
5. Anwer, M.S., Kroker, R. and Hegner, D. (1976). Cholic acid uptake into isolated rat hepatocytes. *Hoppe Seyler's Z. Physiol. Chem.*, **357**, 1477-86
6. Scharschmidt. B.F. and Stephens, J.E. (1981). Transport of sodium, chloride, and taurocholate by cultured rat hepatocytes. *Proc. Natl. Acad. Sci. USA*, **78**, 986-90
7. Schwarz, L.R., Burr, R., Schwenk, M., Pfaff, E. and Greim, H. (1975). Uptake of taurocholic acid into isolated rat-liver cells. *Eur. J. Biochem.*, **55**, 617-23
8. Paumgartner, G. and Reichen, J. (1975). Different pathways for hepatic uptake of taurocholate and indocyanine green. *Experientia*, **31**, 306-7
9. Blitzer, B.L. and Donovan, C.B. (1984). A new method for the rapid isolation of basolateral plasma membrane vesicles from rat liver. Characterisation, validation, and bile acid transport studies. *J. Biol. Chem.*, **259**, 9295-301
10. Duffy, M.C., Blitzer, B.L. and Boyer, J.L. (1983). Direct determination of the driving forces for taurocholate uptake into rat liver plasma membrane vesicles. *J. Clin. Invest.*, **72**, 1470-81
11. Inoue, M., Kinne, R., Tran, T. and Arias, I.M. (1982). Taurocholate transport by rat liver sinusoidal membrane vesicles: Evidence of sodium cotransport. *Hepatology*, **2**, 572-9
12. Ruifrok, P.G. and Meijer, D.K.F. (1982). Sodium ion-coupled uptake of taurocholate by rat-liver plasma membrane vesicles. *Liver*, **2**, 28-34
13. Wieland, T., Nassal, M., Kramer, W., Fricker, G., Bickel, U. and Kurz, G. (1984). Identity of hepatic membrane transport systems for bile salts, phalloidin, and antamanide by photoaffinity labeling. *Proc. Natl. Acad. Sci. USA*, **81**, 5232-6
14. von Dippe, P. and Levy D. (1983). Characterisation of the bile acid transport system in normal and transformed hepatocytes. *J. Biol. Chem.*, **258**, 8896-901
15. von Dippe, P., Ananthanarayanan, M., Drain, P. and Levy, D. (1986). Purification and reconstitution of the bile acid transport system from hepatocyte sinusoidal plasma membranes. *Biochim. Biophys. Acta*, **862**, 352-60
16. Strange, R.C., Cramb, R., Hayes, J.D. and Percy-Robb, I.W. (1977). Partial purification of two lithocholic acid-binding proteins from rat liver 100,000 g supernatants. *Biochem. J.*, **165**, 425-9
17. Strange, R.C., Nimmo, I.A. and Percy-Robb, I.W. (1977). Binding of bile acids by 100,000 g supernatants of rat liver. *Biochem. J.*, **162**, 659-64
18. Stolz, A., Sugiyama, Y., Kuhlenkamp, J. and Kaplowitz, N. (1984). Identification and purification of a 36 kDa bile acid binder in human hepatic cytosol. *FEBS Lett.*, **177**, 31-5
19. Sugiyama, U., Yamada, T. and Kaplowitz, N. (1983). Newly identified bile acid binders in rat liver cytosol. Purification and comparison with glutathione S-transferases. *J. Biol. Chem.*, **258**, 3602-7
20. Erlinger, S., Dumont, M., Zouboulis-Vafiadis, I. and De Couët, G. (1984). The importance of conjugation in biliary secretion of ursodeoxycholate and 7-ketolithocholate in the rat. *Clin. Sci.*, 487-91
21. Vessey, D.A., Whitney, J. and Gollan, J.L. (1983). The role of conjugation reactions in enhancing biliary secretion of bile acids. *Biochem. J.*, **214**, 923-7

22. Zouboulis-Vafiadis, I., Dumont, M. and Erlinger, S. (1982). Conjugation is rate limiting in hepatic transport of ursodeoxycholate in the rat. *Am. J. Physiol.*, **243**, G208-13
23. Lamri, Y., Roda, A., Dumont, M., Feldmann, G. and Erlinger, S. (1987). Immunoperoxidase localisation of bile salts in rat liver cells. *J. Hepatol.*, **5**, 539 (abstract)
24. Groothuis, G.M.M., Hardonk, M.J., Keulemans, K.P.T., Nieuwenhuis, P. and Meijer, D.K.F. (1982). Autoradiographic and kinetic demonstration of acinar heterogeneity of taurocholate transport. *Am. J. Physiol.*, **243**, G455-62
25. Suchy, F.J., Balistreri, W.F., Hung, J., Miller, P. and Garfield, S.A. (1983). Intracellular bile acid transport in rat liver as visualised by electron microscope autoradiography using a bile acid analogue. *Am. J. Physiol.*, **245**, G681-9
26. Goldsmith, M.A., Huling, S. and Jones, A.L. (1983). Hepatic handling of bile salts and protein in the rat during intrahepatic cholestasis. *Gastroenterology*, **84**, 978-86
27. Simion, A.F., Fleischer, B. and Fleischer, S. (1984). Two distinct mechanisms for taurocholate uptake in subcellular fractions from rat liver. *J. Biol. Chem.*, **259**, 10814-22
28. Dubin, M., Maurice, M., Feldmann, G. and Erlinger, S. (1980). Influence of colchicine and phalloidin on bile secretion and hepatic ultrastructure in the rat. Possible interaction between microtubules and microfilaments. *Gastroenterology*, **79**, 646-54
29. Inoue, P., Kinne, R., Tran, T. and Arias, I.M. (1984). Taurocholate transport by rat liver canalicular membrane vesicles. Evidence for the presence of an Na^+-independent transport system. *J. Clin. Invest.*, **73**, 659-63
30. Meier, P.J., St. Meier-Abt, A., Barrett, C. and Boyer, J.L. (1984). Mechanisms of taurocholate transport in canalicular and basolateral rat liver plasma membrane vesicles. *J. Biol. Chem.*, **259**, 10614-22
31. Ruetz, S., Fricker, G., Hugentobler, G., Winterhalter, K., Kurz, G. and Meier, P.J. (1987). Isolation and characterisation of the putative canalicular bile salt transport system of rat liver. *J. Biol. Chem.*, **269**, 11324-30
32. Ruetz, S., Hugentobler, G. and Meier, P.J. (1987). Functional reconstitution of the canalicular bile salt transport system of rat liver. *Hepatology*, **7**, 1105

3

Hepatic Biliary Lipid Synthesis and Transport

J.M. Graham, H. Ahmed and T.C. Northfield
Departments of Biochemistry and Medicine
St George's Hospital Medical School
London, SW17 0RE, UK

INTRODUCTION

Bile contains many components including bile pigments, selected cellular and serum proteins, cholesterol, phospholipid and bile acids. The hepatocyte is responsible for secreting all these components into the bile canaliculus. This cell is also engaged in the uptake from the blood of phospholipid, cholesterol and triglyceride (in the form of chylomicron remnants and lipoproteins) and bile acids. It can synthesise all these components *de novo* and it can assemble cholesterol, triglyceride, and phospholipid into VLDL for export into the blood. The hepatocyte thus plays a key role in the manufacture of lipids and bile acids; in their packaging, in their reception from exogenous sources and in marshalling them into the correct transit route. Before considering the possible biochemical defects in this system which occur in cholesterol gallstone disease it is therefore worth reviewing, briefly, the structure and function of the hepatocyte in relation to lipid metabolism and its control.

MEMBRANE STRUCTURES OF THE HEPATOCYTE

The surface of the hepatocyte consists of three well-defined domains which are morphologically and functionally distinct (Figure 1): (a) the sinusoidal membrane which is proximal to the blood supply; (b) the bile canalicular membrane across which biliary components are transported; and (c) the contiguous membrane which connects these two domains. Tight junctions occur close to the peripheries of the sinusoidal and bile canalicular domains, which severely limit the 'leakage' of molecules from blood into bile (and vice versa). Within the cell, the membranes of the rough and smooth endoplasmic reticulum are responsible for the synthesis of proteins and lipids, while the

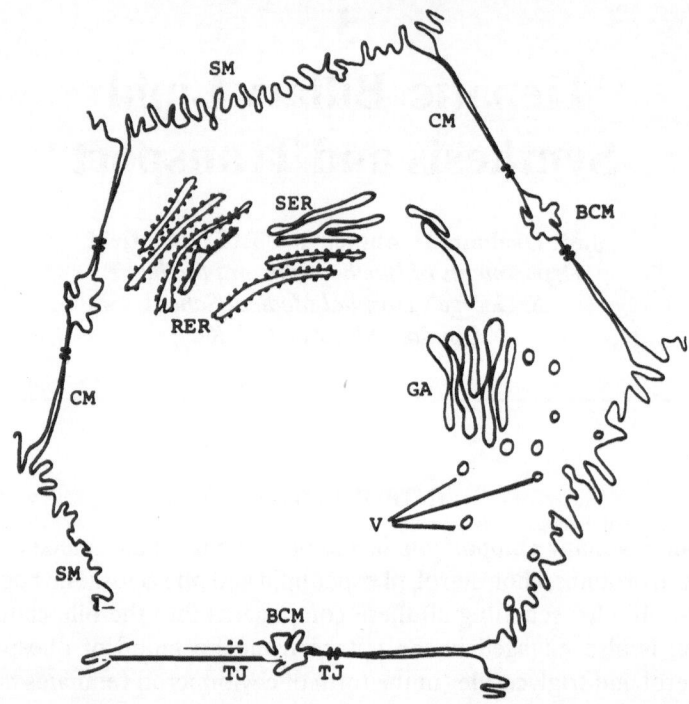

Figure 1 Diagrammatic representation of the hepatocyte to show membranous components involved in the synthesis of plasma membrane domains. SM: sinusoidal membrane, CM: contiguous membrane, BCM: bile canalicular membrane, RER: rough endoplasmic reticulum, SER: smooth endoplasmic reticulum, GA: Golgi apparatus, V: vesicle, TJ: tight junction.

Golgi apparatus is involved in the terminal glycosylation of glycoproteins and glycolipids. These proteins and glycoproteins, lipids and glycolipids, are destined for incorporation into membranes or for secretion. The cytoplasm also contains a huge range of membrane-bound vesicles whose dimensions range from 50 to 500 nm.

LIPIDS IN SERUM, HEPATOCYTE MEMBRANES AND BILE

The main lipids in the body are triglyceride, cholesterol, phospholipid and glycolipid; the cholesterol exists as the free sterol and as the ester. In all hepatocyte membranes the cholesterol is present as the free sterol, which together with phospholipid and glycolipid make up the fluid bilayer characteristic of all membranes. Cholesterol ester is the form in which cholesterol is transported around the body: it exists predominantly in the core of lipoproteins (namely HDL and LDL), at the surface of which cholesterol, phospholipid and glycolipid, together with apoproteins, form a stabilising monolayer. Only in lipoproteins and membranes are proteins known to play an important functional and architectural role. Only in the bile are bile acids involved in solubilising the lipid; in bile a number of different structures have been recognised which contain unesterified cholesterol, phospholipid and bile acid, including mixed micelles, liquid crystals and vesicle-like liposomes[1].

In membranes the phospholipids consist of five major molecular species: phosphatidyl choline, phosphatidyl ethanolamine, sphingomyelins, phosphatidyl serine and phosphatidyl inositol. The first three account for the greater part of the total membrane phospholipid; in rat liver plasma membrane, for example, these phospholipids represent approximately 35%, 19% and 18% respectively of the total: internal membranes have rather less sphingomyelin and rather more of the other two[2]. On the other hand, in lipoproteins the amount of phosphatidyl choline is much higher (60–77%) and the phosphatidyl ethanolamine lower (2–4%)[3]. In bile, phosphatidyl choline, specifically enriched in palmitic and linoleic acids[4,5], is essentially the only phospholipid. Cholesterol levels in bile and the various hepatocyte membranes are also quite distinctive. The plasma membrane, for example, is relatively enriched in cholesterol (when expressed as a mole ratio of phospholipid) compared to both membranes of the internal structures and bile. Moreover, the bile canalicular membrane shows a higher cholesterol:phospholipid ratio than do the other domains of the surface membrane in rat[6], hamster[7] and man (our own data).

The lipids of the biliary compartment are therefore quite unlike those of any other lipid-rich structure (membrane or lipoprotein). Any mechanism which we propose to explain how lipids and bile acids are synthesised and how they are transported into the bile must be consistent with these observations and account for the specific nature of the lipid composition of the various hepatocyte compartments.

LIPID AND BILE ACID SYNTHESIS IN THE HEPATOCYTE

De novo synthesis of all cholesterol, bile acids and phospholipids occurs on the endoplasmic reticulum of the hepatocyte. The starting point for all these syntheses is acetyl CoA. Figure 2 illustrates the conversion of acetyl CoA to cholesterol: the committed step is the conversion of 3-hydroxy-3-methylglutaryl CoA (HMG CoA) to mevalonate by the enzyme HMG CoA reductase. This is the rate-limiting step which is inhibited by the end product – cholesterol[8]. Bile acids are formed from cholesterol in a number of steps involving ring hydroxylation and conversion of the 8-C alkyl side chain to a single carboxyl group (Figure 2). The rate-limiting step is the 7α-hydroxylation reaction[9]. The committed step in the synthesis of fatty acids from acetyl

CoA is the formation of malonyl CoA by the enzyme acetyl CoA carboxylase. Fatty acids are used in the synthesis of both triglycerides and phospholipids.

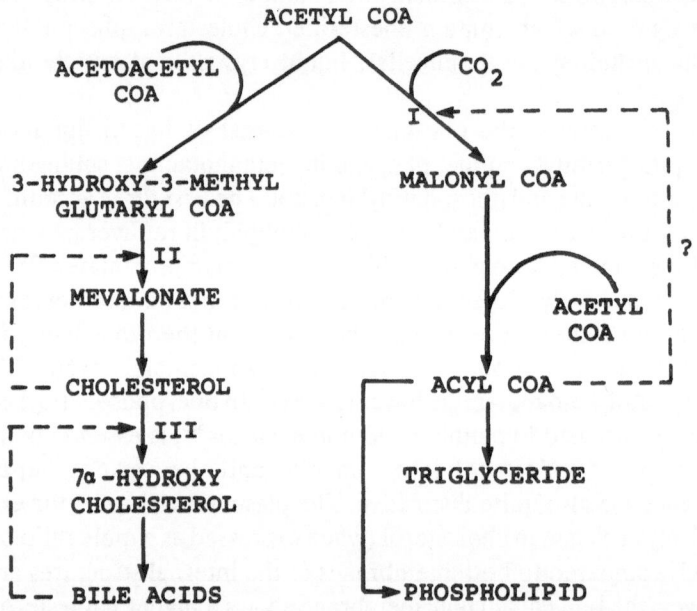

Figure 2   Synthesis of cholesterol and bile acids from Acetyl CoA. I – acetyl CoA carboxylase; II – HMG CoA reductase; III – cholesterol 7α-hydroxylase; (– – –) feedback inhibition.

LIPID AND BILE ACID SYNTHESIS IN CHOLESTEROL GALLSTONE DISEASE AND IN BILE ACID FEEDING

In cholesterol gallstone disease the cholesterol saturation index in the bile is elevated[10,11] and bile acid pool size is often reduced[11,12]. An increase in the rate of synthesis may be due to an increased number of enzyme molecules catalysing the rate-limiting step (i.e. HMG CoA reductase), to activation of the enzyme and/or to its release from end-product inhibition. Coyne *et al.*[13] showed that the level of HMG CoA reductase in liver biopsies from gallstone patients was increased by about 35% (over control patients). On the other hand a study by Ahlberg *et al.*[14] found no increase in hepatic HMG CoA reductase activity in normal weight, non-lipidaemic cholesterol gallstone patients over normals. Our own studies (Figure 3) showed that HMG CoA reductase activity in gallstone patients was clearly obesity related, and even the non-obese patients showed a small but definite increase in HMG CoA reductase over the controls. In experimental animals[15] raised biliary cholesterol has been equated with an elevated HMG CoA reductase. The raised levels of cholesterol synthesis in obesity may reflect an inhibition of the conversion of acetyl CoA to fatty acids with its consequent diversion into the pathway of cholesterol synthesis.

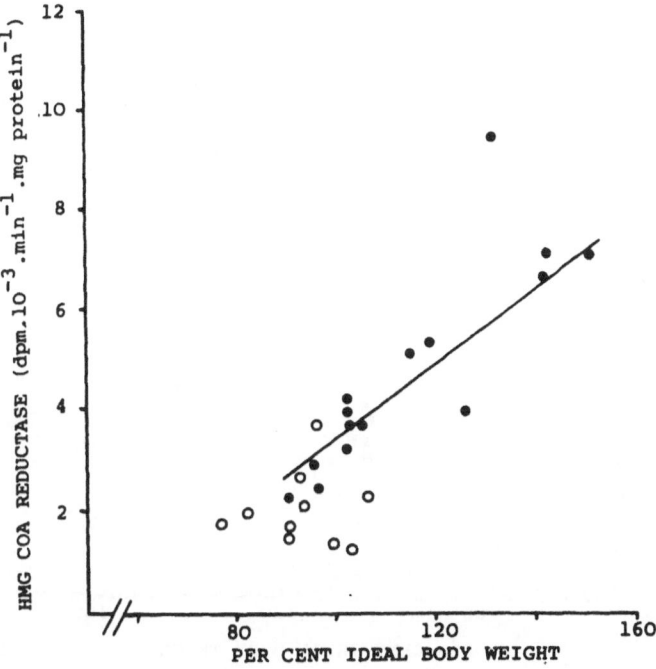

Figure 3 Relation between hepatic HMG CoA reductase and obesity in patients with cholesterol gallstones. o controls; • cholesterol gallstone patients. $p < 0.001$ for gallstone patients.

The reduced bile acid output in gallstone patients has been associated with a reduction in 7α-hydroxylase activity[14]. Ahlberg *et al.*[14] maintained that the reduction in bile acid synthesis was critical in determining biliary cholesterol saturation and that only in untreated gallstone patients and in healthy controls was the HMG CoA reductase related to hepatic biliary cholesterol saturation. Our own data (Figure 4) seem to confirm this inasmuch as all cholesterol gallstone patients showed a similar marked depression of 7α-hydroxylase which was not related to obesity.

Bile acid therapy has demonstrated some interesting effects specific to certain bile acids. Cholesterol desaturation and dissolution of cholesterol gallstones has been achieved by the administration of CDCA and UDCA but not cholic acid[16-19]. In line with this, cholate had no effect on HMG CoA reductase while CDCA resulted in a 40% reduction in enzyme activity[13].

31

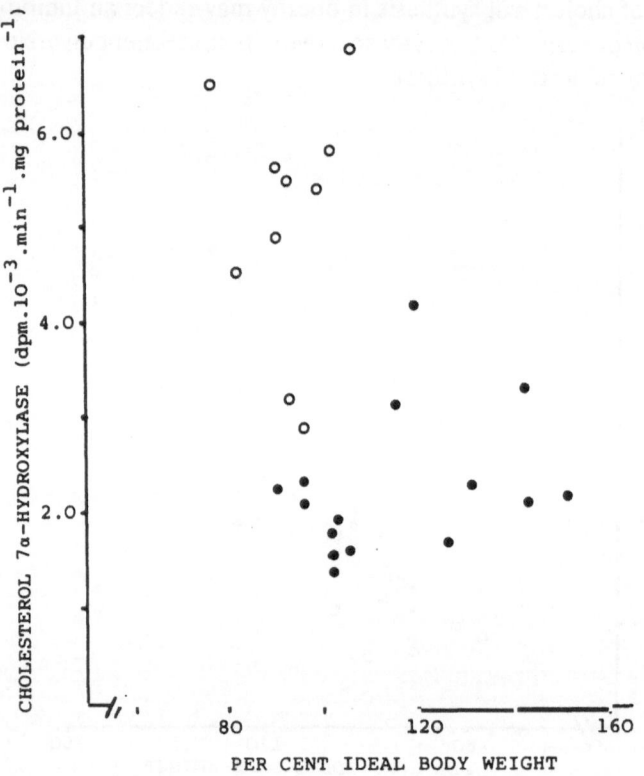

Figure 4 Bile acid synthesis(7α-hydroxylase activity) in control subjects and patients with cholesterol gallstones. o controls; ● cholesterol gallstone patients.

CONTROL OF CHOLESTEROL AND BILE ACID SYNTHESIS

The means by which the rate-limiting enzyme of cholesterol synthesis (HMG CoA reductase) is controlled is far from clear. Its activity *in vitro* is reversibly modulated by phosphorylation and dephosphorylation[20,21] but this has not provided a satisfactory explanation for the *in vivo* control of the enzyme. In cholesterol-fed rats the V_{max} and K_m for the enzyme were both reduced compared to control rats, while in cholestryramine-fed animals both parameters were raised[22] but the state of phosphorylation of the HMG CoA reductase was unaltered; moreover the K_m of the solubilised enzyme did not change[23]. In familial hypercholesterolaemia, the HMG CoA reductase in skin fibroblasts cultured from homozygotes was not inhibited by addition of LDL to the medium while it was inhibited by cholesterol added in a non-lipoprotein form[24]. The defect is now known to be either a lack of receptor

32

for the LDL in the sinusoidal membrane or a fault in the endocytotic pathway for LDL[25]. The enzyme is therefore unaltered: it could respond to cholesterol, but the delivery of cholesterol to the site of action is impaired. Lack of inhibitory action then results in over-production of the enzyme. Modulation of cholesterol levels in microsomes by incubation of these membranes with serum *in vitro* results in the same reciprocal relationship between HMG CoA reductase and microsomal cholesterol as was observed in the *in vivo* feeding experiments[26]. Sabine and James[27] suggested that the fluidity of the microenvironment of the enzyme might be important in modulating its activity: Arrhenius plot analysis of the enzyme in microsomes from normal rat liver showed a phase transition at 27°C which was abolished by feeding a cholesterol diet for 12 h[28]. Other enzymes such as 7α-hydroxylase, although membrane-bound and increased in activity in cholesterol-fed animals, fail to show Arrhenius discontinuities under either dietary regime[29].

The administration of bile acids to experimental animals inhibits both the HMG CoA reductase and 7α-hydroxylase. Experiments with lymphatic fistulae in experimental rats suggest that cholic acid feeding acts on hepatic HMG CoA reductase rather than through intestinal absorption of cholesterol[30]. *In vitro* experiments preclude an allosteric effect of bile acid on the enzyme, rather they suggest a non-specific detergent effect[31].

Using either isolated hepatocytes or hepatocyte cultures, Kubaska *et al.*[32] were unable to show any effect of externally added bile acids on 7α-hydroxylase activity even though the bile acids were clearly taken up by the cells. In most *in vivo* experiments the effect of individual bile acids on bile acid synthesis is complicated by the presence of other bile acids and the enterohepatic circulation: according to Kubaska *et al.*[32] unequivocal demonstration of the repression of 7α-hydroxylase by bile acids is not available. The effect of bile acids on this enzyme is complicated by their effects on cholesterol synthesis. *In vivo* experiments in the hamster[15] showed that cholate inhibited cholesterol synthesis less effectively than bile acid synthesis; CDC, while more inhibitory than cholate on both syntheses, was relatively more effective on cholesterol synthesis. Davis *et al.*[33] suggested that the 7α-hydroxylase activity may be controlled by the availability of cholesterol to the enzyme.

ORGANISATION OF SYNTHETIC MACHINERY

In discussing the synthesis of cholesterol and bile acids thus far, the location of these synthetic events has been allocated to the 'microsomes'. The enzymes of cholesterol and bile acid synthesis are, however, clearly restricted to certain areas of the microsomes. Mitropoulos *et al.*[34] showed that there are a number of separate pools of cholesterol, some of which are readily accessible to cholesterol added *in vitro* and others which are not. Generally the cholesterol in most membranes, including those of the plasma membrane and Golgi, could be complexed with digitonin with a consequent increase in density of the membrane. The 'substrate pool' of cholesterol available to 7α-hydroxylase was, on the other hand, not complexed by digitonin. Moreover the substrate pool and the 7α-hydroxylase and the HMG CoA reductase were closely associated on the same microsomal subfraction[34]. Measurements made on the entire liver[15] which found no correlation between HMG CoA reductase and hepatic cholesterol nor between 7α-hydroxylase and hepatic bile acids in the hamster may not have been precise enough to allow us to determine the availability of cholesterol to the 7α-hydroxylase enzyme. It is worth noting, however, that an increase in hepatic cholesterol was discerned in patients with cholesterol gallstones[14,35], although Ahlberg *et al.*[14] could detect no difference in total microsomal cholesterol. Kubaska *et al.*[32] suggested that bile acids may influence this availability by altering the absorption of cholesterol from the intestine, the uptake of lipoprotein cholesterol by the hepatocyte and rates of cholesterol synthesis and esterification. To this list one should add the possible effects of bile acids on the loss of cholesterol from the hepatocyte into bile.

The reduced activity of 7α-hydroxylase observed in cholesterol gallstone disease could be associated with a reduced synthesis of the enzyme. If it reflects an inhibition of the enzyme activity, then this could be due to an increased sensitivity of the enzyme to end product inhibition, or to the presence of some independent inhibitor, or to the existence of locally high concentrations of bile acid at the site of the enzyme leading to raised end product inhibition, or to a decreased availability of cholesterol.

Organisational defects have also been implicated in certain Morris hepatomas[28]; in contrast to normal liver, feeding of cholesterol to rats to 5123c, 5123tc and 9618A hepatomas failed to abolish the temperature dependent phase transition temperature of the HMG CoA reductase in tumours. Even though cholesterol levels in the microsomes were raised, they failed to show any feedback inhibition of the HMG CoA reductase. Gregg *et al.*[28] postulated that in these hepatomas there was a decreased 'membrane-enzyme' interaction such that they failed to respond to the added cholesterol. There may indeed be a significant dysfunction in membrane organisation and the targeting of newly synthesised molecules to specific areas of the plasma membrane, for in many of these hepatomas the functional specificities of the various domains of the surface membrane become lost (see Graham[36] for review).

TRANSLOCATION AND SECRETION OF LIPIDS AND BILE ACIDS

The raised cholesterol secretion in cholesterol gallstone disease could be due to more efficient transfer of cholesterol from the site of synthesis (or from an exogenous source) to the bile rather than (or in addition to) increased synthesis. Thus, although secretion of biliary lipids and bile acids is considered in detail in Chapters 2 and 4, it is pertinent to mention it here as the ultimate step in the synthesis and movement of cholesterol, phospholipid and bile acids from the hepatocyte into bile. Any proposed mechanism for the transport of these molecules out of the hepatocyte must square with the observation that newly synthesised bile acids appear in bile ahead of both cholesterol and phospholipid[37]. This asynchronous movement precludes the secretion by exocytosis of a pre-formed lipid–bile acid micelle structure in a manner akin to VLDL secretion at the sinusoidal membrane, and certainly it is unlikely that such a structure could be transported through the membrane by a carrier mechanism. Co-transport of cholesterol and phospholipid across the hepatocyte would almost certainly involve a membrane vesicle.

It is well established that the transfer of newly synthesised cholesterol and phospholipid (together with glycolipid, proteins and glycoproteins) to the sinusoidal plasma membrane occurs as part of a membrane vesicle which is formed from the smooth endoplasmic reticulum or Golgi and translocated to the sinusoidal membrane with which it fuses. This process, in addition to

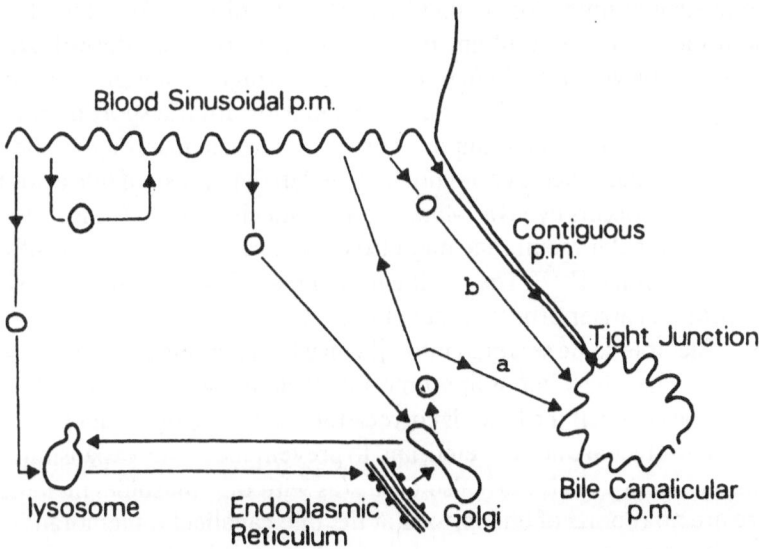

Figure 5 Vesicle pathways within the hepatocyte (modified from Evans[38]).

providing a method for the insertion of new membrane components, also provides the route for the exocytosis of VLDL, which carries the newly synthesised triglyceride into the blood stream.

In the adult, non-dividing hepatocyte, the peripheral flow of membrane vesicles to the sinusoidal membrane must be balanced by an inward flow – this process (endocytosis) is also responsible for the uptake of lipoproteins and chylomicron remnants from the blood for subsequent utilisation. This endocytotic pathway has been the subject of intensive research over the last 5–10 years and is emerging as a very complex process. Some of these pathways are shown in Figure 5. The least well understood aspect of this vesicle traffic is the manner in which specific vesicles are targeted to specific membranes or membrane domains so that, for example, newly synthesised VLDL moves to the sinusoidal membrane rather than the contiguous or bile canalicular membranes, while biliary lipids are directed to the latter rather than the former. The Golgi membranes[39] are thought to be involved in directing the vesicle traffic, but their role in this aspect of membrane translocation is not clear.

Although there is little evidence for a direct vesicular transport from the endoplasmic reticulum or Golgi to the bile canalicular membrane (Route a in Figure 5) there is one vesicular pathway involving the bile canalicular membrane which has been described *viz.* the generation of an endosome from the sinusoidal membrane which subsequently fuses with the bile canalicular membrane (Route b in Figure 5). It may be this route by which certain proteins such as immunoglobulins[40] are shunted directly from blood to bile without the intervention of any other cellular processes. Interestingly, bile acid containing vesicles within or close to the Golgi membranes[41] have now been reported. These vesicles might be responsible for transporting bile acids into bile and/or they may impose some directional marker for bile lipid transport. Certainly vesicles are not involved in the uptake of bile acids from the blood: this occurs by a Na^+-linked carrier mechanism[42]. Transport across the bile canalicular membrane may also be by a carrier mechanism although it is not Na^+-linked[43,44]. The significance of the existence of both a vesicular and a protein carrier process is not clear.

The lipid to be secreted into bile may be a membrane vesicle itself or again it may be a micellar or liposome-like structure within the vesicle which is then exocytosed. If the latter is correct, then the bile canalicular membrane lipids themselves are not secreted, and to prevent indefinite expansion of this membrane endocytosis must also occur (as with the sinusoidal membrane). There are no reports of endocytosis at the bile canalicular membrane.

We have now shown, however, in cholesterol gallstone patients that the synthesis of cholesterol (HMG CoA reductase), the cholesterol:phospholipid ratio in the bile canalicular membrane and cholesterol saturation index of the bile all increase in parallel and are strongly correlated to each other. This shows that the flow of cholesterol from the site of synthesis to bile directly involves the bile canalicular membrane and implies that the secreted lipids are actually incorporated into this membrane prior to secretion. The results support the concept that the source of biliary lipids is the bile canalicular membrane. Colchicine, a drug which interferes with microtubule formation, severely reduces phospholipid and cholesterol secretion in experimental animals[37]. This suggests a vesicular transport for these components. The effect on bile acid transport and secretion is much less well defined. Barnwell et al.[37] showed that colchicine reduced the transport of taurocholate but had no effect on its concentration in bile; while Gregory et al.[5] reported that the reduced output of bile acids in the presence of colchicine was much less marked than the inhibition of cholesterol and phospholipid secretion. What does seem clear is that co-transport of bile acids and lipids does not occur.

HYPOTHETICAL MODEL

Any model of biliary lipid secretion must take account of the following experimental observations:

(1)   Cholesterol and bile acids are synthesised in a specific domain of the endoplasmic reticulum and the rate limiting enzymes of their syntheses are apparently regulated by substrate availability and/or micro-environmental factors.

(2)   The translocation of lipids (cholesterol and phospholipid) within the hepatocyte normally occurs in the form of a membrane vesicle.

(3)   Microtubules are important in vesicular transport and also in biliary lipid secretion.

(4)   The transport of bile acids and lipids into bile are not synchronous.

(5)   Essentially the only phospholipid in bile is phosphatidyl choline whereas membranes contain a mixture of phospholipids.

(6)   In cholesterol gallstone disease increased cholesterol synthesis correlates with a raised cholesterol/phospholipid ratio in both the bile canalicular membrane and in the bile.

(7)   Cholesterol gallstone disease is associated with reduced bile acid pool size.

Figure 6 shows a hypothetical scheme in which cholesterol synthesised on a domain of the endoplasmic reticulum and incorporated along with

37

phospholipid (and protein) into a membrane vesicle, is directed to the bile canalicular membrane by a system of microtubules. Such a unidirectional flow of membrane vesicles would permit not only an efficient lipid transit system but it would also maintain the enzyme specificity of the bile canalicular membrane domain. In this system the synthesis of cholesterol and bile acids is controlled by the availability of cholesterol in the local environment of the

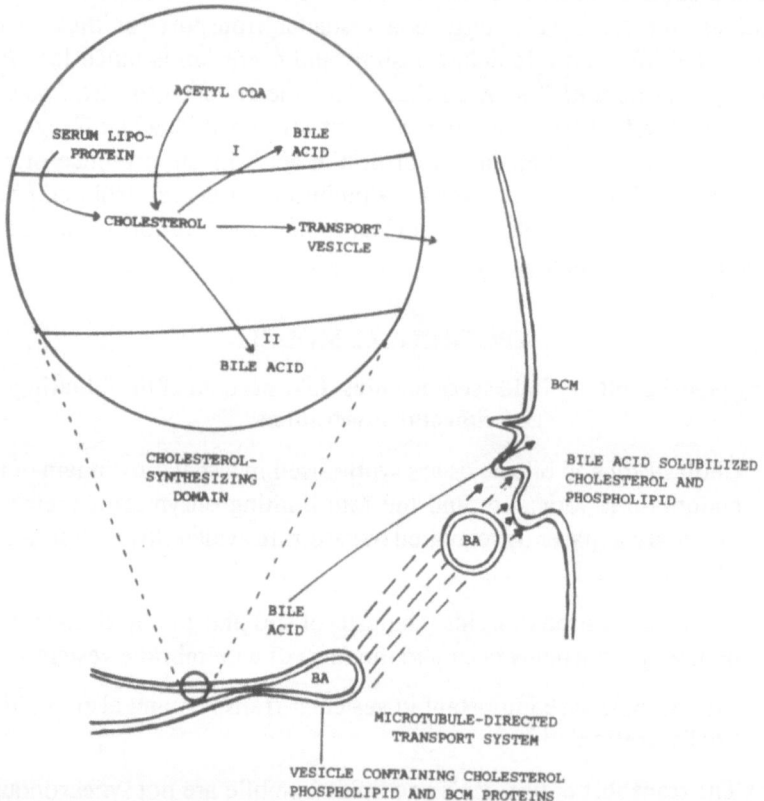

Figure 6 Model for the synthesis and translocation of cholesterol from site of synthesis to bile. Bile acids synthesised from cholesterol take path I for non-vesicular transport; path II for vesicular transport. BA – bile acid.

synthetic domain. The local cholesterol concentration depends upon (a) the delivery to the domain from exogenous sources; (b) the synthetic capability of the domain; and (c) the transport of cholesterol away from the domain.

To account for the preponderance of phosphatidyl choline in bile, either the bile acids must preferentially solubilise this phospholipid from the bile canalicular membrane, or solubilisation must occur from phosphatidyl-choline-rich domains of the membrane: such domains may be derived from the fusion of newly synthesised membrane vesicles. In this context it is pertinent to recall that the lipid secreted at the opposite pole of the hepatocyte (the VLDL) is also highly phosphatidylcholine rich.

Although lipid and bile acid secretion are not synchronous, they are nevertheless probably co-ordinated in the normal situation to maintain the cholesterol in a soluble form in bile. An elevated transfer of cholesterol from the synthetic domain into the bile canalicular membrane in cholesterol gallstone disease would provide the source of raised biliary cholesterol and the reduced availability of cholesterol for bile acid synthesis.

SUMMARY

Cholesterol and bile acids are synthesised on the endoplasmic reticulum of the hepatocyte. Although cholesterol is the precursor of bile acids, the synthetic domains of cholesterol and bile acid synthesis on the endoplasmic reticulum are probably distinct. Transport of cholesterol from the site of synthesis to the bile probably occurs as a membrane vesicle which fuses with the bile canalicular membrane, prior to lipid solubilisation from the membrane by bile acids, which may be transported independently. Since the rate of synthesis of bile acids is probably controlled by the availability of cholesterol to the bile acid synthetic domain, the translocation of cholesterol away from the endoplasmic reticulum may regulate both cholesterol and bile acid synthesis.

We have described a hypothetical model, which predicts that in cholesterol cholelithiasis a more efficient translocation of cholesterol away from the cholesterol synthetic domain will not only release the HMG CoA reductase from feedback inhibition but also reduce the availability of cholesterol for bile acid synthesis.

REFERENCES

1. Carey, M.C. and Cohen, D.E. (1986). Biliary transport of cholesterol in vesicles, micelles and liquid crystals. In: Paumgartner, G., Stiehl, A. and Gerok, W. (eds), *Bile Acids and the Liver*, pp. 287–300 (Lancaster: MTP Press)
2. McMurray, W.C. and Magee, W.L. (1972). Phospholipid metabolism. *Annu. Rev. Biochem.*, **41**, 129–60
3. Skipsi, V.P., Barclay, M., Barclay, R.K., Fetzer, V.A., Good, J.J. and Archibald, F.M. (1967). Lipid composition of human serum lipoproteins. *Biochem. J.*, **104**, 340–352
4. Christie, W.W. (1973). The structure of bile phosphatidyl-choline. *Biochim. Biophys. Acta*, **316**, 204–11
5. Gregory, D.H., Vlahcevic, Z.R., Schatzki, P. and Swell, L. (1975). Mechanism of secretion of bile acids. I. Role of bile canalicular and microsomal membranes in the synthesis and transport of biliary lecithins and cholesterol. *J. Clin. Invest.*, **55**, 105–14
6. Kremmer, T., Wishers, M.H. and Evans, W.H. (1976). The lipid composition of plasma membrane subfractions originating from the three major functional domains of the rat hepatocyte cell surface. *Biochim. Biophys. Acta*, **455**, 655–64
7. Graham, J.M. and Northfield, T.C. (1987). Solubilization of lipids from hamster bile canalicular and contiguous membranes and from human erythrocyte membranes by

39

conjugated bile acids. *Biochem. J.*, **242**, 825–34

8. Dietschy, J.M. and Brown, M.S. (1974). Effect of alterations of the specific activity of the intracellular acetyl CoA pool on apparent rates of cholesterogenesis. *J. Lipid Res.*, **15**, 508–16

9. Mosbach, E.H., Rothschild, M.A., Berkesby, I., Oratz, M. and Mongelli, J. (1971). Bile acid synthesis on the isolated perfused rabbit liver. *J. Clin. Invest.*, **50**, 1720–30

10. Small, D.M. (1976). The etiology and pathogenesis of gallstones. *Adv. Surgery*, **10**, 63–85

11. Shaffer, E.A. and Small, D.M. (1977). Biliary lipid secretion in cholesterol gallstone disease. The effect of cholecystectomy and obesity. *J. Clin. Invest.*, **59**, 828–40

12. Vlahcevic, Z.R., Bell, C.C., Buhac, I., Farrar, J.T. and Swell, L. (1970). Diminished bile acid pool size in patients with gallstones. *Gastroenterology*, **59**, 165–73

13. Coyne, M.J., Bonorris, G.G., Goldstein, L.I. and Schoenfield, L.J. (1976). Effect of chenodeoxycholic acid and phenobarbitol on the rate-limiting enzymes of hepatic cholesterol and bile acid synthesis in patients with gallstones. *J. Lab. Clin. Med.*, **87**, 281–90

14. Ahlberg, J., Angelin, B. and Einarsson, K. (1981). Hepatic 3-hydroxy-3-methylglutaryl coenzyme A reductase activity and biliary lipid composition in man: relation to cholesterol gallstone disease and effects of cholic acid and chenodeoxycholic acid treatment. *J. Lipid Res.*, **22**, 410–22

15. Schoenfield, L.J., Bonnoris, G.G. and Ganz, P. (1973). Induced alterations in rate-limiting enzymes of hepatic cholesterol and bile acid synthesis in the hamster. *J. Lab. Clin. Med.*, **82**, 858–68

16. Danzinger, R.G., Hofmann, A.F., Schoenfield, L.J. and Thistle, J.L. (1972). Dissolution of cholesterol gallstones by chenodeoxycholic acid. *N. Engl. J. Med.*, **286**, 1–8

17. Thistle, J.L. and Hofmann, A.F. (1973). Efficacy and specificity of chenodeoxycholic acid therapy for dissolving gallstones. *N. Engl. J. Med.*, **289**, 655–59

18. Makino, I., Shinozaki, K., Yoshino, K. and Nakagawa, S. (1975). Dissolution of cholesterol gallstones by ursodeoxycholic acid. *Jpn. J. Gastroenterol.*, **72**, 690–702

19. Maton, P.N., Murphy, G.M. and Dowling, R.H. (1977). Ursodeoxycholic acid treatment of gallstones. *Lancet*, **2**, 1297–301

20. Ingebritsen, T.S., Lee, H.S., Parker, R.A. and Gibson, D.M. (1978). Reversible modulation of the activities of both liver microsomal hydroxymethylglutaryl Coenzyme A reductase and its inactivating enzyme. Evidence for regulation by phosphorylation and dephosphorylation. *Biochem. Biophys. Res. Commun.*, **81**, 1268–77

21. Nordstrom, J.L., Rodwell, V.W. and Mitschelsen, J.J. (1977). Interconversion of active and inactive forms of rat liver hydroxymethylglutaryl-CoA reductase. *J Biol Chem*, **252**, 8924–34

22. Mitropoulos, K.A., Knight, B.L. and Reeves, B.E.A. (1980). 3-hydroxy-3-methylglutaryl Coenzyme A reductase: a comparison of the modulation *in vitro* by phosphorylation and dephosphorylation to modulation of enzymic activity by feeding cholesterol- or cholestyramine-supplemented diets. *Biochem. J.*, **185**, 435–41

23. Mitropoulos, K.A. and Venkatesan, S. (1977). The influence of cholesterol on the activity, on the isothermic kinetics and on the temperature-induced kinetics of 3-hydroxy-3-methylglutaryl Coenzyme A reductase. *Biochim. Biophys. Acta*, **489**, 126–42

24. Brown, M.S., Dana, S.E. and Goldstein, J.L. (1974). Regulation of 3-hydroxy-3-methylglutaryl Coenzyme A reductase activity in human fibroblasts. *J. Biol. Chem*, **249**, 789–96

25. Goldstein, J.L. and Brown, M.S. (1977). The low-density lipoprotein pathway and its relation to atherosclerosis. *Annu. Rev. Biochem.*, **46**, 897–930

26. Mitropoulos, K.A., Venkatesan, S., Reeves, B.E.A. and Balasubramaniam, S. (1981). Modulation of 3-hydroxy-3-methylglutaryl-CoA reductase and of acyl-CoA-cholesterol acyl transferase by the transfer of non-esterified cholesterol to rat liver microsomal vesicles. *Biochem. J.*, **194**, 265–71

27. Sabine, J.R. and James, M.J. (1976). The intracellular mechanism responsible for the dietary feedback control of cholesterol synthesis. *Life Sci.*, **18**, 1185–92
28. Gregg, R.G., Sabine, J.R. and Wilce, P.A. (1982). Regulation of 3-hydroxy-3-methylglutaryl Coenzyme A reductase in rat liver and Morris hepatomas 5123c, 9618A and 5123tc. *Biochem. J.*, **204**, 457–62
29. Sipat, A. and Sabine, J.R. (1981). Membrane-mediated control of hepatic β-hydroxy-β-methylglutaryl Coenzyme A reductase. *Biochem. J.*, **194**, 889–92
30. Hamprecht, B., Roscher, R., Waltinger, G. and Nussler, C. (1971). Influence of bile acids on the activity of rat liver 3-hydroxy-3-methylglutaryl Coenzyme A reductase. 2. Effect of cholic acid in lymph fistula rats. *Eur. J. Biochem.*, **18**, 15–9
31. Hamprecht, B., Nussler, C., Waltinger, G. and Lynen, F. (1971). Influence of bile acids on the activity of rat liver 3-hydroxy-3-methylglutaryl Coenzyme A reductase. 1. Effect of bile acids *in vitro* and *in vivo*. *Eur. J. Biochem.*, **18**, 10–4
32. Kubaska, W.M., Gurley, E.C., Hylemon, P.B., Guzelian, P.S. and Vlahcevic, Z.R. (1985). Absence of negative feedback control of bile acid biosynthesis in cultured rat hepatocytes. *J. Biol. Chem.*, **260**, 13459–63
33. Davis, R.A., Hyde, P.M., Kuan, J.-C., Malone-McNeal, M. and Archambault-Schexnayder, J. (1983). Bile acid secretion by cultured rat hepatocytes. Regulation by cholesterol availability. *J. Biol. Chem.*, **258**, 3661–7
34. Mitropoulos, K.A., Venkatesan, S., Balasubramaniam, S. and Peters, T.J. (1978). The submicrosomal localization of 3-hydroxy-3-methylglutaryl-Coenzyme A reductase, cholesterol 7α-hydroxylase and cholesterol in rat liver. *Eur. J. Biochem.*, **82**, 419–29
35. Salen, G., Nicolau, G., Schefer, S. and Mosbach, E.H. (1975). Hepatic cholesterol in patients with gallstones. *Gastroenterology*, **9**, 676–84
36. Graham, J.M. (1979). Surface membrane enzymes in neoplasia. In: Hynes, R.O. (ed.), *Surface of Normal and Malignant Cells*, pp. 199–245. (Chichester: Wiley and Sons)
37. Barnwell, S.G., Lowe, P.J. and Coleman, R. (1984). The effects of colchicine on secretion into bile of bile salts, phospholipids, cholesterol and plasma membrane enzymes: bile salts are secreted unaccompanied by phospholipids and cholesterol. *Biochem. J.*, **220**, 723–31
38. Evans, W.H. (1980). A biochemical dissection of the functional polarity of the plasma membrane of the hepatocyte. *Biochim. Biophys. Acta*, **604**, 27–64
39. Farquar, M.G. (1983). Multiple pathways of exocytosis, endocytosis and membrane recycling: validation of a Golgi route. *Fed. Proc.*, **42**, 2407–13
40. Schiff, J.M., Fisher, M.M. and Underdown, B.J. (1984). Receptor-mediator biliary transport of immunoglobulin A and asialoglycoprotein: sorting and missorting of ligands revealed by two radiolabelling methods. *J. Cell. Biol.*, **98**, 79–89
41. Erlinger, S. (1988). Hepatic bile acid transport and secretion. Chapter 2 (this volume)
42. Petzinger, E., Ziegler, K. and Frimmer, M. (1980). Occurrence of a multispecific transporter for the hepatocellular accumulation of bile acids and various cyclopeptides. In: Paumgartner, G., Stiehl, A. and Gerok, W. (eds.), *Bile Acids and the Liver*, pp. 111–24. (Lancaster: MTP Press)
43. Gonzales, M., Sutherland, E. and Simon, F.R. (1979). Regulation of hepatic transport of bile salts: effects of protein synthesis inhibition on excretion of bile salts and their binding to liver surface membrane fractions. *J. Clin. Invest.*, **63**, 684–95
44. Abberger, H., Bickel, U., Buscher, H.-P., Fuchte, K., Gerok, W., Kramer, W. and Kurz, G. (1981). Transport of bile acids: lipoproteins, membrane polypeptides and cytosolic proteins as carriers. In: Paumgartner, G., Stiehl, A. and Gerok, W. (eds.), *Bile Acids and Lipids*, pp. 233–40. (Lancaster: MTP Press)

4

Biliary Lipid
Secretion and its Control

R. Coleman, K. Rahman, M.E. Bellringer and M. Carrella*
Department of Biochemistry
University of Birmingham
UK
*Institute of Internal Medicine and Metabolic Diseases
University of Naples, II Medical School
Naples, Italy

INTRODUCTION

The processes of biliary lipid secretion are complex and many details are still unknown. This article explores the coupling between bile acid secretion and biliary lipid secretion, and discusses the supply and control of lipid to replenish this biliary lipid outflow.

NATURE AND FORM OF THE BILIARY LIPIDS

The biliary lipids are phospholipids and cholesterol; other lipids, e.g. acylglycerols, fatty acids and cholesterol esters, which are common in plasma, are normally present in bile in only trace amounts. Occasionally some fatty acids and lysophosphatidylcholine may be present due to phospholipid breakdown resulting from contamination of the bile with pancreatic juice[1].

Phosphatidylcholine is the predominant biliary phospholipid (80–95% of the total). Biliary phosphatidylcholine has a distinct fatty acid profile, with the majority being the $C_{16:0}$, $C_{18:2}$, $C_{18:1}$ and $C_{20:4}$ species. Most membrane phosphatidylcholine samples show a much broader fatty acid profile with more important contributions from $C_{18:0}$ and $C_{20:4}$ fatty acids[2,3] (Figure 1).

In bile the phospholipids and cholesterol are found both in vesicles and in bile acid-lipid mixed micelles; the balance between these two forms represents a continuously shifting equilibrium depending upon bile acid concentration and type, storage time etc. In general, at lower bile acid concentrations and with the more hydrophilic bile salts, the proportion of vesicles is

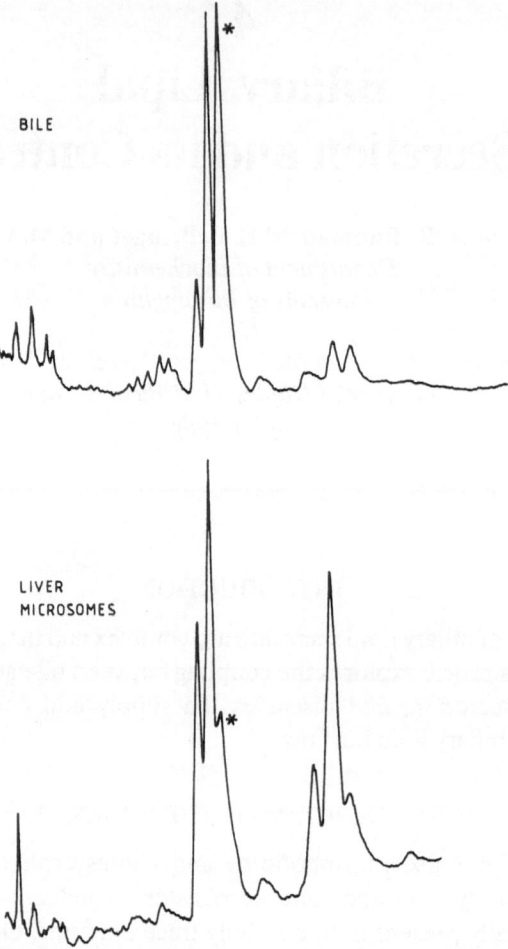

Figure 1   HPLC fractionation of phosphatidylcholine from rat bile and rat liver microsomes. Each peak represents a single component with a specific fatty acid composition. * indicates $C_{16:0}$, $C_{18:2}$. Unpublished data of K. Rahman.

higher; this is consistent with the concept that lipid is initially secreted in vesicles which are subsequently processed by bile acid to bile acid–lipid mixed micelles[2,4,5]. The conversion of vesicles to micelles increases the cholesterol saturation of the bile[4], since lipid vesicles appear to be able to maintain a higher cholesterol:phospholipid ratio than micelles. This increase, compounded by the addition of cholesterol from other sources to bile, may cause the cholesterol to precipitate out around nucleating centres to form cholesterol crystals and, subsequently, cholesterol gallstones[2,4,5].

DEPENDENCE OF BILIARY LIPID SECRETION UPON BILE SALT SECRETION

Under physiological conditions the secretion of biliary lipids is generally dependent upon the secretion of bile salts, so that the concentration of biliary lipids is low when bile salt secretion is low (e.g. during fasting) and increases with increasing bile salt output during feeding[6,7]. Interruption of the enterohepatic circulation (EHC) by T-tube drainage or by a biliary fistula causes a progressive depletion of the bile salt pool down to the level that can be maintained by endogenous synthesis; this decline is accompanied by a corresponding decline in biliary lipids. In these preparations and with the isolated perfused liver, in which the loss can be more rapid and extreme, the subsequent infusion of bile salts causes an increase in the secretion of biliary lipids[8–12]. This rate of lipid secretion can be maintained if bile salt infusion is continuous[12], but peaks and declines if a bolus of bile salt is infused[13].

Using these models of depletion and infusion, the response of biliary lipid secretion to graded rates of bile salt supply can be investigated and the effects of individual, rather than mixed, bile salts can be compared. The response is essentially curvilinear or linear from the basal output at low bile

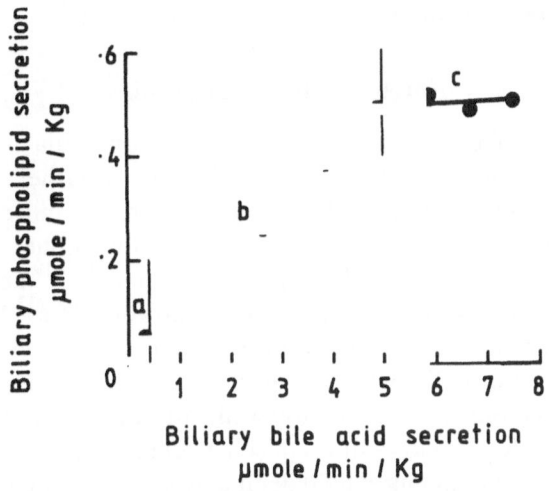

Figure 2 Response of biliary phospholipid secretion to increased bile acid secretion. Taurocholate was infused into isolated perfused rat liver or biliary fistula rats at low (a), medium (b) and high (c) infusion rates up to 12.5 μmol/min/kg body wt. Data derived from 12 and 16.

salt secretion rates[9,11,14,87]; in general three distinct regions to the response can be identified at low, intermediate and high bile salt infusion rates (see Figure 2).

General Features of the Response

The main feature of the response (region b) is the increase in both phospholipid and cholesterol secretion as bile salt infusion rate (and biliary bile acid concentration) increases. Cholesterol and phospholipid secretion often increase in similar proportion so that the cholesterol:phospholipid molar ratio is relatively constant; the ratio differs between species (e.g. dog ≈ 0.033,[14] rat ≈ 0.1[11,16,87] man ≈ 0.3[7,9,87]). At higher bile salt infusion rates (region c) bile acid and biliary lipid secretion rates plateau and then decline at even higher infusion rates, signalling the onset of bile acid toxicity[2]. The maximum rate for rats infused with taurocholate causes a biliary bile acid secretion rate of ≈ 10 μmol/min/kg and a concentration of 80–90 mmol/l[12], plus a maximum phospholipid secretion rate of 0.5 μmol/min/kg (perfused liver) – 0.8 (bile fistula rat) and a biliary concentration of 5–7 mmol/l[12].

At low bile salt secretion rates (region a) or concentrations (< 0.16 μmol/min/kg[9,11] or 3 mmol/l) the relative proportions of cholesterol and phospholipid are different. Phospholipid output declines much more than cholesterol. Cholesterol:phospholipid ratios increase variably (man 0.3–0.5[7,9,87], rat 0.1–0.15[11,16] and dog hardly at all[9,14]). Extrapolation of the cholesterol output to zero bile salt output yields a value which may reflect a mechanism different from that at higher bile salt outputs[11].

Effects of Different Bile Acids

Infusion of single bile acids into animals with a biliary fistula or into isolated perfused livers indicates that bile acids differ greatly in their ability to influence biliary lipid secretion, so that the slopes of lipid vs bile acid secretion rates differ for different bile acids[17,18]. Bile acids with one or more keto groups appear to provoke little biliary lipid secretion[11,17,19] and this is true particularly of the triketo compound taurodehydrocholate[11,13,20,21]. Since many such bile acids are also choleretic, they cause a dilution of bile which reduces the secretion of lipids stimulated by other more effective bile acids[11]. Biliary lipid secretion correlates fairly well with the hydrophobicity of the bile acid; molecules with low critical micellar concentration (cmc) stimulate secretion of greater amounts of lipid per molecule, and act at lower bile acid concentrations, than those with a higher cmc[2,5,11,18]. Dihydroxy bile acids are thus more effective than trihydroxy, 7α-OH bile acids are more effective than 7β-OH[5,18,] and 7-CH$_3$ more effective than 7-H[22].

These differences between individual bile acids partly explain the differences in biliary lipid:bile acid secretion ratio between animal species, and the higher maximum secretion rate with whole rat bile than with taurocholate alone[15]. Other factors, such as different effects on lipid synthesis rates and intracellular transport[20], may also contribute, especially to the cholesterol:phospholipid secretion ratio.

Although different bile acids may stimulate, or be associated with, different lipid secretion rates at moderate rates of infusion (Figure 2, b) maximum lipid secretion rates appear to be similar in all cases so far investigated, thus suggesting that the maximum secretion rate may reflect the maximum rate of lipid synthesis, delivery and secretion[23].

COUPLING OF BILIARY LIPID SECRETION TO BILE ACID SECRETION

During continuous infusion, bile salts stimulate biliary lipid secretion and determine its rate (Figure 2 region b). After secretion, the biliary lipids are found in association with the bile salts as vesicular structures and as mixed micelles. It has been proposed, at various times[24-26], that the association of bile acids and biliary lipids takes place inside the cell, particularly in the formation of mixed micelles perhaps by the interaction of bile acids with intracellular membranes. This is unlikely, however, since intracellular bile acid concentration is around 0.2 mmol/l[27-29], much lower than the micellar range

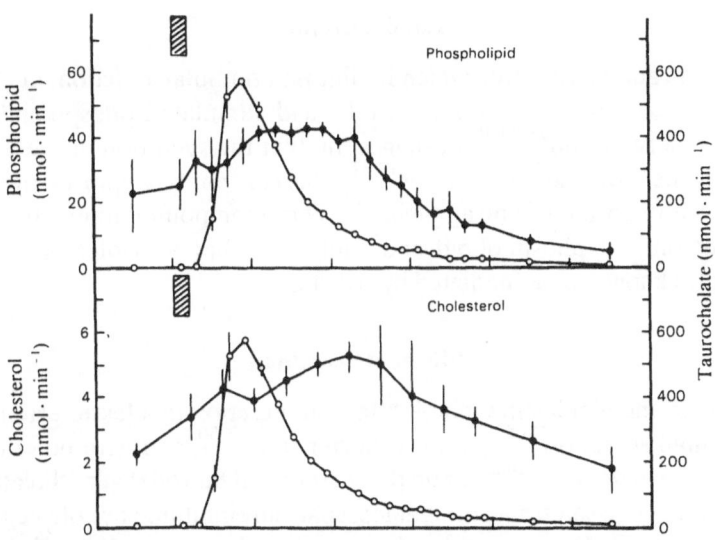

Figure 3   Kinetic response of biliary lipid secretion to a single pulse of bile acid. A pulse of ^{14}C-taurocholate (5 μmol) was infused in one minute (hatched square) under single pass conditions in isolated rat liver. Open circles represent biliary taurocholate secretion, filled circles represent biliary phospholipid and cholesterol secretion. From 31 with permission.

above 2 mmol/l[2-5]. In addition, the recently identified bile acid transporter in the canalicular membrane has an affinity around 10–50 μmol/l[30], i.e. far lower than micellar concentrations. This transporter would therefore be expected to function as a molecular rather than a micellar pump, pumping bile acids into the canaliculus where micelles would form subsequently[2,5]. Bile salts incapable of forming micelles (e.g. the very hydrophilic taurodehydrocholate) can be secreted without accompanying lipid[11,13,21]. Kinetic experiments show more directly the dissociation of bile acid from lipid transport. Thus, although bile acid secretion seems to coincide with biliary lipid secretion when studied using long collection times[13], it precedes it by several minutes when the collection intervals are reduced[31] (Figure 3).

Several molecules seem to separate biliary lipid secretion from bile acid secretion in that they reduce the former but not the latter. These compounds include iodipamide[32,33] ampicillin[34,35], bilirubin conjugates[36-38], sulphobromophthalein[39], valproic acid[40,41], sulphated glycolithocholic acid[42,43], and other sulphated bile acids[44,45]. The effect of these compounds, when studied, appears to be upon secretion of lipids rather than on hepatic uptake[37] or synthesis[34].

INVOLVEMENT OF VESICLE TRANSPORT

Lipid Secretion

Colchicine and vinblastine, which inhibit microtubular function and hence vesicle movement, strongly inhibit bile acid stimulated phospholipid and cholesterol secretion[13,20,46,47], suggesting that the secretion of these lipids requires the movement of vesicles[13,31]. This concept is supported by recent studies with valproate[41] and ampicillin[48]. These compounds inhibit the secretion not only of phospholipid and cholesterol but also of several other molecules known to be mediated by vesicles.

Bile Acid Secretion

Colchicine and vinblastine inhibit bile acid secretion to a lesser extent than biliary lipid secretion[20,47,49], for a shorter time[13,50], and with no effect on basal bile acid secretion[50,51] or on the secretion of taurodehydrocholate[13,20]. The fact that bile salt transport is at least partially inhibited by colchicine and vinblastine has led to suggestions that it may involve microtubules[46,47,51] and therefore vesicle transport[20,51,53]. While this is clearly untrue for taurodehydrocholate[13,20] it should be considered for more hydrophobic bile salts.

Other evidence that appears to support the involvement of vesicles in the secretion of bile salts includes the increase in the number of vesicles around the bile canaliculus during active bile salt transport[53-56] especially of taurodehydrocholate[53], the presence of radiolabelled bile acid activity over intracellular organelles during bile acid secretion[56,57], and the accumulation of fluorescent – labelled bile acid in/over intracellular organelles[58]. The identification of a bile acid transporting system in hepatocyte Golgi fractions[59] suggests an intracellular site where bile acids are not merely associated with vesicular material but may also be pumped into it; vesicular movement to the canaliculus may then follow.

An equal, if not more convincing, body of evidence points, however, in the opposite direction. The transcellular transport of bile acids is much more rapid (<2 min[31]) than vesicle-mediated endocytosis/pinocytosis and subsequent transocytosis[31,60]. It is also shorter than the duration of secretion of radiolabelled bile acid secretion[56] or of the association of fluorescent bile acids (≈ 20 min) with the Golgi apparatus[58]. Furthermore, it is most unlikely that the vesicles observed around the bile canaliculus are transporting bile salts since taurodehydrocholate transport is unaffected by colchicine[13,31] Transport systems for bile acids have been well documented in bile canalicular membrane preparations[30,61-64] and these would compete with the system described for the Golgi apparatus. Valproic acid and ampicillin inhibit many vesicle mediated processes at both poles of the hepatocyte but neither inhibits bile acid transport[41,48]. Finally, physical studies with ^{31}P NMR and fluorescence anisotropy have concluded that vesicular bile acid transport in the cytoplasm is unlikely[66].

SEQUENCE OF EVENTS IN BILE ACID INDUCED LIPID SECRETION

The balance of evidence from studies of kinetics and of the effects of inhibitors etc. suggests that the movements of bile acids and lipids destined for biliary excretion appears to be independent. The initial secretory event appears to be the secretion of bile acids into the bile canaliculus. The bile acids are then joined by biliary lipids, arriving by microtubule-mediated vesicle transport, to form vesicular structures and then mixed micelles in the bile[31,2,5]. These events can be dissected kinetically using a single-pass liver perfusion method, but they will occur in an apparently continuous fashion in a continuous infusion system or *in vivo* and thus the secreted lipid would not necessarily form micelles with the bile acids initially stimulating its secretion[2,5].

This simplified scheme does not, however, indicate how bile acids determine lipid secretion and how they control the amount of lipid secreted. Nor does it explain anomalies such as the localisation of radio- or fluoro-labelled bile acid analogues with membrane structures, the accumulation of vesicles during intensive bile acid transport and the partial inhibition of bile acid transport by colchicine. These anomalies may be explained by con-

49

sidering the processes of lipid supply in more detail.

IMMEDIATE ORIGIN OF BILIARY LIPIDS

The kinetic experiments[31] outlined above (Figure 3) indicate that bile acids enter the bile canaliculus before biliary lipids, so that the only lipids available to the bile acids immediately after their secretion would be those of the bile canalicular membrane or those shed into the lumen by exocytosis.

Models in which cells are treated by adding bile acids externally, at sub-cytolytic concentrations, have demonstrated that small amounts of membrane material are pinched off as microvesicles, and then converted to mixed micelles. The extent and detail of these processes depend on the struc-

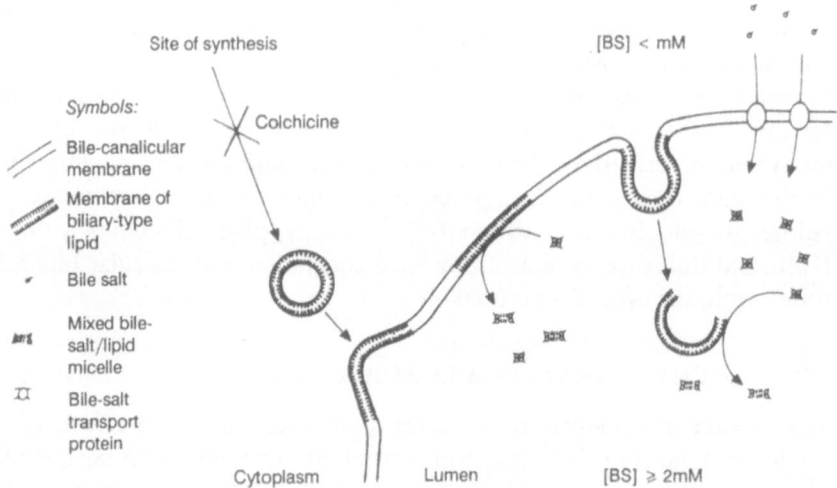

Figure 4 Possible mechanisms for secretion of lipid into bile. Bile acid is secreted by a transport protein. Vesicles composed of biliary-type lipid are moved to and fuse with the bile canalicular membrane by a process that involves the cytoskeleton. The microdomain of lipid thus produced may vesiculate under the influence of the bile acids in the lumen and is then converted to mixed bile acid-lipid micelles. Colchicine inhibits the movement of lipid from within the cell to the canaliculus membrane. From 31 with minor modification, with permission.

ture of the individual bile acids and on the composition and structural order of the membranes involved[5]. The bile canalicular membrane is the least fluid of the plasma membrane domains of the hepatocyte and is rich in sphingomyelin and cholesterol. Microdomains of different fluidity may coexist within this membrane[31], as indicated by studies with probe molecules[67]. Since low fluidity and high cholesterol content militate against intercalation of bile acids into such membrane microdomains[5,66,68], then the following

50

series of events may occur subsequent to the transport of bile salts into the bile canaliculus and their initial build up to micellar concentrations:

(1)   exclusion of bile acids from the less fluid microdomains of the canalicular membrane.

(2)   incorporation of bile acids as reverse micelles into the outer leaflet of a more fluid microdomain of the membrane. This would cause the leaflet to curve outwards to destabilise and fuse, culminating in the pinching off of a microvesicle containing the fluid lipid microdomain leaving a less fluid membrane better able to withstand the bile acid concentration.

(3)   replenishment of the more fluid microdmaines with similar lipid supplied from within the cell in order to avoid ultimate cell damage[2,5,31] (Figure 4).

This concept is supported by observations from the liver and from other systems: (se ref. 5) (i) bile acids are excluded from low fluidity:high cholesterol domains of model membranes; (ii) fluidity probes and chlorpromazine partition selectively into microdomains of different fluidity in different membranes; (iii) biliary lipids are more fluid than hepatocyte plasma membrane lipids they have more $C_{16:0}$, $C_{18:2}$ phosphatidylcholines and less cholesterol; (iv) bile salts extract the more fluid lipids from several membranes; (v) when lipids are removed faster than they are supplied, e.g. at $> SR_{max}$ and as in the presence of colchicine, the membrane is damaged and the cell ultimately lyses.

RESUPPLY OF LIPID TO THE BILE CANALICULUS

A continuous resupply of lipid would be needed to replenish the fluid microdomains processed by bile salts. This lipid could be brought to the canalicular membrane by transfer proteins as components of the membrane or as contents of a vesicle. The experiments with colchicine, vinblastine and valproic acid cited above indicate strongly that vesicular movement is involved. Lipid supply to vesicles destined for the plasma membrane has been described in several cells other than hepatocytes[69-76] whilst in hepatocytes the number of vesicles in the region of the bile canaliculus increases during extensive bile acid transport[53]. These vesicles were originally interpreted as bile acid transporting vesicles[53-55] but they might now be interpreted as vesicles supplying the biliary lipid. This is especially relevant to taurodehydrocholate transport, since this bile acid provokes little lipid secretion so that the accumulating vesicles may represent biliary lipid precursor vesicles 'queuing' close to the site of normal lipid removal[31]. Fusion of the putative biliary lipid-rich vesicles with the plasma membranes would create microdomains of higher fluidity; this would allow intercalation of bile acids and then the pinching off of a vesicle of biliary lipid[5]. Such fusion of vesicles, without a random mixing of their membrane lipids with bulk membrane lipids, has been observed in other cells[31].

The composition of the biliary lipid, i.e. its phosphatidylcholine content, its specific fatty acids and its high cholesterol content, would be expected to be reflected in the composition of the vesicles supplying biliary lipids to the bile canaliculus. Such vesicles have yet to be identified; the abundance of vesicle types in hepatocytes[72,73] and the absence of a suitable protein label makes this task particularly difficult.

Although, at moderate bile acid transport rates, the amount of biliary lipid varies according to the bile acid species, there is now some evidence that the maximum phospholipid secretion rate is similar for several different bile acids. Above this rate, secretory parameters decline and the liver becomes cholestatic. It is interesting that just before the maximum secretory rate, phospholipids other than the biliary type increase slightly in the bile. Plasma membrane preparations made from such cholestatic livers show a reduction in phospholipid:cholesterol ratio, indicating that membrane repair is impaired in the face of maximal lipid removal. The remaining membrane, which would be less fluid and more cholesterol-rich than normal, may then be a less favourable environment for the function of bile acid transport proteins so that overall secretion rates would decline[74-78]. This would in turn cause intracellular bile salt concentrations to rise and promote the onset of a bile salt toxicity[2].

CONTROL OF LIPID SUPPLY

Although the outputs of bile acids and lipids are independent, the rate of bile acid secretion clearly influences that of biliary lipids. The increased output of biliary lipid can moreover be maintained, suggesting the mechanisms of supply and secretion are continuous and regulated[12].

The extent of bile acid transport through the hepatocyte is somehow sensed by the cell, and could affect lipid secretion at several points[2]. These include the provision (i.e. biosynthesis or redistribution) of the lipid, the assembly of the lipid into vesicles, the transport of the vesicles through the cell, and the processing of the lipid at the canalicular membrane[5]. Other authors have generally commented on the facilitation of lipid transport in the cell[79,80] but without indicating the possible location of this effect.

Kinetic studies of bile acid secretion indicate that the control over lipid secretion which it exerts can vary. When small amounts of bile acids are pulsed through the liver the subsequent peaks of lipid vary both in peak definition and time interval. Larger pulses of taurocholate result in some-what better control but variability is still high. A continuous background infusion of the hydrophilic bile acid, taurodehydrocholate, with superimposed pulses of taurocholate seems to bring the lipid delivery and secretion processes under better control in that the lipid peaks become better defined and coincide more closely with the peaks of taurocholate output[81]. Since tauro-dehydrocholate has little detergent effect on membranes[5] these experiments indicate that taurodehydrocholate, or some molecule interacting with it, has controlled the movement of biliary lipids within the cell better[81]. This control could be exercised either on the membrane vesicle itself or on the vesicle:cytoskeletal interaction (Figure 5).

Other studies have shown that bile acids increase the output of lysosomal enzymes into bile[82], stimulate the uptake and secretion of inulin by hepatocytes[83] and increase the polymerisation of tubulin[84]. These all sug-

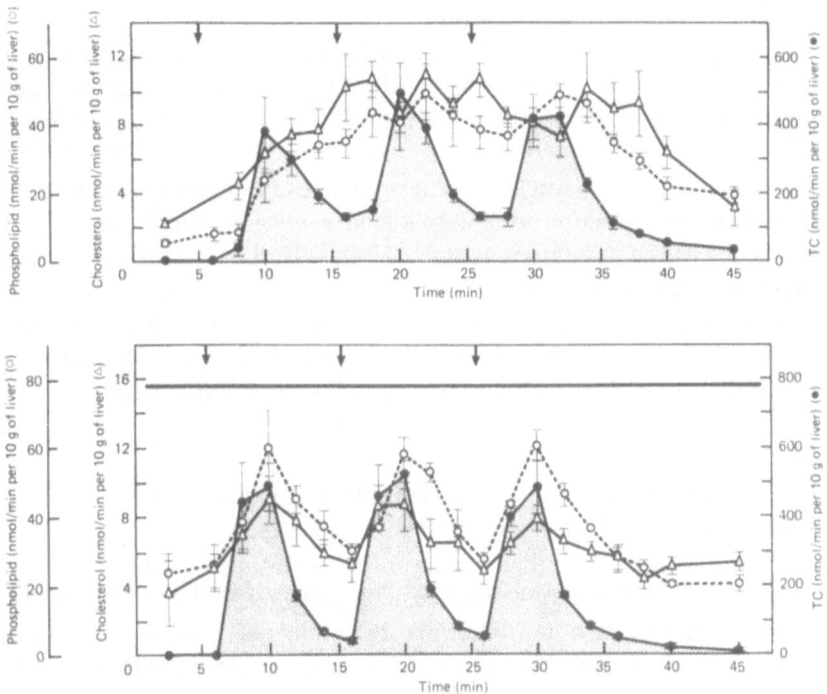

Figure 5 Effect of continuous perfusion of taurodehydrocholate upon the kinetic response of biliary lipids to repeated pulses of bile acid (taurocholate) Upper figure: Three pulses of 2.5 μmole taurocholate (arrows) were infused during single pass perfusion conditions in isolated rat liver. Biliary output of bile acids (filled circles); phospholipid (open circles) and cholesterol (triangles) were then followed. Lower figure: As for above with continuous infusion of taurodehydrocholate (1 μmol/min) throughout the experiment. From 81 with permission.

gest that bile acids stimulate vesicle/cytoskeletal phenomena; they may provide clues to the involvement of bile acids in controlling lipid secretion.

It is also conceivable that bile acids may modulate response through other intracellular signals such as cyclic AMP, calcium protein phosphorylation, phosphoinositides etc. Little is known about the involvement of these messengers in bile secretion. In the dog, dibutyryl cAMP or glucagon have no effect on biliary bile acid secretion but reduce cholesterol secretion[85,86].

DIFFERENTIAL SECRETION OF CHOLESTEROL AND PHOSPHOLIPIDS

In some species, as discussed earlier, cholesterol secretion is appreciable even when biliary bile acid and phospholipid secretion rates are low[7,9,14,16,87]. This cholesterol secretion contributes to the cholesterol: phospholipid ratio of bile at all bile acid secretion rates, and causes variation in the cholesterol:phospholipid ratio.

Several studies have identified differential effects on biliary cholesterol and phospholipid secretions – for instance long term studies of drug administration, feeding, metabolic alteration[88-92]; or acute studies of bile acid administration where metabolic change may contribute little[17,93-96]. It is not clear whether these changes represent changes in the relative contribution of cholesterol secretion at low bile-acid secretion rates[81], the selective processing of the hepatocyte membrane by different bile acids[5] or the different coupling of phospholipid and cholesterol transport and secretion at intermediate bile salt transport rates. The latter would imply that the movement of biliary lipids to the bile canaliculus could involve two types of vesicles – phospholipid-rich and cholesterol-rich. These vesicles would need to be characterised and the factors responsible for their different delivery identified.

Several preliminary experiments have attempted to study the origins of the cholesterol which is present at low bile acid secretion rates. Phalloidin, which polymerises microfilaments, brings about a more substantial inhibition of cholesterol output than of bile acids and phospholipids[88,97]. Perfusion of livers with a pulse of taurodehydrocholate increases the biliary output of cholesterol but not phospholipid, and this can be inhibited with colchicine[13]. Prolonged perfusion of the liver with taurodehydrocholate increases the cholesterol:phospholipid ratio of the biliary lipids[98]. Chloroquine selectively increases biliary cholesterol secretion but has little effect on phospholipids or bile acids[99].

The origin of this component of biliary cholesterol is probably some form of vesicular material since its cholesterol output can be inhibited by the anticytoskeletal agents colchicine and phalloidin[88,97]. Lysosomes are unlikely to be the source, since in perfused liver studies lysosomal enzymes and cholesterol appear in the bile at different times[98-100] indicating that the cholesterol is located either in a distinct population of lysosomes or in some other endosomal or Golgi related compartment[99].

SUMMARY

The principal biliary lipids are phosphatidylcholine and cholesterol. In general, their presence in bile and their secretion rate are determined largely by the rate of bile acid secretion. At high bile acid secretion rates biliary lipid secretion reaches a plateau, the level of which may be determined by a rate limiting step in intracellular processing, in delivery or at the canalicular membrane.

Biliary lipid secretion can, nevertheless, be dissected from bile acid secretion in several ways. These include the selective reduction in lipid secretion caused by compounds such as iodipamide, ampicillin, valproic acid and, to some extent, colchicine, the secretion of taurodehydrocholate with little lipid, and the secretion of bile acids before biliary lipids in rapid kinetic experiments. Studies of vesicular transport inhibition with colchicine and valproic acid suggest that biliary lipids are brought to the canalicular membrane by intracellular vesicle transport, but that this is less likely for bile acids.

Bile acids are probably initially secreted into the bile canaliculus, and then joined by biliary lipids which have been brought to the canalicular membrane by vesicle transport and removed from it by bile salts already in the canaliculus.

Though bile acid secretion and biliary lipid secretion are separate processes, the former normally controls the latter. Kinetic experiments with pulses of bile acid in perfused livers indicate that the degree of this control may vary. Taurodehydrocholate, unable itself to provoke substantial lipid secretion, can improve the control of the biliary lipid delivery and secretion.

In some species cholesterol output is appreciable even when biliary lipid secretion is low. The differential effects of several compounds on biliary cholesterol:phospholipid ratios support a second source of biliary cholesterol.

REFERENCES

1. Billington, D., Rahman, K., Jones, T.W., Coleman, R., Sykes, I.R. and Aulak, K.S. (1986). Phospholipid degradation in, and protein content of, rat fistula bile. *J. Hepatol.*, 3, 233–40
2. Coleman, R. (1987). Biochemistry of bile secretion. *Biochem. J.*, 244, 249–61
3. Cantafora, A., DiBiase, A., Alvaro, D., Angelico, M., Marin, M. and Attili, A.F. (1983). High performance liquid chromatographic analysis of molecular species of phosph-

atidylcholine: development of quantitative assay and its application to human bile. *Clin. Chem. Acta*, **134**, 281–95

4. Somjen, G.J. and Gilat, T. (1986). Changing concepts of cholesterol solubility in bile. *Gastroenterology*, **91**, 772–75

5. Coleman, R. (1987). Bile salts and biliary lipids. *Biochem. Soc. Trans.*, **15**, 685–805

6. Northfield, T.C. and Hofmann, A.F. (1975). Biliary lipid output during three meals and an overnight fast. *Gut*, **16**, 1–7

7. Mok, H.Y.I., von Bergman, K. and Grundy, S.M. (1978). Effects of interruption of enterohepatic circulation on biliary lipid secretion in man. *Digest. Dis.*, **23**, 1067–75

8. Balint, J.A., Beeler, D.A., Kyriakides, E.C. and Treble, D.H. (1971). The effect of bile salts upon lecithin synthesis. *J. Lab. Clin. Med.*, **77**, 122–33

9. Wagner, C.I., Trotman, B.W. and Soloway, R.D. (1976). Kinetic analysis of biliary lipid excretion in man and dog. *J. Clin. Invest.*, **57**, 473–7

10. Wheeler, H.O. (1972). Secretion of bile acids by the liver and their role in the formation of hepatic bile. *Arch. Intern. Med.*, **130**, 533–41

11. Hardison, W.G. and Apter, J.T. (1972). Micellar theory of biliary cholesterol secretion. *Am. J. Physiol.*, **222**, 61–7

12. Rahman, K., Hammond, T.G., Lowe, P.J., Barnwell, S.G., Clark, B. and Coleman, R. (1986). Control of biliary phospholipid secretion. *Biochem. J.*, **234**, 421–27

13. Barnwell, S.G., Lowe, P.J. and Coleman, R. (1984). The effects of colchicine on secretion into bile of bile salts, phospholipids, cholesterol and plasma membrane enzymes: bile salts are secreted unaccompanied by phospholipids and cholesterol. *Biochem. J.*, **220**, 723–31

14. Wheeler, H.O., May, R.J. and Loeb, P.M. (1973). Determinants of biliary lipid secretion. In Preisig, R. and Bircher, J. (eds.) *The Liver: Quantitative Aspects of Structure and Function.* pp. 368–75 (Basle: Karger)

15. Hardison, W.G.M., Hatoff, D.E., Mayal, K. and Weiner, R.G. (1981). Nature of bile acid maximum secretory rate in the rat. *Am. J. Physiol.*, **241**, G337–G343

16. Rahman, K. and Coleman, R. (1986). Selective biliary lipid secretion at low bile salt output rates in the isolated perfused liver: effects of phalloidin. *Biochem. J.*, **237**, 301–4

17. Sewell, R.B., Hoffman, N.E., Smallwood, R.A. and Cockbain, S. (1980). Bile acid structure and bile formation: a comparison of hydroxy and keto bile acids. *Am. J. Physiol.*, **238**, G10–G17

18. Gurantz, D. and Hofmann, A.F. (1984). Influence of bile acid structure on flow and biliary lipid secretion in the hamster. *Am. J. Physiol.*, **247**, G736–G748

19. Hoffman, N.E., Sewell, R.B. and Smallwood, R.A. (1978). Bile acid structure and biliary lipid secretion: a comparison of three hydroxy and two keto acids. *Am. J. Physiol.*, **234**, E637–41

20. Berken, C.A., Hartman, C.B. and Gollan, J.L. (1983). Microtubules and the excretion of bile acids and biliary lipid. *Gastroenterology*, **84**, 1103

21. O'Maille, E.R.L. and Hofmann, A.F. (1986). Relatively high biliary secretory maximum for non-micelle forming bile acid. Possible significance for mechanism of secretion. *Q. J. Exp. Physiol.*, **71**, 475–82

22. Kuroki, S., Mosbach, E.H., Stenger, R.J., Cohen, B.I. and McSherry, C.K. (1987). Comparative effects of deoxycholate and 7-methyldeoxycholate in the hamster. *Hepatology*, **7**, 229–34

23. Barnwell, S.G. (1987). Evidence that sequential solubilisation of the bile canalicular membrane occurs during the onset of bile acid-induced cholestasis. *Biochem. Soc. Trans.*, **15**, 480

24. Small, D.M. (1970). The formation of gallstones. *Adv. Intern. Med.*, **16**, 243–64

25. Forker, E.L. (1977). Mechanisms of hepatic bile formation. *Annu. Rev. Physiol.*, **39**, 323–47

26. Reuben, A. and Allen, R.M. (1986). Intrahepatic sources of biliary-like micelles. *Biochim. Biophys. Acta*, **876**, 1–12

27. Okishio, T. and Nair, P.P. (1966). Studies on bile acids. Some observations on the intracellular localisation of major bile acids in rat liver. *Biochemistry*, 5, 3662–8

28. Oh, S.Y. and Dupont, J. (1975). Identification and quantitation of cholanoic acids in hepatic and extra-hepatic tissues of rat. *Lipids*, 10, 340–7

29. Erlinger, S. (1985). Hepatic transport of bile acids: intracellular events. In Barbara, L. *et al.* (eds.) *Recent Advances In Bile Acid Research*, pp. 5–9 (New York: Raven Press)

30. Meier, P.J., Meier-Abt, A. St., Barret, C. and Boyer, J.C. (1984). Mechanism of taurocholate transport in canalicular and basolateral rat liver plasma membrane vesicles. *J. Biol. Chem.*, 259, 10614–22

31. Lowe, P.J., Barnwell, S.G. and Coleman, R. (1984). Rapid kinetic analysis of the bile-salt-dependent secretion of phospholipid, cholesterol and a plasma membrane enzyme into bile. *Biochem. J.*, 222, 631–37

32. Apstein, M.D. and Robins, S.J. (1981). A model to dissociate bile salt from cholesterol and phospholipid secretion. The effects of iodipamide on biliary lipid synthesis and secretion. *Gastroenterology*, 80, 1326

33. Apstein, M.D. and Robins, S.J. (1982). Effect of organic anions on biliary lipids in the rat. *Gastroenterology*, 83, 1120–26

34. Apstein, M.D. and Roxbury, W. (1984). The relationship of biliary lecithin (PC) secretion to hepatic PC stores. In *Enterohepatic Circulation of Bile Acids and Sterol Metabolism*, (Lancaster: MTP Press)

35. Apstein, M.D. and Russo, A.R. (1985). Ampicillin inhibits biliary cholesterol secretion. *Digestive Dis. Sci.*, 30, 253–56

36. Apstein, M.D. (1982). Inhibition of biliary phospholipid and cholesterol secretion by bilirubin in the Sprague–Dawley and Gunn rat. *Hepatology*, 2, 143

37. Apstein, M.D. (1984). Inhibition of biliary phospholipid and cholesterol secretion by bilirubin in the Sprague–Dawley and Gunn rat. *Gastroenterology*, 87, 634–38

38. Apstein, M.D. and Roxbury, W. (1986). Bilirubin is a competitive inhibitor of biliary cholesterol and phospholipid secretion. In *Bile Acids and the Liver*, (Lancaster: MTP Press)

39. Shaffer, E.A. and Preshaw, R.M. (1981). Effects of sulphobromophthalein excretion on biliary lipid secretion in humans and dogs. *Am. J. Physiol.*, 240, G85–G89

40. Jezequel, A.M., Bonazzi, P., Novelli, G., Venturini, C. and Orlandi, F. (1984). Early structural and functional changes in liver of rats treated with a single dose of valproic acid. *Hepatology*, 4, 1159–66

41. Bellringer, M.E., Rahman, K. and Coleman, R. (1987). Sodium valproate inhibits the movement of secretory vesicles in rat hepatocytes. *Biochem. J.*, 249, 513–519

42. Kuipers, F., Havinga, R. and Vonk, R.J. (1985). Cholestasis induced by sulphated glycolithocholic acid in the rat: protection by endogenous bile acids. *Clin. Sci.*, 68, 127–34

43. Kuipers, F., Derksen, J.P.T., Gerding, A., Scherphof, G.L. and Vonk, R.A. (1987). Biliary lipid secretion in the rat: the uncoupling of biliary cholesterol and phospholipid secretion from bile acid secretion by sulphated glycolithocholic acid. *Biochim. Biophys. Acta*, 922, 136–144

44. Mathis, U., Karlaganis, G. and Preisig, R. (1983). Monohydroxy bile acid sulphates: tauro 3β hydroxy 5 cholenoate-3-sulphate induces intrahepatic cholestasis in rats. *Gastroenterology*, 85, 674–81

45. Yousef, I.M., Barnwell, S.G., Tuchweber, B., Weber, A. and Roy, C.C. (1987). Effect of complete sulphonation of bile acids on bile formation in rats. *Hepatology*, 7, 535–42

46. Dubin, M., Maurice, M., Feldman, G. and Erlinger, S. (1980). Influence of colchicine and phalloidin on bile secretion and hepatic ultrastructure in the rat. *Gastroenterology*, 79, 646–54

47. Gregory, D.H., Vlahceviv, Z.R., Prugh, M.F. and Swell, L. (1978). Mechanism of secretion of biliary lipids: role of a microtubular system in hepatocellular transport of biliary lipids in the rat. *Gastroenterology*, 74, 93–100

48. Bellringer, M.E., Steele, N.J., Rahman, K. and Coleman, . (1988). Ampicillin inhibits the movement of biliary secretory vesicles in rat hepatocytes. *Biochim. Biophys. Acta* (In press).

49. Sewell, R.B., Barham, S.S., Zinsmeister, A.R. and La Russo, N.L. (1984). Microtubule modulation of biliary excretion of endogenous and exogenous hepatic lysosomal constituents. *Am. J. Physiol.*, **246**, G8–G15

50. Erlinger, S., Dubin, M. and Dumont, M. (1981). The cytoskeleton and secretion of biliary lipids. In *Bile Acids and Lipids*, 147–152. (Lancaster: MTP Press)

51. Berken, C.A., Hartmann, C.B. and Gollan, J.L. (1982). Microtubule dependent biliary secretion of micelle forming bile acids. *Hepatology*, **2**, 715

52. Erlinger, S. (1985). Hepatic transport of bile acids: intracellular events. In Barbara, L. *et al.* (eds.) *Recent Advances in Bile Acid Research*, 5–9 (New York: Raven Press)

53. Boyer, J.L., Itabashi, M. and Hruben, Z. (1979). Formation of canalicular vesicles during sodium dehydrocholate choleresis: a mechanism for bile salt transport. In Preisig, R. and Bircher, J. (eds.) *The Liver: Quantitative Aspects of Structure and Function*, 163–67 (Basle: Karger)

54. Jones, A.L., Schmucker, D.L., Mooney, J.S. and Ockner, K. (1979). Alterations in hepatic pericanalicular cytoplasm during enhanced bile secretory activity. *Lab. Invest.*, **40**, 512–17

55. Goldsmith, M., Huling, S. and Jones, A.L. (1983). Hepatic handling of bile salts and protein in the rat during intrahepatic cholestasis. *Gastroenterology*, **84**, 978–86

56. Suchy, R., Balistreri, W.F., Hung, J., Miller, P. and Garfield, S.A. (1983). Intracellular bile acid transport in rat liver as visualised by electron microscope autoradiography using a bile acid analogue. *Am. J. Physiol.*, **245**, G681–G689

57. Jones, A.L., Schmucker, D.L., Reuston, R.H. and Murakami, I. (1980). The architecture of bile secretion: a morphological perspective of physiology. *Digestive Dis. Sci.*, **25**, 609–29

58. Dixit, V., Sherman, I.A. and Fisher, M.M. (1986). Vesicular transport of bile acids by isolated rat hepatocytes. *Hepatology*, **6**, 1131

59. Simion, F.A., Fleischer, B. and Fleischer, S. (1984). Two distinct mechanisms for taurocholate uptake in subcellular fractions from rat liver. *J. Biol. Chem.*, **259**, 10814–822

60. Lowe, P.J., Kan, K.S., Barnwell, S.G., Sharma, R.K. and Coleman, R. (1985). Transcytosis and paracellular movements of horseradish peroxidase across liver parenchymal tissue from blood to bile. *Biochem. J.*, **229**, 529–37

61. Meier, P.J., Sztul, E.S., Reuben, A. and Boyer, J.L. (1984). Structural and functional polarity of canalicular and basolateral membrane vesicles isolated in high yield from rat liver. *J. Cell. Biol.*, **98**, 991–1000

62. Inoue, M., Kinne, R., Tran. T. and Arias, I.M. (1984). Taurocholate transport by rat liver canalicular membrane vesicles: evidence for the presence of an Na^+ independent transport system. *J. Clin. Invest.*, **73**, 659–63

63. Boyer, J.L. (1986). Mechanisms of bile formation: recent studies on the role of ion transport. In Elias, E. and Murphy, G. (eds.) *Bile in Health and Disease*, 32–7. (Welwyn Garden City, Herts. UK: SKF Laboratories)

64. Meier, P.J., Reutz, G., St. Fricker, G. and Landmann, L. (1987). Characterisation of the canalicular bile acid transport system of rat liver. In *Bile Acids and the Liver*. (Lancaster: MTP Press)

65. Arias, I.R. (1986). Mechanisms and consequences of ion transport in the liver. *Prog. Liver Dis.*, **8**, 145–59

66. Schubert, R., Beyer, K., Wolburg, H. and Schimdt, K.H. (1986). Structural studies in membranes of large unilamellar vesicles after binding of sodium cholate. *Biochemistry*, **25**, 5263–69

67. Schroeder, F. (1983). Lipid domains in plasma membranes from rat liver. *Eur. J. Biochem.*, **132**, 509–16

68. Carey, M.C. (1985). Physical and chemical properties of bile acids and their salts. In Danielsson, H. and Sjovall, J. (eds.) *Sterols and Bile Acids*, pp. 345–402. (Amsterdam: Elsevier)

69. DeSilva, N.S. and Siu, C-H. (1981). Vesicle-mediated transfer of phospholipids to plasma membrane during cell aggregation of Dictostelium discoideum. *J. Biol. Chem.*, **256**, 5845–50

70. DeGrella,. R.F. and Simoni, R.D. (1982). Intracellular transport of cholesterol to the plasma membrane. *J. Biol. Chem.*, **257**, 14256–262

71. Lange, Y. and Matthias, J. (1984). Transfer of cholesterol from its site of synthesis to the plasma membrane. *J. Biol. Chem.*, **259**, 14624–630

72. Evans, W.H. and Flint, N. (1985). Subfractionation of hepatic endosomes on Nycodenz gradients and by free-flow electrophoresis: separation of ligand-transporting and receptor-enriched membranes. *Biochem. J.*, **232**, 25–32

73. Evans, W.H. and Hardison, W.G.M. (1985). Phospholipid, cholesterol, polypeptide and glycoprotein composition of hepatic endosome fractions. *Biochem. J.*, **232**, 33–36

74. Barnwell, S.G., Tuchweber, B. and Yousef, I.M. (1986). The extent of biliary phospholipid secretion and canalicular membrane solubilisation may be common determinants for the secretory rate maximum (SRm) of bile acids. *Gastroenterology*, **90**, 1710

75. Barnwell, S.G., Yousef, I.M., Tuchweber, B., Weber, A. and Roy, C.C. (1986). Pathogenesis of bile and induced cholestasis. *Hepatology*, **6**, 772

76. Barnwell, S.G., Tuchweber, B. and Yousef, I.M. (1987). In Davison, J.S., Schaffer, E.A., Boyer, J.L. and Sachs, G. (eds.) *Mechanisms of Gastrointestinal Secretion*, (University of Calgary Press) (In Press)

77. Barnwell, S.G. (1987). Evidence that sequential solubilisation of the bile canalicular membrane occurs during the onset of bile acid induced cholestasis. *Biochem. Soc. Trans.*, (In Press)

78. Yousef, I.M., Barnwell, S.G., Gratton, F., Tuchweber, B., Weber, A. and Roy, C.C. (1987). Liver cell membrane solubilisation may control the maximum secretory rate of cholic acid in the rat. *Am. J. Physiol.*, **252**, G84–G91

79. Gregory, D.H., Vlahcevic, Z.R., Schatzki, P. and Swell, L. (1975). Mechanism of secretion of biliary lipids. 1. Role of bile canalicular and microsomal membranes in the synthesis and transport of biliary lecithin and cholesterol. *J. Clin. Invest.*, **55**, 105–17

80. Montet, J.C. and Gerolami, A. (1978). Intrahepatic metabolism and secretion of biliary lipids. *Digestion*, **17**, 346–64

81. Rahman, K. and Coleman, R. (1987). Biliary lipid secretion and its control: effect of taurodehydrocholate. *Biochem. J.*, **245**, 531–36

82. Marinelli, R.A., Luquita, M.G. and Garay, E.A.R. (1986). Bile salt related secretion of acid phosphatase in rat bile. *Can. J. Physiol.*, **64**, 1347–52

83. Lorenzini, I., Sakisaka, S., Meier, P.J. and Boyer, J.L. (1986). Demonstration of a transcellular vesicle pathway for biliary excretion of inulin rat liver. *Gastroenterology*, **91**, 1278–88

84. Andreu, Torre and Carrascosa, (1986). Interaction of Tubulin with octylglycoside and deoxycholate. 2. Protein conformation, binding of colchicine ligands and microtubule assembly. *Biochemisty*, **25**, 5230

85. Bickerstaff, K.I., Garberoglio, C.A., Baker, A.L. and Moosa, A.R. (1983). Hormonal control of biliary lipid secretion in dogs. *Ann. Surg.*, **198**, 168–71

86. Kortz, W.J., Meyers, W.C., Schirmer, B.D. and Jones, R.S. (1984). Effects of dibutyryl cyclic AMP and theophylline on biliary cholesterol secretion. *J. Surg. Res.*, **36**, 62–70

87. Turley, S.D. and Dietschy, J.M. (1982). Cholesterol metabolism and excretion. In Arias, I., Popper, H., Schachter, D. and Shafritz, D.A. (eds.) *The Liver: Biology and Pathobiology*, pp. 467–92 (New York: Raven Press)

88. Dubin, M. and Erlinger, S. (1980). Effect of phalloidin on biliary lipid secretion in rats. *Clin. Sci.*, **53**, 545–48

89. Nervi, F., Bronfman, M., Allalon, W., Depiereux, E. and Del Pozo, R. (1984). Regula-

tion of biliary cholesterol secretion in the rat: role of hepatic cholesterol esterification. *J. Clin. Invest.*, **74**, 2226–2237

90. Stone, B., Erickson, S.K., Craig, W.Y. and Cooper, A. (1985). Regulation of rat biliary cholesterol secretion by agents that alter intrahepatic cholesterol metabolism: evidence for a distinct biliary precursor pool. *J. Clin. Invest.*, **76**, 1773–81

91. Kempen, H.J.M., De Lange, J., Vos van Holstein, M.P.M., Van Wachem, P., Havinga, R. and Vonk, R.J. (1984). Effect of ML-236B (compactin) on biliary excretion of bile salts and lipids and on bile flow in the rat. *Biochim. Biophys. Acta*, **794**, 435–43

92. Bonazzi, P., Amabali, P., Freddara, U., Jezequel, A.M., Novelli, G. and Orlandi, F. (1983). Study on the lipid composition of rat bile during choleresis induced by diethyl maleate. *Digestion*, **27**, 218–26

93. Loria, P., Medici, G., Salvioli, G.F., Iori, R., and Carulli, N. (1984). Effect of ursocholic acid on biliary lipid secretion in man. In *Enterohepatic Circulation of Bile Acids and Sterol Metabolism*, (Lancaster: MTP Press)

94. Hoffman, N.E., Sewell, R.E. and Smallwood, R.A. (1978). Bile acid structure and biliary lipid secretion: II: a comparison of three hydroxy and two keto bile salts. *Am. J. Physiol.*, **234**, E637–E640

95. Pellicciari, R., Cecchetti, S., Natalini, B., Roda, B., Grigoli, B. and Roda, E. (1983). Preparation and biological properties of a cyclopropylog of ursodeoxycholic acid. *Hepatology*, **3**, 820

96. Gurantz, B., Gilmore, I.T., Hofmann, A.F. and Kozmary, S. (1981). Biliary lipid secretion in the hamster: greater cholesterol secretion induced by unconjugated bile acids. *Hepatology*, **1**, 513

97. Rahman, K. and Coleman, R. (1986). Selective biliary lipid secretion at low bile-salt output rates in the isolated perfused rat liver: effects of phalloidin. *Biochem. J.*, **237**, 301–4

98. Rahman, K. and Coleman, R. (1987). Output of lysosomal contents into bile can be stimulated by taurodehydrocholate. *Biochem. J.*, **245**, 289–92

99. Rahman, K. and Coleman, R. (1987). Effect of chloroquine on biliary lipid and lysosomal enzyme output in the isolated perfused rat liver at low bile salt output rates. *Biochim. Biophys. Acta*, **922**, 395–397

100. del Pino, V.H., and La Russo, N.F. (1981). Dissociation of bile flow and biliary lipid secretion from biliary lysosomal enzyme output in experimental cholestasis. *J. Lipid. Res.*, **22**, 229–35

5
Lipid Solubilisation in Bile

M.C. Carey
Department of Medicine, Harvard Medical School
Brigham and Women's Hospital and
Harvard Digestive Diseases Center
Boston, MA 02115, USA

INTRODUCTION

Bile is an optically-clear, lipid-rich solution composed principally of two insoluble lipids, cholesterol and phosphatidycholine (lecithin), and two soluble lipids, bile salts and bilirubin conjugates[1]. The insoluble lipids interact with each other and with the soluble lipids to become dispersed in a number of colloid-chemical states in bile. An understanding of the interactions of individual biliary lipids with water, and with each other in water, is central to the comprehension of the physical chemistry of cholesterol and phosphatidylcholine solubilisation in native bile[2]. It gives us an insight into the subtle imbalances in these interactions that lead to the nucleation and precipitation from bile of cholesterol monohydrate and calcium bilirubinates, the principal components of human gallstones[3]. Because cholesterol stones are the most common human gallstones[3], I will focus in this chapter upon cholesterol monohydrate solubility in model and native biles. Little systematic information is available yet on the physical chemistry of bile pigments or of calcium bilirubinate solubility in bile[4].

First, I will describe the bulk equilibrium interactions of bile salts, cholesterol and phosphatidylcholine individually with water[5,6] and then, in detail, the equilibrium behaviour of binary lipid mixtures with water[6-8], and the characteristics of bile salt–phosphatidylcholine–cholesterol–water systems[9-12]. I will show how an appreciation of the complex behaviour of this model bile system, at both metastable and true equilibria, helps one understand the behaviour of native bile[2]. Throughout the chapter, I will concentrate on the most recent work. For more detailed background on the physical chemistry of bile, I refer the reader to three comprehensive reviews[13-15] and an entire supplement to the journal *Hepatology*[16].

BINARY SYSTEMS

Bile Salt–Water Interactions

Despite being bulky lipid molecules, fully ionised common bile salts are extremely water soluble. For example, sodium cholate and sodium deoxycholate have solubility limits of $\approx$56 and 34 g/dl in water at room temperature, respectively[17]. This important property results from self-association of the bile salt monomers to form polymolecular aggregates (micelles) above critical micellar concentrations (CMC) that range from 1 to 12 mmol/l[17]. The crucial role of self-aggregation in the solubility behaviour of bile salts is further illustrated by sodium lithocholate, the commonest monohydroxy bile salt, which is very insoluble at ambient temperatures. Lithocholate molecules readily enter aqueous solution at a characteristic temperature where the monomeric solubility of the bile salt reaches the CMC value. This is called the critical micellar temperature[13]. Taurine-conjugated common bile salts are much more soluble than the unconjugated species, and glycine conjugates exhibit intermediate solubility values[17]. Most calcium salts of the common bile acids are much less soluble than the alkali salts, but systematic studies are lacking[14].

When bile salts are unionised, they become bile acids. Bile acids exhibit only sparing solubilities in water; however, micellar solutions of bile salts can solubilise bile acids as mixed micelles[13,15]. The extent to which bile salts solubilise bile acids depends upon the bile salt species, their state of conjugation and the physical-chemical conditions[13–15]. Small concentrations of bile acids are found in gallstones[18] but it is not known what proportion of these precipitate as calcium salts. Bile acids precipitate in bile only in pathophysiological situations when an excess of unconjugated species is secreted from the liver, a rare event, or when conjugated bile salts are deconjugated by bacteria in the biliary tree, a common event in one form of pigment gallstone disease[19].

Above their solubility limits, bile salts form two-phase systems of bile salt hydrates in equilibrium with saturated micellar phases[6,17]. The size and shape of the micelles vary with bile salt species, temperature, solute concentration and ionic strength[20]. In dilute solutions, bile salts form spherical micelles with aggregation numbers (average number of monomers per micelle) of 2–20. In concentrated solutions, bile salt micelles become rod-shaped, and their aggregation numbers grow to several hundred molecules[20]. Investigators have yet to determine the precise packing of bile salt monomers in spherical or rod-shaped micelles. Liquid–crystalline phases do not occur in bile salt–water systems, but aqueous gel phases of unknown structure form with certain dihydroxy bile salts under conditions of low pH, low temperature and in the presence of high concentrations of added electrolyte[17].

Phosphatidylcholine–Water Interactions

Native biles are rich in the most hydrophilic phosphatidylcholines found in liver cell membranes[21]. About 80% of biliary phosphatidylcholines have 16:0 fatty acids in the *sn*-1 position and 18:1, 18:2 or 20:4 fatty acids in the *sn*-2 position[21,22]. Compared with *sn*-1 16:0 molecular species, the paucity of *sn*-1 18:0 phosphatidylcholines in bile may reflect slow desorption of the more hydrophobic molecular species from liver cell membranes[15]. Because bile and egg yolk phosphatidylcholines have similar chemical compositions[23,24], their physical-chemical interactions with water are essentially the same. Due to the high degree of unsaturation of the *sn*-2 fatty acids[25], these phosphatidylcholines have melted fatty acid chains at all ambient temperatures. Water penetrates and hydrates the zwitterionic phosphatidylcholine polar groups and the crystalline lattice swells in water, thereby forming a lamellar liquid–crystalline phase[5,25]. The packing structure of the hydrated lattice consists of phosphatidylcholine bilayers interleaved with layers of water. In both dry and slightly hydrated states, the fatty acid chains of phosphatidylcholine molecules become stiff at very low temperatures, forming a liquid–crystalline gel phase[5,25]. At very high temperatures, the molecules become molecularly dispersed[25]. The lamellar liquid–crystalline phase becomes maximally swollen with $\approx$35–45% w/w water at ambient temperatures. With further additions of water, a two-phase system of fully hydrated liquid–crystalline lamellae in excess water forms[5]. The application of external energy folds these lamellae into multilamellar and unilamellar vesicles[26]. The aqueous monomeric solubility of natural phosphatidylcholines is of the order of 10^{-12} molar. Because of this, and their bulk interactions with water, described above, D.M. Small classified phosphatidylcholines as insoluble swelling amphiphiles[25].

Cholesterol–Water Interactions

The aqueous monomeric solubility of cholesterol is also very low (3×10^{-8} mol/l at 37°C[25]). Cholesterol–water systems cannot, therefore, form micelles, nor do they form liquid crystals; hence, cholesterol is an insoluble non-swelling amphiphile[5,25]. The phase diagram of cholesterol in water is dominated by a two-phase system composed of crystals of cholesterol monohydrate in equilibrium with excess water containing monomers of cholesterol monohydrate[5,25]. The non-physiological anhydrous cholesterol has different solubility properties and temperature-dependent phase behaviour[27,28].

TERNARY SYSTEMS

Bile Salt–Cholesterol–Water Interactions

Cholesterol can be solubilised in a stable solution in gallbladder bile in a 1 million-fold higher concentration than its solubility in water[10]. This increase in solubility is due principally to its solubilisation in mixed bile salt–phosphatidylcholine micelles. Bile salts, rather than phosphatidylcholines, are the most important binders of cholesterol in bile. The addition of phosphatidylcholine increases cholesterol solubility by, at most, 3–4-fold over that in pure bile salt micelles[10]. Sterols that resemble cholesterol (i.e. with 3β-OH groups and 27 carbon atoms), have micellar solubilities similar to that of cholesterol[29], but more hydrophobic sterols, with longer side chains, have much lower solubilities[29]. This suggests that the aqueous monomeric solubility of a sterol is the main determinant of its solubilisation in bile salt micelles. Furthermore, 3α-OH and 3β-SH analogues of cholesterol (epicholesterol and thiocholesterol, respectively) are also solubilised poorly by common bile salt micelles. These observations have suggested that hydrogen bonding between the 3β-OH group of the sterol and an alpha-oriented OH group on the hydrophilic surfaces of bile salt micelles, as well as hydrophobic interactions, are important in bile salt–sterol binding[14,30]. The observation that the capacity of different bile salts to solubilise cholesterol at equimolar concentrations depends upon the hydrophilic/hydrophobic balance of the bile salt (hydrophobic bile salts > hydrophilic bile salts) further supports this concept[31].

There is a linear inverse relationship between the capacity of a bile salt to solubilise cholesterol and the elution order of its monomer on a reverse-phase HPLC column[31]. The cholesterol solubilising capacity decreases in the order deoxycholate > chenodeoxycholate > cholate > ursodeoxycholate > ursocholate and unconjugated > glycine-conjugated > taurine-conjugated bile salts[31]. Since the interior hydrophobic surface of the micelle should be similar for different bile salts, this suggests that cholesterol binds by both hydrophobic and hydrophilic interactions to the *exterior* surface of micelles[30]. Precisely where solubilised cholesterol molecules lie in or on the micelle is unknown, since we do not know exactly how bile salt molecules pack in simple micelles[14]. Earlier self-diffusion studies suggested that cholesterol solubilisation dramatically increases the aggregation numbers of bile salt micelles[32], but more recent non-invasive studies have established that it induces only small (≈ 1–2 Å) increases in mean micellar size[11]. This suggests strongly that the solubilised sterol does not perturb pre-existing micellar size or structure.

Cholesterol–Phosphatidylcholine–Water Interactions

At equilibrium, the lamellar liquid–crystalline phase of egg yolk phosphatidylcholine can incorporate a maximum of 1 mole of cholesterol per mole of phosphatidylcholine and up to 35–45% (w/w) of water[8,33]. With excess cholesterol, a two-phase system is present, composed of cholesterol monohydrate crystals in equilibrium with the lamellar phase. With higher water content, an excess water phase separates from the lamellar phase. Between these two-phase regions, there is an extensive three-phase zone that contains a cholesterol- and water-saturated lamellar phase, an aqueous phase and a crystalline cholesterol monohydrate phase[8]. Within the lamellar phase, the orientation of the cholesterol molecules is normal to the bilayer interface, with the steroid ring system and side chain lying parallel to the acyl chains of the phosphatidylcholine molecules[33]. The sterol's OH group, located at the boundary of the aqueous layer, then 'hydrates', in part, the polar groups of the phosphatidylcholine molecules[34]. The acyl chain mobility, i.e. bilayer fluidity, decreases markedly with incorporation of cholesterol[34] and, hence, the bilayer thickness increases[35]. The Phase Rule predicts two degrees of freedom in the lamellar phase. Cholesterol molecules are therefore probably not homogeneously mixed with the phosphatidylcholine molecules within the liquid crystals. When cholesterol-to-phosphatidylcholine ratios are < 1, kinetic and spectroscopic studies suggest lateral phase separation, in that patches of cholesterol-rich and pure phosphatidylcholine domains coexist[36,37].

In small unilamellar vesicles, it is possible to disperse, by sonication, as many as four cholesterol molecules for each phosphatidylcholine molecule in a non-equilibrium state[38]. These systems are very metastable and eventually fuse, precipitate cholesterol monohydrate crystals, and separate into stable 1:1 cholesterol–phosphatidylcholine multilamellae[38].

Bile Salt–Phosphatidylcholine–Water Interactions

Figure 1 displays the general characteristics of the important bile salt (sodium cholate)–phosphatidylcholine (egg yolk lecithin)–water phase diagram[7]. The inset (Figure 2) shows the details at low (< 12%) total lipid (i.e. > 88% H_2O), relevant to the physical state of hepatic and gallbladder biles[15].

The base axis of the triangle represents the binary water-phosphatidylcholine system. With water contents < 12%, this system is complex and is dominated by the structure of the slightly hydrated phosphatidylcholine crystal phase ('dry' lecithin). Between 12 and 45% water, the liquid–crystalline lamellar phase of phosphatidylcholine becomes increasingly swollen up to a maximum of 45% water. At higher water contents, an excess

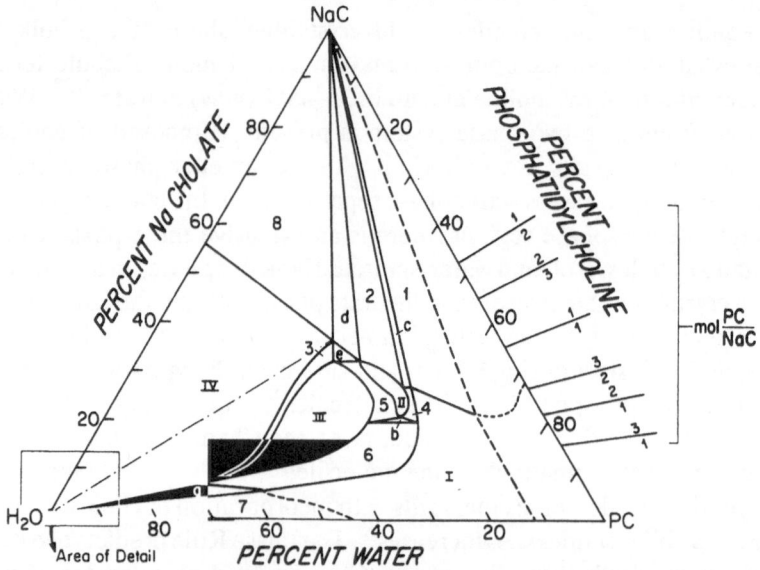

Figure 1 Sodium cholate (NaC)–egg yolk phosphatidylcholine (PC)–water phase diagram with axes plotted in weights (w) per cent (pH 10.0; 20 °C; 1 atm). *Roman numerals* indicate one-phase zones: I-lamellar liquid–crystalline phase; II-cubic liquid–crystalline phase; III-hexagonal liquid–crystalline phase; IV-micellar phase. *Arabic numerals* represent two-phase zones: 1-lamellar phase plus NaC crystals; 2-cubic phase plus NaC crystals; 3-hexagonal phase plus micellar phase; 4-lamellar phase plus cubic phase; 5-cubic phase plus hexagonal phase; 6-lamellar phase plus hexagonal phase; 7-lamellar phase plus aqueous NaC monomeric phase; 8-micellar phase plus NaC crystals. Alphabet letters (a–e) represent invariant three-phase zones. All three-phase zones are triangles. The compositions and physical nature of the three phases are indicated by the apices of the triangles. The dot at about 0.5% (w/w) on the H2O–NaC axis represents the CMC of NaC in water ($\cong$ 10 mol/l). Molar ratios of PC to NaC are indicated on the NaC–PC axis of the triangle. The interrupted line crossing the micellar phase (IV) is the 'coexistence limit' discussed in the text. The area of detail shown in the box is displayed in Figure 2. [Adapted from reference 7 with permission].

water phase separates from the lamellar phase. The left axis of the triangle represents the binary water–sodium cholate (NaC) system. The dot at about 0.5% (10 mmol/l) NaC represents the CMC of the bile salt[14]. Between this point and 56% NaC, the length of the line represents the extent of the binary micellar phase[6]. At higher NaC concentrations, the system contains two phases: NaC hydrate, in equilibrium with a saturated NaC micellar phase[6]. The right axis of the triangle represents the binary dry mixtures of NaC and phosphatidylcholine, whose structures are unknown.

Within the triangular diagram (Figure 1), all points represent mixtures of the three components: H2O, NaC and phosphatidylcholine, in different proportions. Such mixtures may form one homogeneous phase (Roman numerals I–IV), or separate into zones of two phases (Arabic numerals 1–8) or three phases (letters a-e). By X-ray diffraction and polarised light microscopy[7], Zone I is a lamellar liquid–crystalline phase, Zone II a cubic liquid–crystalline phase, Zone III a hexagonal liquid–crystalline phase, and Zone IV a micellar phase. By applying the Phase Rule, each one-phase zone has two degrees of freedom. This means that one can vary independently the composition of two of the components; each composition falling within a one-phase zone will then have different physical-chemical characteristics. The interrupted diagonal line drawn through Zone IV depicts an important example of this heterogeneity. The line runs upwards to the right from the CMC of NaC in H_2O (dot on the left axis) to the apex of the zone close to the epicenter of the triangle. This line intersects with the NaC-phosphatidylcholine axis at a constant phosphatidylcholine-to-NaC molar ratio of 1:2. Compositions within Zone IV falling above this line form a micellar system with coexisting simple NaC plus mixed (NaC + phosphatidylcholine) micelles in varying proportions[39]. Compositions below the line contain only mixed micelles in which two of the components can vary independently without a phase change occurring[39].

The physical states in Zones 1–8, where two phases separate, are described elsewhere[15] and in the legend to Figure 1. In these regions, there is only one degree of freedom. A variation in the composition of one of the phases therefore automatically defines the composition of the other phase. A straight tie-line connects the overall composition of any mixture in a two-phase zone with the corresponding compositions of the phases. These compositions fall on the opposing phase boundaries of the zone[15]. Separate triangles represent all five three-phase zones (a–e) in the phase diagram (Figure 1). Since the Phase Rule dictates that mixtures falling into these zones have no degree of freedom, the systems are invariant. The apices of the triangles give the compositions of the three coexisting phases, and their values are not changeable. For a system to remain within a three-phase zone, relative proportions of each phase can change, but not their compositions[15].

Figure 2 shows the physiologically important area of detail from Figure 1 (square box). This area encloses the H_2O apex of the phase diagram and defines the physical-chemical states of the systems at high water contents, typical of hepatic (≈ 3 g/dl total lipids) and gallbladder (≈ 10 g/dl total lipids) biles[10]. This figure shows the phase relations that occur within the three-component phase diagram between the binary systems, H_2O-NaC and H_2O-phosphatidylcholine. As inferred from Figure 1, the biggest zone in Figure 2 is Zone IV, the micellar zone. This zone is heterogeneous and exists at all compositions between the CMC of NaC and the micellar solubility limit of phosphatidylcholine. It begins at the H_2O–NaC boundary, fans into the triangle, and ends at the micellar phase limit, 2 mol phosphatidylcholine to 1 mol NaC (Figures 1 and 2). While it may appear from Figure 1 that, at high phosphatidylcholine contents, the phase boundary of Zone IV is also a phase boundary of the invariant three-phase zone (a), Figure 2 shows that this is not the case. The two-phase zone, where mixed micellar and hexagonal phases coexist (no. 3 in Figure 1), sends a long sliver between Zone IV and Zone a, which extends as far as the position of the CMC dot on the H2O–

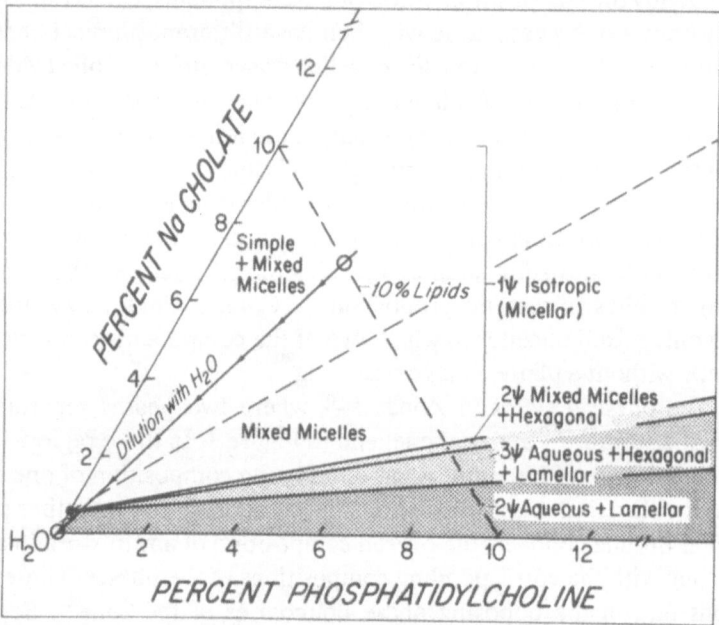

Figure 2 Area of detail from sodium cholate–egg yolk phosphatidylcholine–water phase diagram at high H2O concentrations (same conditions as in Figure 1). The left axis shows weight per cent Na cholate, with the dot at 0.5% w/w Na cholate representing the CMC of the bile salt ($\cong 10$ mmol/l). The base axis shows weight per cent phosphatidylcholine increasing from left to right. This is equivalent to weight per cent H2O from right to left, as displayed in Figure 1. Parts of the one-phase isotropic (micellar) region IV, two-phase mixed micelle plus hexagonal region no. 3, three-phase aqueous plus hexagonal plus lamellar region, a, and two-phase aqueous plus lamellar region no. 7 (see Figure 1) are shown. The dashed (coexistence limit) line bisecting region IV is the same as in Figure 1. It falls along a lipid composition of 1 mol phosphatidylcholine to 2 mol NaC. This is a pseudophase boundary separating regions of the micellar phase where simple and mixed micelles coexist and the region where only mixed micelles are found. The line at 10% lipids crosses all phase regions as phosphatidylcholine-to-NaC ratio is varied from 0 to 1. The arrowed line connecting the open circle on the 10% lipid line to the H2O apex of the triangle represents an H2O dilution path. This shows that all five regions of the phase diagram are also crossed when a micellar solution containing a physiological phosphatidylcholine and Na cholate composition is diluted with H2O (further discussed in text). [Modified from reference 15 with permission].

NaC axis (Figure 2)[15]. The tie-lines within this narrow zone are probably parallel to the base axis of the triangle, as they are at higher total lipid concentrations[15].

As one approaches the H_2O-phosphatidylcholine axis, the system passes from this two-phase zone into an invariant three-phase zone (a, in Figure 1), where an aqueous phase coexists with hexagonal and lamellar liquid–crystalline phases. The apices of the triangle (Figure 1) give each composition and physico-chemical state. This shows that the composition of the aqueous phase must have a monomeric NaC concentration at the CMC (dot on the H_2O–NaC axis) (Figure 2). The phase diagram then passes into a two-phase zone (no. 7 in Figure 1) where aqueous NaC monomers coexist with a lamellar liquid–crystalline phase. As shown by the systematic changes along the interrupted line, when phosphatidylcholine-to-NaC ratios vary from 0 to 1 (between 10% NaC and 10% phosphatidylcholine), each of these zones is entered in sequence at constant total lipid concentration. Moreover, as shown by the arrowed line connecting the open circle at 10% lipid and the H_2O apex of the triangle, we also encounter each zone when a micellar solution of phosphatidylcholine and NaC (open circle in Zone IV, Figure 2) is diluted with water[15].

As one dilutes the model system at point 0 through the micellar zone, the physical state of the system first changes from that of a coexistence of simple plus mixed micelles to a pure mixed micellar region. The dilution path passes close to the apex of the two-phase hexagonal plus mixed micellar zone (which includes NaC monomers at the CMC). Further dilution passes close to the apex of the three-phase zone, composed of an aqueous phase (including NaC monomers at the CMC), a hexagonal phase, and a lamellar phase before finally entering a two-phase zone, composed of aqueous plus lamellar phases (Figure 2). The phase considerations in Figure 2 suggest that only in the final two-phase aqueous plus lamellar zone will the monomeric concentration of NaC fall below its CMC. In fact, the tie-lines in this zone (not shown) connect the H_2O–NaC axis with the phase boundary of Zone I (the lamellar phase, Figure 1)[15] and their directions parallel the upper and lower boundaries of the two-phase aqueous plus lamellar zone. Hence, within this zone, as the dilution curve comes closer to the H_2O apex, the 'CMC' of NaC should fall progressively. Recent experiments have verified this prediction[40].

Figure 3 shows an experiment using quasielastic light scattering to monitor the mean hydrodynamic radius ($\overline{R}_h$) of the particles found in such an aqueous-dilution experiment[41]. For graphing convenience, we begin this experiment with a sodium taurocholate (NaTC)-phosphatidylcholine composition which falls in the mixed micellar region of the micellar zone. Other dilution experiments, beginning with 10 g/dl lipids and relative compositions falling within the coexistence region (Figure 2), showed no appreciable change in particle sizes until the compositions entered the mixed micellar region[39,40]. This verifies that, as water dilutes the system, the smaller simple micelles (which contribute least to the scattered light intensity) dissociate to maintain the CMC, and the mixed micellar sizes do not change[39]. Once the dilution path enters the pure mixed micellar region of this zone, each addi-

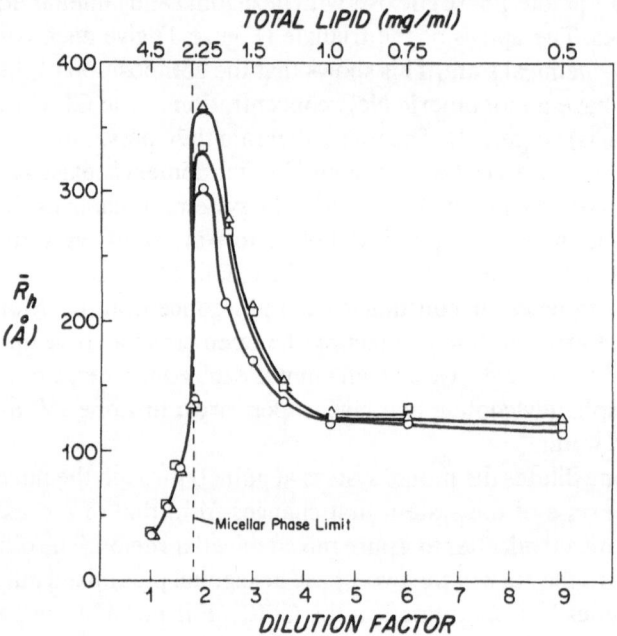

Figure 3 Mean hydrodynamic radius ($\bar{R}_h$) in Å of sodium taurocholate (TC) egg phosphatidylcholine (PC) mixtures as a mixed micellar solution (weight ratio 2.4:1, total lipid concentration 4.5 mg/ml) was serially diluted with 0.15 mol/l NaCl, at 37 °C (pH 7.0). The data points represented by circles, squares and triangles represent measurements, at 30 min, 24 h, and 48 h, respectively, following each dilution. The micellar phase limit is shown by the dashed vertical line. The upper abscissa displays the total lipid concentration, the lower abscissa displays the dilution factor. The $\bar{R}_h$ values at time-dependent peaks in the curves probably represent the sizes of fragments of the hexagonal phase in the two- and three-phase regions of Figure 2. The horizontal part of the curves represents the two-phase lamellar plus aqueous region in Figure 2. The lamellar phase is present as small unilamellar vesicles that spontaneously form upon dilution (see text for further discussion). [Modified from reference 41 with permission].

tional dilution step (Figure 3) results in a significant increase in mixed micellar sizes, consistent with the mixed-disc model for the micellar structure[39]. The three data points for each dilution within the mixed micellar zone clearly show that equilibrium was attained by 30 min (open circles); no further changes occurred at 24 h (open squares) or at 48 h (open triangles). This observation sets the limit for the boundary of the micellar phase at a dilution factor of ≈ 2 where micellar $\overline{R}_h$ values were $\approx 130–140$ Å. The next dilution step produced particles of nearly 3-fold larger $\overline{R}_h$ values whose sizes were strongly time-dependent, increasing from 300 Å at 30 min to ≈ 360 Å at 48 h. These sizes are too large for micelles and probably represent precipitates of the hexagonal phase in the two-phase mixed micellar plus hexagonal zone or in the three-phase aqueous, hexagonal, and lamellar zone[15]. At higher dilutions, the particle sizes decrease progressively and become less time-dependent, although their growth is still in an upward direction. Once the particle sizes level off at ≈ 120 Å $\overline{R}_h$, there exists a two-phase zone composed of aqueous NaC monomers plus a lamellar phase[40]. As shown by other techniques, this lamellar liquid–crystalline phase is, in fact, a dispersion of small unilamellar vesicles that form spontaneously without the need for external energy[42,43]. The light scattering variances are also low in this region, consistent with a monodisperse vesicle system[39,40]. In contrast, at the peak of the curves where two- or three-phase dispersions that include rod-like fragments of the hexagonal phase exist (Figure 2), the variances are approximately 80–100%[39].

These concepts are highly relevant to the formation of bile. As inferred from quasielastic light scattering studies on model bile, the addition of cholesterol causes only small changes in the size or structure of bile salt–phosphatidylcholine micelles or vesicles at true and metastable equilibria[11]. Whether or not all three lipids are secreted into the canaliculus from liver cells in monomeric or aggregated state, they must become concentrated during passage along the biliary tree. Hence, during bile formation, there should be a reversal in the dilution curves shown in Figures 2 and 3. It is probable, therefore, that a dispersed hexagonal phase forms as an intermediate (as in the two- or three-phase region of Figure 2) during the complex processes by which secreted biliary lipids attain the physical-chemical state of physiological bile.

QUATERNARY SYSTEMS

Bile Salt–Phosphatidylcholine–Cholesterol–Water Interactions

Model systems composed of bile salt, phosphatidylcholine and cholesterol in water are a logical starting place to gain insight into the solubility of cholesterol in native bile[10]. I represent the phase diagram of this four-component system at constant temperature and pressure as a regular tetrahedron (Figure 4, inset)[44]. Each apex of the tetrahedron represents 100% of each component, each edge a binary system of the two components at opposite ends, and each face the appropriate ternary system, i.e. bile salt–cholesterol–water, bile salt–phosphatidylcholine–water, phosphatidylcholine–

cholesterol–water and the dry mixtures, bile salt–cholesterol–phosphatidyl-choline. All points inside the tetrahedron represent mixtures containing four components in different proportions. The Phase Rule predicts that such mixtures may form one homogeneous phase or separate into zones of two, three

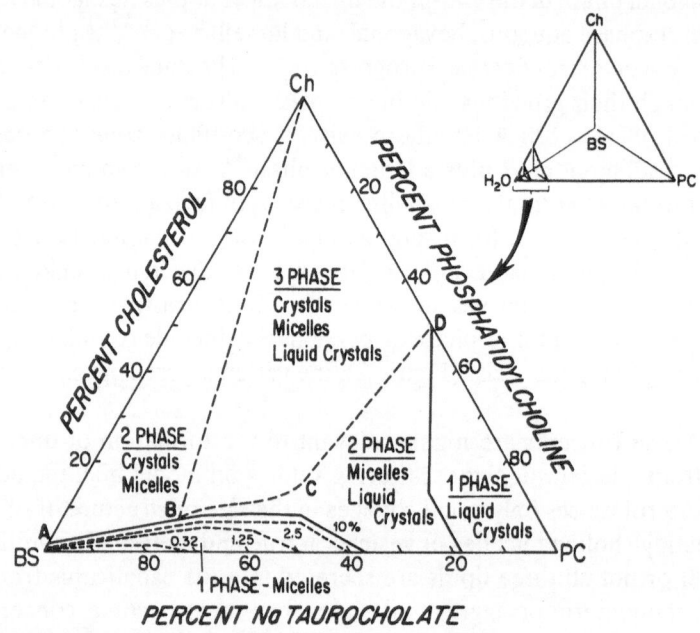

Figure 4 Sodium taurocholate (NaTC)–egg yolk phosphatidylcholine (PC)–cholesterol–water phase diagram with axes plotted in moles per cent (0.2 mol/l Na$^+$, pH 7.4, 37 °C). The triangle is a cut, at constant H$_2$O content, of the insetted regular tetrahedron that represents the bile salt (BS)–phosphatidylcholine–cholesterol–water system. At 10% lipid there are two one-phase zones in the bile salt–cholesterol–phosphatidylcholine phase diagram. A micellar phase at the bottom is bounded by a solid line and a lamellar liquid–crystalline phase at high phosphatidylcholine contents is also bounded by a solid line. The interrupted micellar zone lines represent the micellar phase boundaries with decreases in total lipid concentrations between 10 and 0.32 g/dl. The interrupted phase boundaries above and to the right of the micellar phase have been derived for 10% lipids but probably vary, especially at point B, with dilution. In the left two-phase region, cholesterol monohydrate crystals are in equilibrium with a cholesterol-saturated micellar solution. Above phase boundary B–C–D, there are three phases in equilibrium, each with invariant compositions: cholesterol monohydrate crystals, cholesterol–phosphatidylcholine liquid crystals with a 1:1 molar composition (point D) and cholesterol-saturated micelles with a composition given by point B. In the two-phase region below B–C–D there are lamellar liquid crystals and mixed micelles of variable composition (see text for further discussion). [Redrawn from reference 10 with permission].

and four phases. Although a systematic definition of the complete system is lacking, systems with water held constant at the dilute corner of the tetrahedron have been defined (Figure 4, inset). By holding the water component constant and varying the other three components, the systems are graphically represented by a *triangular* phase diagram, as discussed for the water-containing ternary systems such as bile salt-phosphatidylcholine-water. These cuts, employed for physical-chemical modelling of hepatic and gallbladder biles (shown in Figure 4), are cuts of the regular tetrahedron parallel to the bile salt–phosphatidylcholine–cholesterol 'dry' system. Because the proportion of water is fixed, one cannot consider it a component or one of the coexisting 'phases', even though it contains a monomeric bile salt concentration[44]. Since the system is reduced to three components, the Phase Rule predicts that a maximum of three phases is present. Figure 4 presents the superimposed phase diagrams for sodium taurocholate (NaTC), egg yolk phosphatidylcholine and cholesterol systems at four concentrations of water (90, 97.5, 98.75, 99.68%), that is, for constant total lipid concentrations of 10, 2.5, 1.25 and 0.32 g/dl, respectively[10].

In these diagrams there are two one-phase zones. One is an isotropic micellar region which sets limits for phosphatidylcholine solubility on the bile salt–phosphatidylcholine axis, cholesterol solubility on the bile salt–cholesterol axis and along a line within the triangle. The other one-phase region contains anisotropic liquid–crystalline droplets that are the lamellar phase of phosphatidylcholine–water systems with incorporated bile salt and cholesterol molecules. The lamellar phase (Figure 4) can incorporate approximately twice the number of cholesterol molecules as bile salt molecules.

As the total lipid concentration decreases, less cholesterol and phosphatidylcholine are solubilised in the micellar phase[10]. When the total lipid concentration falls to 0.16 g/dl, the micellar phase disappears. The lipid concentration at which the micellar phase vanishes and the extent of contraction with dilution are not the same for each bile salt, since they depend upon the magnitude of the CMC[45,46]. With the taurine conjugates of the more hydrophobic deoxycholate and chenodeoxycholate, the micellar zone demonstrates less concentration-dependent changes[47], and does not disappear until lower concentrations as predicted by the low CMC values of these bile salts[30].

Above and to the right of the micellar zone (Figure 4), there are three regions where other phases separate. Interrupted lines, which are fairly exact for the system with 10% lipids, separate these regions[10]. However, analogous phase boundaries are lacking for lower total lipid concentrations. With cholesterol contents above the micellar phase at line A–B, there are two phases in equilibrium, cholesterol monohydrate crystals and a cholesterol-saturated micellar phase. The tie-lines in this two-phase region extend upward from variable points on line A–B to the 100% cholesterol apex of the triangle[44]. With cholesterol contents above interrupted line B–C–D, three phases separate at equilibrium. These phases are cholesterol monohydrate crystals, lamellar liquid crystals and cholesterol-saturated micelles. The Phase Rule predicts that this region is invariant, i.e. has no degree of freedom; therefore, the three co-existing phases have fixed compositions at points B, D and the cholesterol apex of the triangle. Above and to the right of the micellar zone, toward the phosphatidylcholine side of the diagram, liquid crystals composed of phosphatidylcholine, cholesterol and bile salts are in equilibrium with a saturated micellar phase. The Phase Rule predicts that this two-phase zone exhibits one degree of freedom. This means that the composition of one phase, such as on the micellar phase boundary, fixes the composition of the other phase on the liquid–crystalline phase boundary[44]. The tie-lines are known only for the region below line segment B–C, and run slightly upwards from the micellar phase boundary to reach the liquid–crystalline phase boundary on the right[44].

I have discussed the phase relations of the bile salt–phosphatidylcholine–cholesterol–water system at equilibrium. I will now focus on the same system in the non-equilibrium or metastable state[11]. Figure 5 displays the phase relations of the sodium taurocholate–phosphatidylcholine–cholesterol system under non-equilibrium conditions. On this truncated triangular diagram, the solid line encloses the micellar zone; above and to the right of this zone are the equilibrium two- and three-phase regions described for Figure 4. This diagram displays schematically the continuum of micellar sizes and structures as the composition progresses from left to right within the micellar phase, that is, as the phosphatidylcholine-to-bile salt ratio increases. Simple bile salt-cholesterol micelles form in the absence of phosphatidylcholine; at intermediate phosphatidylcholine-to-bile salt ratios, there is a coexistence of simple (bile salt–cholesterol) and mixed (bile salt–phosphatidylcholine–cholesterol) micelles; and at high lipid ratios near the phase limit, only pure 'mixed-disc' (bile salt-phosphatidylcholine-cholesterol) micelles exist[11,39].

When such lipid mixtures are hydrated following co-precipitation from an organic solvent, the micellar systems reach equilibrium so fast that metastable particles are difficult to observe. However, micellar particles can become transiently supersaturated with either phosphatidylcholine or cholesterol[10,11,39]. With passage of time, the phosphatidylcholine-supersaturated micelles and cholesterol-supersaturated micelles evolve into a two-phase system of micelles coexisting with small unilamellar vesicles (≈ 250 Å to 1500 Å in diameter)[11]. Like vesicles produced by sonication of phospholipid dispersions, these vesicles are metastable, tending to fuse and evolve into other structures[2]. In dilute model bile, vesicles are surprisingly stable; in concentrated model bile, they are very unstable, fusing rapidly[11]. It is now well established that vesicles are the transport particles for excess (supramicellar) cholesterol in native hepatic and gallbladder biles[49]. Ap-

74

parently, in concentrated gallbladder biles, bile proteins are responsible for the metastability of vesicles, preventing their rapid fusion. Hence, vesicles may remain in the gallbladder as discrete cholesterol-solubilising units for prolonged periods, such as during fasting[49].

To the left of the dashed semivertical line, cholesterol-saturated micelles and cholesterol monohydrate crystals are the equilibrium phases. Vesicles in this region tend, therefore, to fuse quickly and nucleate their cholesterol as cholesterol monohydrate crystals. This will occur irrespective of whether the cholesterol-to-phosphatidylcholine ratio is > 1 or not. Mixed micelles dissolve the remaining phosphatidylcholine. Between the two dashed lines, liquid crystals are one of the equilibrium phases in the three-phase region and, at equilibrium, their cholesterol-to-phosphatidylcholine ratio equals 1[8]. In this region, therefore, vesicles will fuse and nucleate cholesterol monohydrate crystals only if their vesicle cholesterol-to-phosphatidylcholine ratio is > 1[38]. If the relative lipid composition falls outside the micellar phase but below the dashed curved line, phosphatidylcholine-rich vesicles separate and, by definition, these cannot nucleate cholesterol monohydrate crystals. However, in concentrated systems, they may fuse to form microscopically visible myelin figures[11]. A reworking of published experimental data employing model vesicle systems[50,51] shows that these phase diagram predictions are correct.

In summary, native bile that contains > 75 moles per cent common bile salts and supramicellar concentrations of cholesterol will separate into cholesterol–phosphatidylcholine vesicles in the metastable state. These vesicles disappear in time, nucleating cholesterol monohydrate crystals, and the remaining phosphatidylcholine dissolves in phosphatidylcholine-unsaturated micelles. If the bile contains < 75 moles per cent bile salt and supramicellar concentrations of cholesterol, vesicles also separate. Depending upon the relative cholesterol content, these vesicles will have different compositions and properties. With modest relative excesses of cholesterol (e.g. < 12 moles per cent), the vesicles will be phosphatidylcholine-rich. In dilute bile, these will remain stable; in concentrated bile, they may fuse to form myelin figures. Because their compositions fall within a two-phase region of the phase diagram, cholesterol monohydrate crystals cannot nucleate from such vesicles. With cholesterol contents > 12 moles per cent, the fate of separated vesicles will depend upon their cholesterol-to-phosphatidylcholine ratios. Vesicles cannot nucleate cholesterol monohydrate crystals if the cholesterol-to-phospholipid ratio is < 1, although fusion can occur to form large liposomes (liquid crystals). However, vesicles with lipid ratios > 1 will, in time, fuse and nucleate cholesterol monohydrate crystals.

It is clear from Figure 5 that unilamellar vesicles are a form of the lamellar liquid–crystalline phase reduced to its smallest dimension and, as

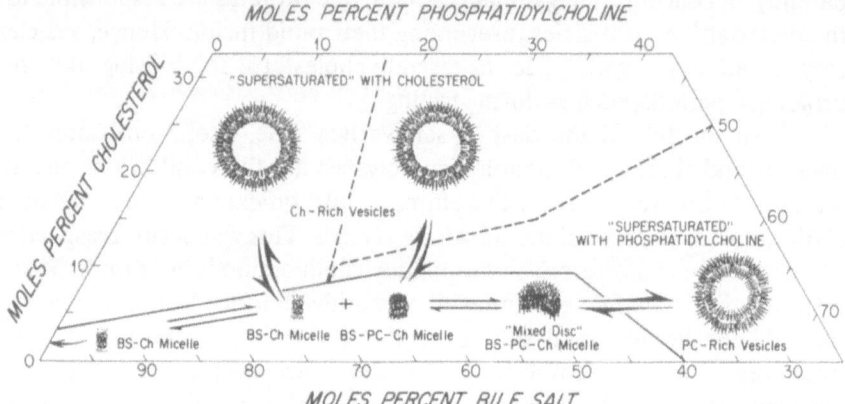

Figure 5 Schematic triangular diagram of sodium taurocholate, egg phosphatidylcholine–cholesterol interactions in water to display metastable phases. Within the micellar zone there is a continuum of micellar structures of different sizes and compositions. In the absence of phosphatidylcholine, only bile salt (BS)–cholesterol (Ch) micelles are present. With physiological bile salt-to-phosphatidylcholine compositions, there is a coexistence of simple bile salt–cholesterol and mixed bile salt–phosphatidylcholine (PC)–cholesterol micelles. At higher phosphatidylcholine contents, there are only mixed bile salt–phosphatidylcholine–cholesterol micelles. Above the micellar zone, excess cholesterol is dispersed in cholesterol-rich small unilamellar vesicles of phosphatidylcholine with only traces of bile salt. Just above and to the right of the micellar zone, similar sized vesicles are present, but these are phosphatidylcholine-rich (see text for further description). [Modified from reference 2 with permission].

such, act as solubilising agents in bile[2,15]. The thermodynamic instability of vesicles drives them to form larger particles; their degree of supersaturation with cholesterol and their position in the phase diagram may drive them to nucleate cholesterol monohydrate crystals. Clearly, if one could enlarge the area of the phase diagram in which vesicles (unilamellar or multilamellar liquid–crystalline liposomes) are stable, then the transport of cholesterol in vesicles or liquid crystals would not be potentially hazardous. Such a phase change occurs in human bile when ursodeoxycholic acid is chronically ingested to effect dissolution of cholesterol gallstones[12]. It is instructive, therefore, to examine the phase diagrams of the hydrophilic–hydrophobic series of common bile salts with egg phosphatidylcholine and cholesterol – all at 90% H_2O (0.15 mmol/l NaCl).

Figure 6 displays the ternary phase diagrams for individual taurine-conjugated bile salts at 10 g/dl total lipid[12,52]. In each triangle, there is a central three-phase region surrounded by two-phase regions and a one-phase micellar region (the liquid–crystalline one-phase regions are undefined). The number and location of the phase regions are similar for all five bile salts, but two of the boundaries change. In the micellar zones, we note that cholesterol

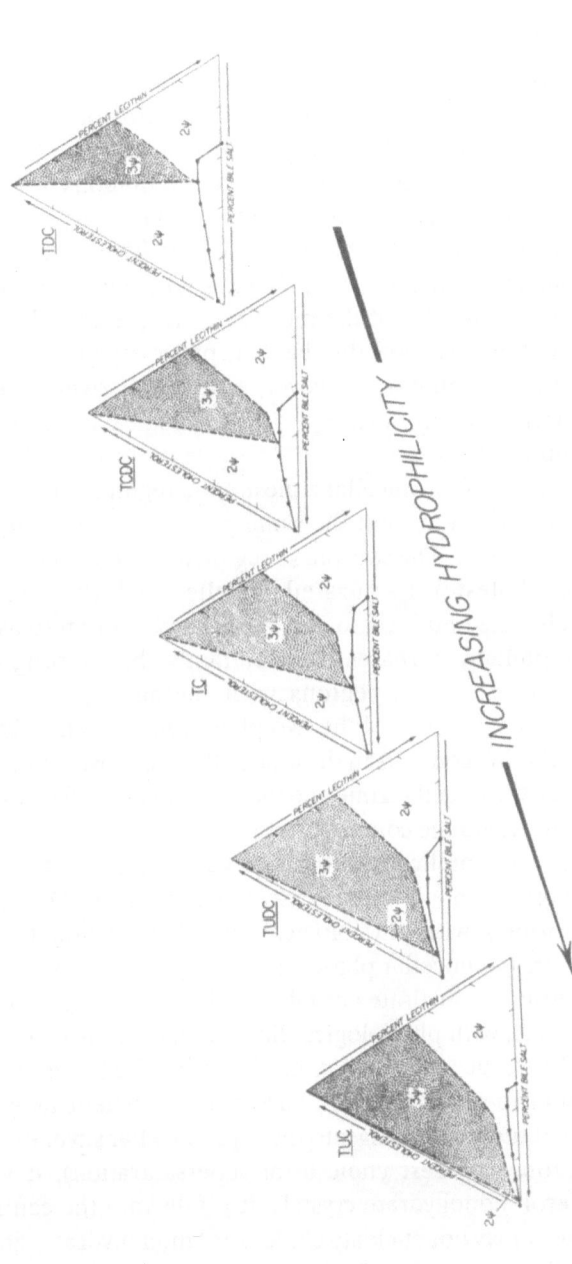

Figure 6 Phase diagrams of tauroursocholate (TUC)-, tauroursodeoxycholate (TUDC)-, taurocholate (TC)-, taurochenodeoxycholate (TCDC)-, and taurodeoxycholate (TDC)-egg phosphatidylcholine (lecithin)-cholesterol systems in 0.15 mol/l NaCl (10% w/w lipids, pH 7.0, 37 °C). The axes are plotted in moles per cent. As the hydrophilicity of the bile salt increases, the two-phase zone on the left contracts and is replaced by expansion of the central three-phase region. A narrow sliver of the two-phase region on the right separates the central three-phase region from the micellar phase. The widths of these projections above the micellar phases are wider than previously reported (see refs. 2 and 12). The solid line represents the limits of the micellar phase. The maximum amount of cholesterol that can be solubilised in the micellar phase decreases progressively as the hydrophilicity of the bile salt increases. Further details and pathophysiological implications are given in the text. [From references 12 and 52].

solubility in simple bile salt micelles, i.e. the data point on the percent cholesterol axis, decreases progressively with increasing hydrophilicity of the bile salt. With the most hydrophobic bile salt, taurodeoxycholate (TDC, 10 g/dl), only about 20 molecules of bile salt are required to solubilise one molecule of cholesterol[10]. With an identical concentration of tauroursocholate (TUC), the most hydrophilic bile salt, nearly 2000 molecules are required to solubilise one molecule of cholesterol[52]. With increasing hydrophilicity of the bile salt, phosphatidylcholine solubility in each bile salt system, i.e. the data points on the percent bile salt axes, changes in a discontinuous fashion. With TDC and phosphatidylcholine, the molar ratio at the phase limit is $\approx 1{:}1.6$; with taurochenodeoxycholate (TCDC) it is $\approx 1{:}1.7$; with taurocholate (TC) it is 1:2; with tauroursodeoxycholate (TUDC) it is 1:1.5; and with TUC it is 1:1. As shown by the overall size of the micellar zone, the equilibrium cholesterol solubilitys limit in mixed micelles become progressively reduced with increasing bile salt hydrophilicity. However, as noted elsewhere, TC, TCDC and TDC systems do not differ markedly at physiological bile salt-to-phosphatidylcholine compositions[10].

Above and to the right of the micellar zone are the regions where two and three phases separate. These exhibit the same physical states, at equilibrium, as discussed for Figure 4. The two-phase region at the left (high bile salt content) contains cholesterol-saturated micelles and cholesterol monohydrate crystals. The size of this region varies, becoming progressively smaller as bile salt hydrophilicity increases. Concomitantly, there is progressive expansion of the three-phase regions with increasing bile salt hydrophilicity. As this occurs, a wedge of the two-phase region on the right, i.e. at high phosphatidylcholine contents in the case of the more hydrophobic bile salts, extends between the micellar zone and the three-phase zone. Since, at physiological phosphatidylcholine contents, there is now a two-phase zone above the micellar phase, its implications become very important for the stability of metastable vesicles in bile. In the case of TDC- and TCDC-containing biles, vesicles forming with physiological phosphatidylcholine and cholesterol contents above the micellar phase will be unstable, always tending to nucleate cholesterol monohydrate crystals to achieve the equilibrium two-phase state. In contrast, with physiological lipid compositions in TUC- and TUDC-containing biles, the vesicles that form in either the three-phase zone or in the right-hand two-phase zone will have different kinetic fates. If the overall composition of such a bile falls into the supramicellar sliver of the right-hand two-phase zone (modest cholesterol supersaturation), it will never nucleate cholesterol monohydrate crystals. If it falls into the central three-phase zone, it may or may not nucleate cholesterol monohydrate, since liquid crystals with cholesterol-to-phosphatidylcholine ratios of 1:1 are an equilibrium phase in this zone.

SUMMARY

The foregoing discussion has presented rigorous thermodynamic and phase equilibria criteria for cholesterol solubilisation in human bile at equilibrium. It is clear that, in relation to native biles, the stability of biles with excess cholesterol is thermodynamically and kinetically controlled. Cholesterol gallstones are, therefore, simply a manifestation of a metastable state that has evolved into an equilibrium system. It is unlikely that the myriad other 'minor' components of bile, such as divalent ions, soluble proteins, gelled glycoproteins, bile pigments, etc. have important influences on the phase behaviour of bile at equilibrium. Nevertheless, these factors undoubtedly have large influences on the kinetic behaviour of 'supersaturated' bile. Not only are proteins possible stabilising factors, but certain proteins may be nucleating factors. Much more kinetic, biochemical and physico-chemical work on these aspects of bile is still required.

Acknowledgements

Supported in part by Grants DK36588 and DK34854 from the National Institutes of Health (US Public Health Service). I am especially grateful to Ms. Rebecca Ankener, who edited and word-processed the manuscript, and to Drs. D.J. Cabral and D.M. Small for generously allowing me to read their unpublished review (ref 15) which greatly influenced the writing of this chapter.

REFERENCES

1. Carey, M.C. and Robins, S.J. (1987). Bile production and secretion. In Stein, J.H. (ed.) *Internal Medicine, 2nd Edition*. pp. 28–34. (Boston: Little Brown)
2. Carey, M.C. and Cohen, D.E. (1987). Biliary transport of cholesterol in vesicles, micelles and liquid crystals. In Paumgartner, G., Stiehl, A. and Gerok W. (eds.) *Bile Acids and the Liver*. pp. 287–300. (Lancaster: MTP Press)
3. Berman, M.D., Angelico, M. and Carey, M.C. (1987). Biliary tract stones and associated disease. In Stein, J.H. (ed.) *Internal Medicine, 2nd Edition*. pp. 245–57. (Boston: Little Brown)
4. Carey, M.C. and Spivak, W. (1986). Physical chemistry of bile pigments and porphyrins with particular reference to bile. In Ostrow, J.D. (ed.) *Bile Pigments and Jaundice: Molecular, Metabolic and Medical Aspects*. pp. 81–132. (New York: Marcel Dekker).
5. Small, D.M. (1967). Phase equilibria and structure of dry and hydrated egg lecithin. *J. Lipid Res.* **8**, 551–9
6. Small, D.M. (1968). A classification of biological lipids based upon their interactions in aqueous systems. *J. Am. Oil Chem. Soc.*, **45**, 108–19
7. Small, D.M., Bourgès, M.C. and Dervichian, D.G. (1966). The biophysics of lipidic associations. I. The ternary systems lecithin–bile salt–water. *Biochim. Biophys. Acta*, **125**, 563–80
8. Bourgès, M., Small, D.M. and Dervichian, D.G. (1967). Biophysics of lipidic associations. II. The ternary systems cholesterol–lecithin–water. *Biochim. Biophys. Acta*, **137**, 157–67

9. Bourgès, M., Small, D.M. and Dervichian, D.G. (1967). Biophysics of lipid association. III. The quaternary systems lecithin–bile salt–cholesterol–water. *Biochim. Biophys. Acta*, **144**, 189–201

10. Carey, M.C. and Small, D.M. (1978). Physical chemistry of cholesterol solubility in bile. Relationship to gallstone formation and dissolution in man. *J. Clin. Invest.*, **61**, 998–1026

11. Mazer, N.A. and Carey, M.C. (1983). Quasielastic light scattering studies of aqueous biliary lipid systems. Cholesterol solubilisation and precipitation in model bile solutions. *Biochemistry*, **22**, 426–42

12. Salvioli, G., Igimi, H. and Carey, M.C. (1983). Cholesterol gallstone dissolution in bile: dissolution kinetics of crystalline cholesterol monohydrate by conjugated chenodeoxycholate–lecithin and conjugated ursodeoxycholate–lecithin mixtures. Dissimilar phase equilibria and dissolution mechanisms. *J. Lipid Res.*, **24**, 701–20

13. Small, D.M. (1971). The physical chemistry of cholanic acids. In Nair, P.P. and Kritchevsky, D. (eds.) *The Bile Acids, Vol I*. pp. 249–356. (New York: Plenum Press)

14. Carey, M.C. (1985). Physical chemical properties of bile acids and their salts. In Danielsson, H. and Sjövall, J. (eds.) *Sterols and Bile Acids*. pp. 345–403. (Amsterdam: Elsevier)

15. Cabral, D.J. and Small, D.M. (1988). The physical chemistry of bile. In Forte, J.G. (ed.) *Handbook of Physiology*. (Washington, D.C.: American Physiological Society) (in press)

16. Hofmann, A.F. (ed.) (1984). The physical chemistry of bile. *Hepatology* (Supplement), **4**, S1–S252

17. Carey, M.C. and Small, D.M. (1972). Micelle formation by bile salts. Physical chemical and thermodynamic considerations. *Arch. Intern. Med.*, **130**, 506–27

18. Schoenfield, L.J., Sjövall, J. and Sjövall, K. (1966). Bile acid composition of gallstones from man. *J. Lab. Clin. Med.*, **68**, 186–94

19. Akiyoshi, T. and Nakayama, F. (1988). Role of bile acids in the formation of brown pigment stones (calcium bilirubinate stones). *Dig. Dis. Sci.*, (In press)

20. Mazer, N.A., Carey, M.C., Kwasnick, R.F. and Benedek, G.B. (1979). Quasielastic light scattering studies of aqueous biliary lipid systems. Size, shape and thermodynamics of bile salt micelles. *Biochemistry*, **18**, 3064–75

21. Ahlberg, J., Curstedt, T., Einarsson, K. and Sjövall, J. (1981). Molecular species of biliary phosphatidylcholine in gallstone patients: The influence of treatment with cholic acid and chenodeoxycholic acid. *J. Lipid Res.*, **22**, 404–9

22. Cantafora, A., Angelico, M., DiBiase, A., Pierche, U., Bracci, F., Attili, A.F. and Capocaccia, L (1981). Structure of biliary phosphatidylcholine in cholesterol gallstone patients. *Lipids*, **16**, 589–92

23. Montet, J.-C. and Dervichian, D.G. (1971). Solubilisation micellaire du cholesterol par les sels biliaires et les lecithins extraits de la bile humaine. *Biochimie*, **53**, 751–4

24. Cantafora, A., DiBiase, A., Alvaro, D., Angelico, M., Marin, M. and Attili, A.F. (1983). High performance liquid chromatographic analysis of molecular species of phosphatidylcholine; development of quantitative assay and its application to human bile. *Clin. Chim. Acta*, **134**, 281–5

25. Small, D.M. (1986). *The Physical Chemistry of Lipids*. pp. 1–672. (New York: Plenum Press)

26. Huang, C.-H. (1969). Studies on phosphatidylcholine vesicles. Formation and physical characteristics. *Biochemistry*, **8**, 344–51

27. Loomis, C.R., Shipley, G.G. and Small, D.M. (1979). The phase behaviour of hydrated cholesterol. *J. Lipid Res.*, **20**, 525–35

28. Igimi, H. and Carey, M.C. (1981). Cholesterol gallstone dissolution in bile: dissolution of kinetics of crystalline (anhydrate and monohydrate) cholesterol with chenodeoxycholate, ursodeoxycholate and their glycine and taurine conjugates. *J. Lipid Res.*, **22**, 254–70

29. Armstrong, M.J. and Carey, M.C. (1987). Thermodynamic and molecular determinants of sterol solubilities in bile salt micelles. *J. Lipid Res.*, **28**, 1144–55

30. Carey, M.C., Montet, J.-C., Phillips, M.C., Armstrong, M.J. and Mazer, N.A. (1981). Thermodynamic and molecular basis for dissimilar cholesterol solubilising capacities by micellar solutions of bile salts: cases of sodium chenodeoxycholate and sodium ursodeoxycholate and their glycine and taurine conjugates. *Biochemistry*, **20**, 3637–48

31. Armstrong, M.J. and Carey, M.C. (1982). The hydrophobic–hydrophilic balance of bile salts: Inverse correlation between reverse-phase high performance liquid chromatographic mobilities and micellar cholesterol solubilising capacities. *J. Lipid Res.*, **23**, 70–80

32. Woodford, F.P. (1969). Enlargement of taurocholate micelles by added cholesterol and monoolein. Self-diffusion measurements. *J. Lipid Res.*, **10**, 539–45

33. Lecuyer, H. and Dervichian, D.G. (1969). Structure of aqueous mixtures of lecithin and cholesterol. *J. Mol. Biol.*, **45**, 39–57

34. Huang, C.-H. (1977). A structural model for the cholesterol–phosphatidylcholine complexes in bilayer membranes. *Lipids*, **12**, 348–56

35. Small, D.M. and Bourgès, M. (1966). Lyotropic paracrystalline phases obtained with ternary systems of amphiphilic substances in water. *Mol. Cryst. Liq. Cryst.*, **1**, 541–61

36. Darke, A., Finer, E.G., Flook, A.G. and Phillips, M.C. (1972). Nuclear magnetic resonance study of lecithin–cholesterol interactions. *J. Mol. Biol.*, **63**, 265–79

37. McLean, L.R. and Phillips, M.C. (1982). Cholesterol desorption from clusters of phosphatidylcholine in unilamellar vesicle bilayers during lipid transfer or exchange. *Biochemistry*, **21**, 4053–9

38. Collins, J.J. and Phillips, M.C. (1982). The stability and structure of cholesterol-rich codispersions of cholesterol and phosphatidylcholine. *J. Lipid Res.*, **23**, 291–8

39. Mazer, N.A., Benedek, G.B. and Carey, M.C. (1980). Quasielastic light scattering studies of aqueous biliary lipid systems. Mixed micelle formation in bile salt–lecithin solutions. *Biochemistry*, **19**, 601–15

40. Schurtenberger, P., Mazer, N. and Känzig, W. (1985). Micelle to vesicle transition in aqueous solutions of bile salt and lecithin. *J. Phys. Chem.*, **89**, 1042–9

41. Donovan, J.M., Benedek, G.B. and Carey, M.C. (1987). Formation of mixed micelles and vesicles of human apolipoprotein A-I and A-II with synthetic and natural lecithins and the bile salt, sodium taurocholate: Quasielastic light scattering studies. *Biochemistry*, **26**, 8125–33

42. Stark, R.E., Gosselin, G.J., Donovan, J.M., Carey, M.C. and Roberts, M.S. (1985). Influence of dilution on the physical state of model bile systems: Nuclear magnetic resonance and quasielastic light scattering investigation. *Biochemistry*, **24**, 5599–5605

43. Brunner, J., Skrabel, P. and Hauser, H. (1976). Single bilayer vesicles prepared without sonication. Physical chemical properties. *Biochim. Biophys. Acta*, **455**, 322–31

44. Carey, M.C. (1983). Measurement of the physical chemical properties of bile salt solutions. In Barbara, L., Dowling, R.H., Hofmann, A.F. and Roda, E. (eds.) *Bile Acids in Gastroenterology*. pp. 19–56. (Lancaster: MTP Press)

45. Duane, W.C. (1975). The intermicellar bile salt concentration in equilibrium with the mixed micelles of human bile. *Biochim. Biophys. Acta*, **398**, 275–86

46. Duane, W.C. (1977). Taurocholate– and taurochenodeoxycholate–lecithin micelles: The equilibrium of bile salt between aqueous phase and micelle. *Biochem. Biophys. Res. Commun.*, **74**, 223–9

47. Carey, M.C. and Ko, G. Unpublished observations

48. Sömjen, G.J. and Gilat, T. (1986). Changing concepts of cholesterol solubility in bile. *Gastroenterology*, **91**, 772–5

49. Holzbach, R.T., Kibe, A., Thiel, E., Howell, J.H., Marsh, M. and Hermann, R.E. (1984). Biliary proteins: Unique inhibitors of cholesterol crystal nucleation in human gallbladder bile. *J. Clin. Invest.*, **73**, 33–45

50. Kibe, A., Dudley, M.A., Halpern, Z., Lynn, M.P., Breuer, A.C. and Holzbach, R.T. (1985). Factors affecting cholesterol monohydrate crystal nucleation time in model systems of supersaturated bile. *J. Lipid Res.*, **26**, 1102–11

81

51. Halpern, Z., Dudley, M.A., Lynn, M.P., Nader, J.M., Breuer, A.C. and Holzbach, R.T. (1986). Vesicle aggregation in model systems of supersaturated bile: Relation to crystal nucleation and lipid composition of the vesicular phase. *J. Lipid Res.*, **27**, 295–306
52. Salvioli, G., Igimi, H., Carey, M.C. and Ko, G. Unpublished observations.
53. Carey, M.C. and Cahalane, M.J. (1988). Whither biliary sludge? *Gastroenterology* (In press)

6
Gallbladder Motor Function in Man

A. Lanzini and T.C. Northfield
Department of Medicine
St. George's Hospital Medical School
London, SW17 0RE, UK

INTRODUCTION

Ivy summarised the physiology of gallbladder motor function in 1934[1] with the concept that 'the gallbladder stores much of the bile formed during the interdigestive period to evacuate it during the early part of the following digestive period'. According to this classical concept, gallbladder motor function can be likened to a slow pump, with an emptying phase after meals and a storage phase between meals.

Improved research techniques have led us to hypothesise a new concept of gallbladder motor function in which the gallbladder behaves like a bellows rather than a pump[2] – represented in Figure 1. The 'bellows' con-

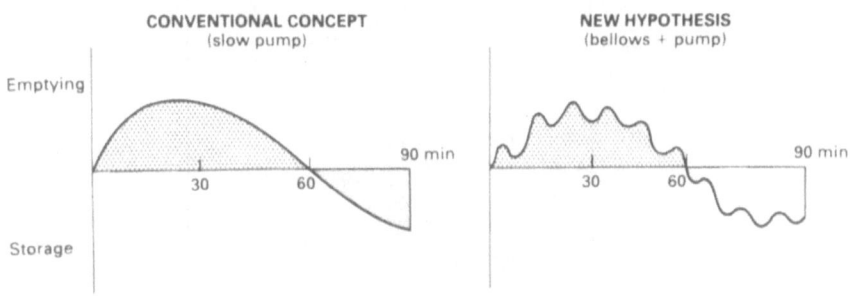

Figure 1 Concepts of gallbladder motor function.

cept envisages a rapid pump mechanism with frequent alternations in gallbladder expansion and contraction (absolute storage and emptying) over short time intervals, which is superimposed on the classical slow pump mechanism representing the net result of these rapid alternations over a longer time interval.

The bellows, like the gallbladder, is a hollow structure with a single narrow exit and entry; it achieves its effect by rapid alternations of filling and emptying that perturb the surrounding air. There must be a corresponding perturbation of the air within the bellows and, by analogy, of bile within the gallbladder.

Concepts of gallbladder (GB) function depend upon the methods used to observe it. Conventional methods of measuring GB motility have supported the slow pump concept of GB motor function, but when applied with certain modifications they have provided clues to the new hypothesis. This chapter will review the contribution of different methods and of different applications of the same method to the understanding of GB motor function in man.

ASSESSMENT OF GALLBLADDER MOTOR FUNCTION

(a) Cholecystography and Ultrasonography

Both these methods enable GB volume to be measured at fixed time inter-

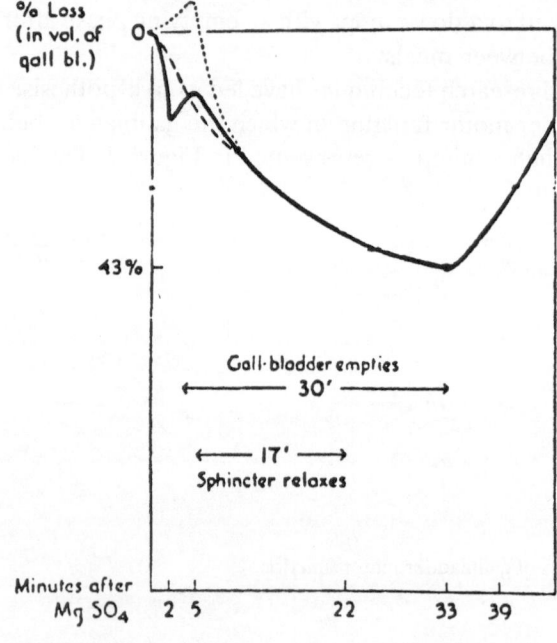

Figure 2 Changes in gallbladder volume measured by cholecystography in ten healthy subjects following oral administration of magnesium sulphate (modified from reference 7, with permission). Rapid alternation of storage and emptying was detected in two-thirds of the subjects (solid and dotted lines) during frequent measurements of gallbladder volume (2–3 minute intervals). Slow and smooth emptying and storage phases were detected sequentially during measurements carried out at longer time intervals (about 15 minutes).

vals; changes of GB volume over time are assumed to reflect GB motor function. These methods do not, however, measure only GB motor function, because GB volume is also influenced by absorption and secretion of fluid within the GB.

They cannot distinguish whether a change in GB volume over a period of time reflects GB storage or emptying alone, or a combination of the two within the period. Both methods can therefore provide only measurements of net GB motor function. Conventional application of these techniques, every 30 minutes or more, has supported the slow pump concept of GB motor function, but increasing the frequency of measurement has pointed to the new hypothesis.

Cholecystography was first applied by Boyden[3-7] to the systematic study of GB motor function, and the method he devised for measurement of GB volume[4] was later improved by De Paula E Silva[8]. At that time, the major concern about radiation hazard was that 'the Roentgen ray could produce erythema', and this enabled Boyden to use many radiographs (16–20 per hour) in his human studies, most of them in the first 15 minutes following a meal. This high frequency enabled Boyden to observe that postprandial GB emptying was 'intermittent in character' with an initial response of two minutes with maximum GB emptying, followed by a '2 minute pause' charac-

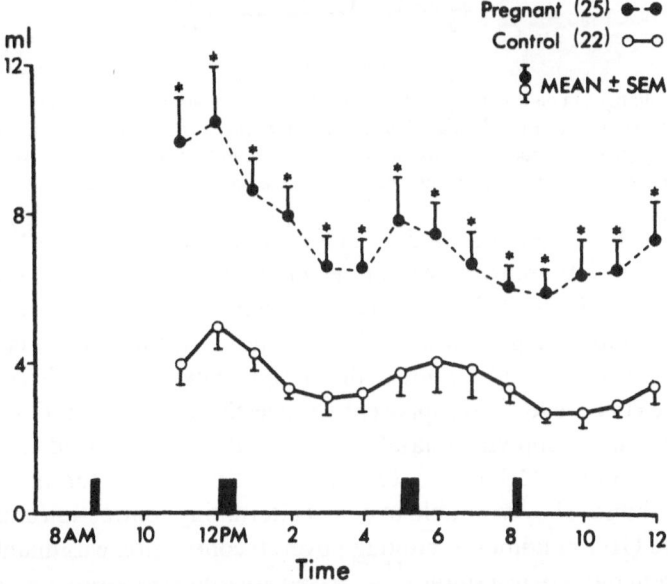

Figure 3 Changes in gallbladder volume measured by ultrasonography at 60 minute intervals in normal and pregnant women during intermittent administration of meals (solid bars) (from reference 22 with permission). The changes in gallbladder volume illustrate the classical slow pump concept of gallbladder motor function.

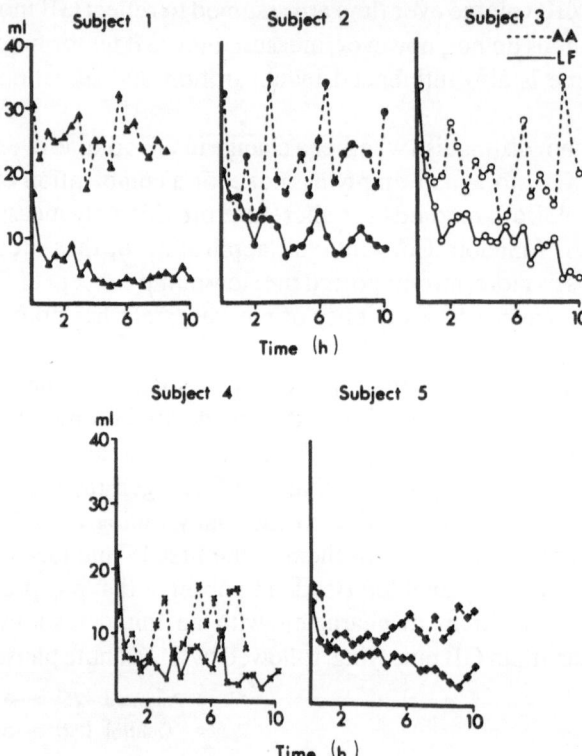

Figure 4 Changes in gallbladder volume measured by ultrasonography in five healthy subjects during continuous intraduodenal administration of essential aminoacid (AA) or lipid formula (LF) (from reference 34 with permission). Fluctuations in gallbladder volume were present in each individual, and during intraduodenal administration of each nutrient.

terised by GB storage, followed by a new phase of GB emptying[4,7] This intermittency in GB emptying was not evident when radiographs were taken only every 15 minutes (Figure 2). Paul Edholm in 1960[9] took three successive X-ray films during the first 7 minutes after intravenous cholecystokinin and observed many 'small humps' in the GB emptying curve; 'in three of these humps the curves even rose, apparently suggesting a short period of refilling during the major emptying phase'. Torsoli et al. in 1960[10] used cineradiography to monitor GB motor function continuously after intravenous cholecystokinin. They were able to detect alternating contraction and relaxation in the GB infundibulus, although overall contraction was mainly tonic. More recent radiological studies[11-17] based, for ethical reasons, on a reduced number of radiographs, have failed to show this rapid alternation of emptying and storage.

Real time ultrasonography provides a simpler and safer method than cholecystography for assessment of GB volume[18]. The technique has been

validated *in vitro* by Everson *et al.*[19], and a direct comparison *in vivo* with
cholecystography gave reproducible results for GB volume[19].
Ultrasonographic studies are conventionally carried out at no less than 10
minute intervals, and under these conditions support the conventional concept of GB motor function[19–32] (Figure 3). Howard *et al.*[33], however, took
advantage of the safety of the procedure and performed ultrasound scanning
at 2 minute intervals after a meal. They found rapid fluctuations of GB
volume consistent with the new hypothesis. Recently Everson *et al.*[34] have
used ultrasonography to assess the effect of continuous duodenal infusion of
either an amino acid or lipid formula meal on GB motor function. GB volume
fluctuated in each individual subject during duodenal infusion of both
nutrients, by as much as 20 ml during amino acid infusion (Figure 4). The
authors interpret these fluctuations as alternating GB filling and emptying.
These studies show that the human GB responds to both intermittent[33] or

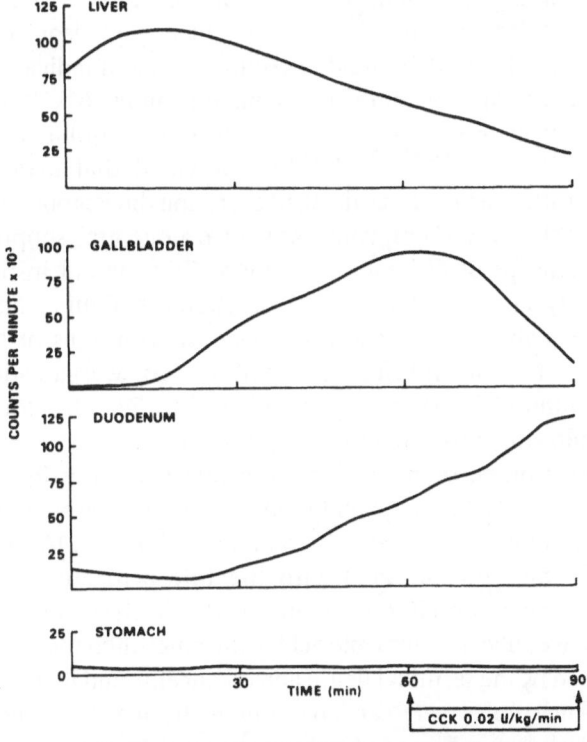

Figure 5 Sequential measurement of gallbladder storage and emptying function in one individual subject with single isotope cholescintigraphy (from reference 54 with permission).
The pattern of ^{99m}Tc-HIDA time–activity curve illustrates the classical slow pump concept
of gallbladder motor function.

continuous feeding[34] by alternating storage and emptying, rather than by tonic contraction.

(b) Cholescintigraphy

Englert and Chiu[35] were the first to assess GB storage and emptying of a cholephilic gamma labelled substance by external scanning. Many substances have since been used[35–50], and ^{99m}Tc-labelled imido diacetic acid derivatives found to be best because of their specific uptake by the liver, their high hepatic excretory efficiency and very low urinary excretion, their short half life and low radiation exposure[48–52]. Cholescintigraphy allows GB storage or emptying to be measured[53–74] separately during any given time interval if a single radiolabelled agent is used (Figure 5). Since this method cannot measure both functions simultaneously, it is not suitable for testing the bellows hypothesis, and has overall supported the classical slow pump concept.

Combining cholescintigraphy with naso-duodenal intubation and collection of GB bile sample[71,72] has extended single isotope cholescintigraphy to the study of biliary lipid physiology, but still indicates only net GB storage and has not contributed to the understanding of GB dynamics.

GB emptying can, however, be measured in absolute terms by cholescintigraphy[35,36,53,54,57,60,63,64,66–69,73,74] provided that measurements are started only after the liver has finished excreting the isotope. In most cholescintigraphic studies GB emptying has been exponential, supporting the conventional concept of GB motor function. Close visual inspection of GB time–activity curves after a meal or cholecystokinin administration, however, reveals frequent and short-lived interruptions of GB emptying, consistent with frequent brief refilling of the GB. Mesgarzadeh et al.[60], for instance, found 40% GB emptying followed by 7% GB storage within 21 minutes following intravenous cholecystokinin.

Dual isotope scanning[75] has recently made possible simultaneous measurement of GB storage and emptying during the same short time intervals (1 minute). Jazrawi et al.[75] combined ^{99m}Tc-HIDA (as a non-absorbable GB emptying marker) with the bile acid analogue ^{75}Se tauro homocholic acid (^{75}Se-HCAT – as an absorbable GB storage marker). ^{75}Se-HCAT behaves like a natural bile acid in the enterohepatic circulation in that it is absorbed by the terminal ileum and is concentrated in the GB in the fasting state. The studies were carried out in the fasting state. The GB area was delineated on gamma-camera scans using a light pen. GB emptying was stimulated by intramuscular CCK-octapeptide and time activity curves for both isotopes were constructed following simultaneous continuous gamma-camera scanning using a dual isotope probe. They found that GB emptying of Tc-HIDA and storage of Se-HCAT occurred during the same postpran-

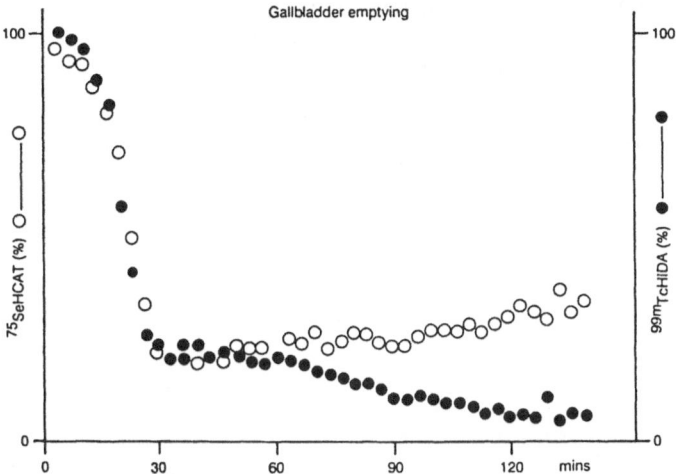

Figure 6 Simultaneous measurement of gallbladder storage and emptying function in one individual subject with a dual isotope technique. Time–activity curves of both ^{99m}Tc-HIDA (non-absorbable biliary marker) and of ^{75}Se-HCAT (absorbable biliary marker) were similar during a first rapid postprandial phase and then diverged, indicating gallbladder storage (^{75}S-HCAT curve) and emptying (^{99m}Tc-HIDA curve) during the same short time intervals.

dial time interval in a study of eight healthy subjects. (Figure 6). This study seems to support the new hypothesis of GB motor function: the only way to explain what appears to be 'simultaneous' GB storage of Se-HCAT and emptying of Tc-HIDA is to postulate rapid alternations of storage and emptying.

(c) Duodenal Perfusion Techniques

Duodenal perfusion techniques provide an alternative method of measuring GB motor function; they are not influenced by GB absorption or secretion and therefore specifically indicate GB motor function. Whether they provide net or absolute measurements of GB storage and emptying depends on the experimental conditions, and particularly on whether a GB bile marker, a hepatic bile marker or both are used in addition to a duodenal recovery marker.

Duane and Hanson[74] measured absolute GB emptying using an intravenous bolus of indocyanine green, (ICG) as a GB bile marker. They found that GB emptying of ICG followed the typical exponential 'slow pump' pattern seen in cholescintigraphic studies.

Measurement of the duodenal output of a substance excreted by the liver at a constant rate indicates only *net* GB storage and emptying[77–81]; a duodenal recovery of less than 100% of the hepatic excretion rate indicating

89

net GB storage, and vice versa. This technique cannot therefore be used to test the 'bellows' concept. Mok et al.[77] used bilirubin as an endogenous hepatic bile marker and found about 50% net GB storage of hepatic bile during nocturnal fasting. Van Berge Henegouwen and Hofmann[78] used a continuous intravenous infusion of indocyanine green (ICG) as an exogenous

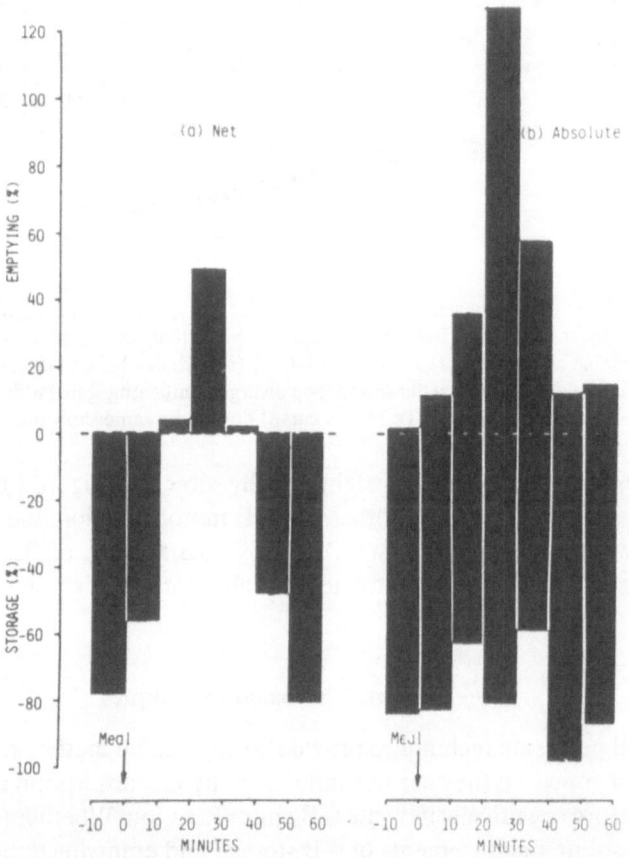

Figure 7 Median gallbladder storage and emptying of indocyanine green (ICG) in six subjects at 10 minute intervals during the first postprandial hour showing a comparison between net gallbladder storage and emptying of ICG (a) and absolute gallbladder storage and emptying of ICG (b) (from reference 80 with permission). Absolute values indicate that both storage and emptying occur during the same 10 minute intervals, supporting the 'bellows' hypothesis of gallbladder motor function.

hepatic bile marker. They found during nocturnal fasting about 50% net GB storage of hepatic bile with an occasional burst of net GB emptying, and after a meal net GB emptying ranging from 30% to 250% of the ICG intravenous infusion rate. This pattern of net storage between meals, and net emptying after meals is consistent with the 'slow pump' concept.

Lanzini et al.[80] have recently developed a duodenal perfusion techni-que involving the simultaneous use of a hepatic bile marker and a GB bile marker in order to measure both GB storage and emptying simultaneously within the same short time interval. They used continuous intravenous in-fusion of ICG (as a hepatic bile marker) and intravenous bolus of ^{99m}Tc-HIDA (as a GB bile marker) together with duodenal perfusion of polyethylene glycol as a intestinal recovery marker. This allows calculation of the mass of ICG entering the GB (absolute GB storage) and leaving the GB (absolute GB emptying) during each time interval, together with the net results of these absolute changes in storage and emptying. GB ejection frac-tion of ^{99m}Tc-HIDA can also be measured. This technique has therefore al-lowed quantitative testing of the 'bellows' concept in man. Results based on duodenal recovery during the first postprandial hour of ICG only (Figure 7 on the left) are consistent with the classical concept of a storage phase before the meal and an emptying phase postprandially. Incorporation of the Tc-HIDA data indicates that the net storage and net emptying phases for ICG were both composed of two components: absolute storage and absolute emptying, both of which occurred during each time interval. The amount of absolute GB storage of ICG secreted from the liver during each 10 minute postprandial interval was on average about 70%. This storage was combined with emptying of almost half the Tc-HIDA in the GB during the first postprandial hour. Since the GB has a single narrow channel for entry and exit of bile, the occurrence within 10 minute intervals of both absolute storage and emptying of ICG indicates that the two phenomena must alternate rapid-ly by a mechanism which is more analogous to a 'bellows' effect than to a slow pump effect. It is tempting to speculate that these alternations may have the same frequency (once every 10–20 seconds) as for pressure changes in the human sphincter of Oddi[82], and that they may contribute to mixing of GB bile. During nocturnal fasting, net GB storage of ICG occurred during each hourly interval, and absolute measurements indicated that GB storage of ICG was virtually complete. These findings indicate that most of the hepatic bile enters the GB both after meals and during fasting, and that the GB is not quiescent during nocturnal fasting.

SUMMARY

A new concept of GB motor function envisages a rapid pump, with frequent alternations in absolute storage and emptying, superimposed on a slow pump that reflects the net changes in storage and emptying over a longer time course. Conventional application of methods available for assessment of GB motor function in man can only detect these latter net changes in GB storage and emptying, and thus cannot be used to test the new concept. By contrast, radiology[3-10] and ultrasonography[32-34] carried out at short time intervals, scanning using two isotopes[75], and duodenal perfusion techniques combining a hepatic and a GB bile marker[80] are able to detect rapid alternation of GB storage and emptying, and supporting the 'bellows' concept of GB motor function. These latter techniques cannot determine the frequency of the alternating bouts of GB storage and emptying, although the perfusion technique can assess their size.

REFERENCES

1. Ivy, A.C. (1934). The physiology of the gallbladder. *Physiol. Rev.*, **14**, 1–102
2. Lanzini, A., Jazrawi, R.J. and Northfield, T.C. (1983). Does the gallbladder function as a pump or as a bellows? *Gut*, **24**, A475
3. Boyden, E.A. (1926). A study of the behaviour of the human gallbladder in response to the ingestion of food; together with some observations on the mechanism of the expulsion of bile in experimental animals. *Anat. Rec.*, **33**, 201–56
4. Boyden, E.A. (1928). An analysis of the reaction of the human gallbladder to food. *Anat. Rec.*, **40**, 147–89
5. Boyden, E.A. and Grantham, S.A. (1936). Evacuation of the gallbladder in old age. *Surg. Gynecol. Obstet.*, **62**, 34–42
6. Gerdes, M.M. and Boyden, E.A. (1938). The rate of emptying of the human gallbladder in pregnancy. *Surg. Gynecol. Obstet.*, **66**, 145–56
7. Boyden, E.A., Bergh, G.S. and Layne, J.A. (1943). An analysis of the reaction of the human gallbladder and sphincter of Oddi to magnesium sulphate. *Surgery*, 723–33
8. De Paula E Silva, G.S. (1949). A simple method for computing the volume of human gallbladder. *Radiology*, **52**, 94–102
9. Edholm, P. (1960). Gallbladder evacuation in the normal male induced by cholecystokinin. *Acta Radiol.*, **53**, 257–65
10. Torsoli, A., Ramorino, M.L., Colagrande, C. and Demaio, G. (1960). Experiments with cholecystokinin. *Acta Radiol.*, **55**, 193–205
11. Rose, D.J. (1959). Serial cholecystography. *Arch. Surg.*, **78**, 56–66
12. Nilsson, S. and Stattin, S. (1967). Gallbladder emptying during the normal menstrual cycle. *Acta Chir. Scand.*, **133**, 648–52
13. Nathan, M.H., Newman, A., Murray, D.J. *et al.* (1970). Cholecystokinin cholecystography. *Am. J. Roentgenol.*, **110**, 240–51
14. Park, C.Y., Pae, Y.S. and Hong, S.S. (1970). Radiological studies on emptying of human gallbladder. *Ann. Surg.*, **171**, 294–9
15. Sacchetti, G., Mandelli, V., Roncoroni, R. *et al.* (1973). Influence of age and sex on gallbladder emptying induced by a fatty meal in normal subjects. *Am. J. Roentgenol. Radium Ther. Nucl. Med.*, **119**, 40–5
16. Davidsen, D. and Jorgensen, J. (1981). Gallbladder emptying with ceruletide in oral cholecystography. *Acta Radiol. Diagnos.*, **22**, 165–69
17. Morewood, D.J.W. and Whitehouse, G.H. (1984). Ceruletide cholecystography: dose response and gallbladder function. *Br. J. Radiol.*, **57**, 439
18. Ornstein, M.H.,, Palframan, A. and Meire, H. (1978). Real-time ultrasound – a new method for investigating gallbladder dynamics. *Gut*, **19**, A971
19. Everson, G.T., Braverman, D.Z., Johnson, L. and Kern Jr., F. (1980). A critical evaluation of real-time ultrasonography for the study of gallbladder volume and contraction. *Gastroenterology*, **79**, 40–6
20. Braverman, D.Z., Johnson, M.L. and Kern, F. (1980). Effect of pregnancy and con-

traceptive steroids on gallbladder function. *N. Engl. J. Med.*, 302, 362–4

21. Kern, Jr., F., Everson, G.T., DeMark, B., McKinley, C., Showalter, R., Braverman, D.Z., Szczepanik-Van Leeuwen, P. and Klein, P.D. (1982). Biliary lipids, bile acids, and gallbladder function in the human female: effects of contraceptive steroids. *J. Lab. Clin. Med.*, 99, 798–805

22. Everson, G.T., McKinley, C., Lawson, M., Johnson, M. and Kern, Jr., F. (1982). Gallbladder function in the human female: effect of the ovulatory cycle, pregnancy and contraceptive steroids. *Gastroenterology*, 82, 711–19

23. Thompson, J.C., Gried, G.M., Ogden, W.D., Fagan, C.J., Inoue, K., Wiener, I. and Watson, L.C. (1982). Correlation between release of cholecystokinin and contraction of the gallbladder in patients with gallstones. *Ann. Surg.*, 195, 670–75

24. Lawson, M., Everson, G.T., Klingensmith, W. and Kern, Jr. F. (1983). Coordination of gastric and gallbladder emptying after ingestion of a regular meal. *Gastroenterology*, 85, 866–70

25. Hansen, W.E., Maurer, H., Vollmar, J. and Brauning, C. (1983). Guar gum and bile: effects on postprandial gallbladder contraction and on serum bile acids in man. *Hepato-Gastroent.*, 30, 131–33

26. Gullo, L., Bolondi, L., Priori, P., Casanova, P. and Labo, G. (1984). Inhibitory effect of atropine on cholecystokinin-induced gallbladder contraction in man. *Digestion*, 29, 209–13

27. Ladas, S.D., Isaacs, P.E.T., Murphy, G.M. and Sladen, G.E. (1984). Comparison of the effects of medium and long chain triglyceride containing liquid meals on gallbladder and small intestinal function in normal man. *Gut*, 25, 405–11

28. Walker, J.P., Khalil, T., Wiener, I., Fagan, C.J., Townsend, C.M., Greeley, G.H. and Thompson, J.C. (1985). The role of neurotensin in human gallbladder motility. *Ann. Surg.*, 201, 678–83

29. Liddle, R.A., Goldfine, I.D., Rosen, M.S., Tapliz, R.A. and Williams, J.A. (1985). Cholecystokinin bioactivity in human plasma. Molecular forms, responses to feeding, and relationship to gallbladder contraction. *J. Clin. Invest.*, 75, 1144–52

30. Hopman, W.P.M., Rosenbusch, G., de Long, A.J.L. and Lamers, C.B.H.W. (1985). Gallbladder contraction: effects of fatty meals and cholecystokinin. *Radiology*, 157, 37–9

31. Khalil, T., Walker, J.P., Wiener, I. Fagan, C.J., Townsend, C.M., Greeley, G.h. and Thompson, J.C. (1985). Effect of aging in gallbladder contraction and release of cholecystokinin-33 in humans. *Surgery*, 98, 423–29

32. Lilja, P., Fagan, C.J., Wiener, I., Inoue, K., Watson, L.C., Rayford, P.L. and Thompson, J.C. (1982). Infusion of pure cholecystokinin in humans. Correlation between plasma concentrations of cholecystokinin and gallbladder size. *Gastroenterology*, 83, 256–61

33. Howard, P., Murphy, G.M. and Dowling, R.H. (1985). Is gallbladder emptying really exponential? *Gut*, 26, A1147

34. Everson, T.G., Lawson, M.J., McKinley, C., Showalter, R. and Kern. Jr. F. (1983). Gallbladder and small intestinal regulation of biliary lipid secretion during intraduodenal infusion of standard stimuli. *J. Clin. Invest.*, 71, 596–603

35. Englert, jr. E. and Chiu, V.S.W. (1966). Quantitative analysis of human biliary evacuation with radioisotopic techniques. *Gastroenterology*, 50, 506–18

36. Chapple, M.J., Dowsett, L., Low-Beer, T.S., et al. (1975). Gallbladder emptying measured by a radioisotopic method. *Br. J. Radiol.*, 48, 19–22

37. Low-Beer, T.S., Harvey, R.H. Davies, E.R. and Read, A.E. (1975). Abnormalities of serum cholecystokinin and gallbladder emptying in celiac disease. *N. Engl. J. Med.*, 292, 961–63

38. Harvey, E., Lobert, M. and Cooper, M. (1975). ^{99m}Tc-HIDA, a new radiopharmaceutical for hepatobiliary imaging. J. Nucl. Med., 16, 533

39. Loberg, M.D., Cooper, M., Harvey, E., et al. (1976). Development of new radiopharmaceutical based on N substitution of iminodoacetic acid. *J. Nucl. Med.*, 17, 633–38

40. Wistow, B.W., Subramanian, G., Van Heertum, R.L. *et al.* (1977). An evaluation of Tc-99m-labelled hepatobiliary agents. *J. Nucl. Med.*, **18**, 455–61

41. Baker, R.G. and Marion, M.A. (1977). Biliary scanning with Tc-99m pyridoxylidene glutamate: the effect of food in normal subjects. *J. Nucl. Med.*, **18**, 793–95

42. Lobert, M., Callery, P., Porter, D., *et al.* (1979). Chemistry of technetium radiopharmaceuticals derived from bifunctional chelating agents. *J. Labelled Compds.*, **16**, 77–79

43. Yeh, S.H., Liu, O.K. and Huang, M.J. (1980). Sequential scintigraphy with technetium-99m pyridoxylideneglutamate in the detection of intrahepatic lithiasis: concise communication. *J. Nucl. Med.*, **21**, 17–21

44. Berk, E. (ed.) (1980). *Developments in Digestive Disease*. Functional scintigraphy: diagnostic application in gastroenterology in developments in digestive disease. Vol. 3, p. 139–64. (Philadelphia: Lea and Febiger)

45. Schoubye, J., Oester-Jorgensen, E. and Pedersen, S.A. (1981). The use of (99m Tc) (2,6-diethylacetanilide)-iminodiacetic acid ((99m Tc)HIDA) in evaluating normal hepatobiliary dynamics. *Scand. J. Clin. Lab. Invest.*, **41**, 127–34

46. Nunn, A.D., Loberg, M.D. and Conley, R.A. (1983). A structure–distribution-relationship approach leading to the development of Tc-99m-mebrofenin: an improved cholescintigraphic agent. *J. Nucl. Med.*, **24**, 423–30

47. Denkhaus, S.P.H., Montz, R. and Klapdor, R. (1983). Quantification and tracer kinetics in Intra- and extrahepatic bile ducts and of gallbladder filling rates in hepatobiliary dynamic scintigraphy using 99m Tc-HIDA derivates. *Nucl. Med.*, **22**, 181–6

48. Bobba, V.R., Krishnamurthy, G.T., Kingston, E. *et al.* (1983). Comparison of biokinetics and biliary imaging parameters of four Tc-99m iminodiacetic acid derivatives in normal subjects. *Clin. Nucl. Med.*, **8**, 70–5

49. Klingensmith III, W.C., Fritzberg, A.R., Spitzer, V.M., Kuni, C.C., Williamson, M.R. and Gerhold, J.P. (1983). Work in progress: Clinical evaluation of Tc-99m-trimethylbromo-HIDA and Tc-99m-diisopropyl-IDA for hepatobiliary imaging. *Radiology*, **146**, 181–4

50. Harvey, E., Loberg, M., Ryan, J., Sikorski, S., Faith, W. and Cooper, M. (1979). Hepatic clearance mechanism of Tc-99m-HIDA and its effect on quantitation of hepatobiliary function. *Concise Comm. J. Nucl. Med.*, **20**, 310–13

51. Smith, E.M. (1965). Internal dose calculation for Tc-99m. *J. Nucl. Med.*, **6**, 231–51

52. Brown, P.H., Krishnamurthy, G.T., Bobba, V.R. *et al.* (1982). Radiation dose calculation for five Tc-99m IDA hepatobiliary agents. *J. Nucl. Med.*, **23**, 1025–30

53. Spellman, S.J., Shaffer, E.A. and Rosenthall, L. (1979). Gallbladder emptying in response to cholecystokinin. A cholescintigraphic study. *Gastroenterology*, **77**, 115–20

54. Shaffer, E.A., McOrmond, P. and Duggan, H. (1980). Quantitative cholescintigraphy: assessment of gallbladder filling and emptying and duodenogastric reflux. *Gastroenterology*, **79**, 899–906

55. Klingensmith, III, W.C., Spitzer, V.M., Fritzberg, A.R., *et al.* (1981). The normal fasting and postprandial diisopropyl-IDA-Tc-99m-hepatobiliary study. *Radiology*, **141**, 771–76

56. Shaffer, E.A. (1981). The effect of vagotomy on gallbladder function and bile composition in man. *Ann. Surg.*, **195**, 413–18

57. Krishnamurthy, G.T., Bobba, V.R. and Kingston, E,. (1981). Radionucleide ejection fraction: a technique for quantitative analysis of motor function of the human gallbladder. *Gastroenterology*, **80**, 482–90

58. Fisher, R.S., Stelzer, F., Rock, E., and Malmud, L.S. (1982). Abnormal gallbladder emptying in patients with gallstones *Dig. Dis. Sci.*, **27**, 1019–24

59. Krishnamurthy, G.T., Bobba, V.R., McConnel, E., *et al.* (1983). Quantitative biliary dynamics: introduction of a new non-invasive scintigraphic technique. *J. Nucl. Med.*, **24**, 217–23

60. Mesgarzadeh, M., Krishnamurthy, G.T., Bobba, V.R. and Langrell, K. (1983). Filling postcholecystokinin emptying, and refilling of normal gallbladder: effects of two dif-

ferent doses of CCk on refilling: concise communication. *J. Nucl. Med.*, **24**, 666–71

61. Van der Linden, W., and Kempi, W. (1984). Filling of the gallbladder as studied by computer assisted Tc-99m HIDA scintigraphy: concise communication. *J. Nucl. Med.*, **25**, 292–98

62. Shaffer, E.A., Taylor, P.J., Logan, K., Gadomski, S. and Corenblum. B. (1984). The effect of a progestin on gallbladder function in young women. *Am. J. Obstet. Gynecol.*, **148**, 504–7

63. Kraglund, K. Hjermind, J., Jensen, F.T., Stodkilde-Jorgensen, H., Oster-Jorgensen, E. and Pedersen S.A. (1984). Gallbladder emptying and gastrointestinal cyclic motor activity in humans. *Scand. J. Gastroenterol.*, **19**, 990–94

64. Svenberg, T., Nilsson, I., Samuleson, K. and Welbourn, R.D. (1984). Studies on the relationship between gallbladder emptying and motilin release in man, *Acta Chir. Scand. Suppl.*, **520**, 59–61

65. Williams, W., Krishnamurthy, G.T. Brar, H.S. and Bobba, V.R. (1984). Scintigraphic variations of normal biliary physiology. *J. Nucl. Med.*, **25**, 160–65

66. Sarva, R.P., Shreiner, D.P., Van-Thiel, D. and Yingvorapant, N. (1985). Gallbladder function: methods for measuring filling and emptying. *J. Nucl. Med.*, **26**, 140–44

67. Fisher, S.R., Rock, E. and Malmud, L.S. (1986). Gallbladder emptying response to sham feeding in humans. *Gastroenterology*, **90**, 1854–57

68. Svenberg, T., Christofides, N.D. Fitzpatrick, M.L., Bloom, S.R. and Welbourn, R.B. (1985). Oral water causes emptying of the human gallbladder through actions of vagal stimuli rather than motilin. *Scand. J. Gastroenterology*, **20**, 775–78

69. Fisher, R.S., Rock, E. and Malmud, L.S. (1985). Cholinergic effects on gallbladder emptying in humans. *Gastroenterology*, **89**, 716–22

70. Tooluli, J., Bushell, M., Stevenson, G., Dent. J., Wycherley, A. and Iannos, J. (1986). Gallbladder emptying in man related to fasting migrating motor contractions. *N.Z. J. Surg.*, **56**, 625–30

71. Jazrawi, R.P., Kupfer, R.M., Bridges, C., Joseph, A. and Northfield, T.C. (1983). Assessment of gallbladder storage function in man. *Clin. Sci.*, **65**, 185–91

72. Jazrawi, R.P., Brown, C. and Northfield, T.C. (1984). Measurement of biliary lipid mass within the gallbladder in health and in ileal Crohn's disease. *Gut*, **25**, A1141

73. Baxter, J.N., Grime, J.S., Critchley, M. and Shields R. (1985). Relationship between gastric emptying of solids and gallbladder emptying in normal subjects. *Gut*, **26**, 342–51

74. Krishnamurthy, G.T., Bobba, V.R., Kingston, E. and Turner, F. (1982). Measurement of gallbladder emptying sequentially using a single dose of 99m Tc-labelled hepatobiliary agent. *Gastroenterology*, **83**, 773–76

75. Jazrawi, R.P., Lanzini, A., Britten, A., Meller, S.T. and Northfield, T.C. (1984). Dynamics of gallbladder function and of the enterohepatic circulation studied by gamma labelled bile acid. *Clin. Sci.*, **66**, 10P

76. Duane, W.C. and Hanson, K.C. (1978). Role of gallbladder emptying and small bowel transit in regulation of bile acid pool size in man. *J. Lab. Clin. Med.*, **92**, 858–72

77. Mok, H.Y.I., Von Bergman, K. and Grundy, S.M. (1980). Kinetics of the enterohepatic circulation during fasting: biliary lipid secretion and gallbladder storage. *Gastroenterology*, **78**, 1023–33

78. Van Berge Henegouwen, G.P. and Hofmann, A.F. (1979). Nocturnal gallbladder storage and emptying in gallstone patients and healthy subjects. *Gastroenterology*, **75**, 879–85

79. Bjornsson, O.G., Adrian, T.E. Dawson, J., McCloy, R.F. Greenberg, G.R., Bloom, S.R. and Chadwick, V.S. (1979). Effects of gastrointestinal hormones on fasting gallbladder storage patterns in man. *Eur. J. Clin. Invest.*, **9**, 293–300

80. Lanzini, A., Jazrawi, R.P. and Northfield, T.C. (1987). Simultaneous quantitative measurements of absolute gallbladder storage and emptying during fasting and eating in man. *Gastroenterology*, **92**, 852–61

81. Bjornsson, O.G., Maton, P.N., Fletcher, D.R. and Chadwick, V.S. (1982). Effects of

duodenal perfusion with sodium taurocholate on biliary and pancreatic secretion in man. *Eur. J. Clin. Invest.*, **12**, 97–105

82. Greenen, G.E., Hogan, W., Dodds, W.J., Stewart, E.T. and Arndorfer, R.C. (1980). Intraluminal pressure recording from the human sphincter of Oddi. *Gastroenterology*, **78**, 317–24

SECTION B
PATHOGENESIS OF CHOLESTEROL GALLSTONE DISEASE

7

Pathogenesis of Cholesterol Gallstone Disease: The Secretory Defect

K. Einarsson and B. Angelin
Division of Gastroenterology and Metabolism Unit,
Department of Medicine,
Karolinska Institutet at Huddinge University Hospital,
S-141 86 Huddinge,
Sweden

INTRODUCTION

Most patients with cholesterol gallstone disease have supersaturated gallbladder bile, i.e. the amount of cholesterol is in excess of what can theoretically be kept in solution. Saturated bile is also more common among races and populations with a high frequency of gallstones[1,2]. The development of supersaturated bile appears to be a necessary step for the subsequent precipitation of cholesterol, and may thus be considered a major risk factor for cholesterol gallstones. Many individuals without gallstone disease, however, also have supersaturated bile[3,4] (Figure 1). It has therefore become evident that other factors are required for crystallisation of cholesterol and aggregation of the crystals to occur. This chapter summarises and discusses recent studies of the mechanisms leading to the supersaturation of bile in situations where cholesterol gallstones are common.

PREDISPOSING FACTORS

Age

Gallstones are more common in older people and in women[5] (Figure 2). We investigated the relationship between age and biliary lipid composition in a large number of non obese gallstone-free healthy subjects[6], all of whom had normal serum lipids. There was a clear increase in the cholesterol saturation of bile with age in both sexes (Figure 3), and this correlation between age and saturation was independent of body weight. This may well explain the

99

increase in the prevalence of gallstone disease with age. Whether or not an ageing individual develops gallstones presumably depends on other factors, such as the presence of nucleating agents or lack of stabilising factors in gallbladder bile, and impairment of gallbladder function.

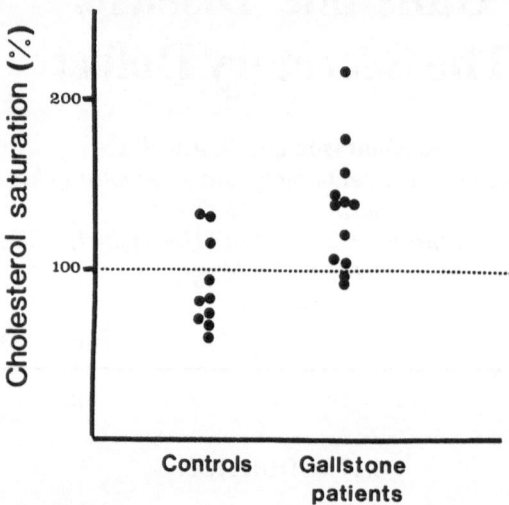

Figure 1 Cholesterol saturation of gallbladder bile in gallstone-free subjects and patients with cholesterol gallstones[11].

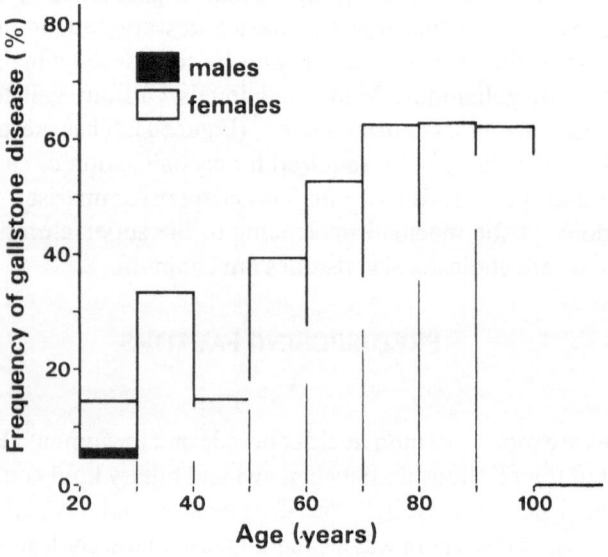

Figure 2 Frequency of gallstone disease (cholecystectomy or cholelithiasis) at autopsy in various age groups[5].

cholesterol saturation of bile (%)

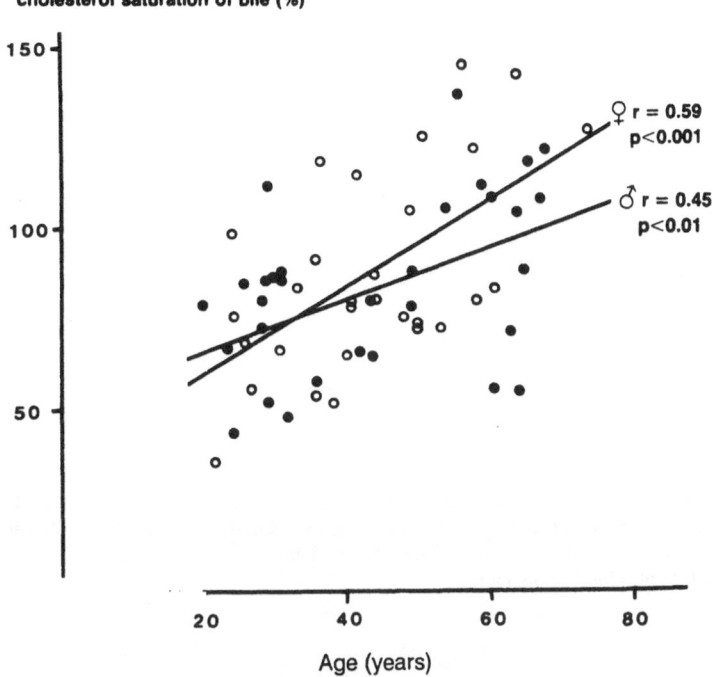

Figure 3 Relation between age and cholesterol saturation of bile[6]. Open circles denote females (n = 29) and closed circles males (n = 31). All subjects were gallstone-free, nor-molipidaemic and less than 120% of ideal body weight.

Obesity

Cholesterol gallstones are common in obese subjects and most obese subjects with or without gallstones have supersaturated gallbladder bile[1]. In a detailed study[7] gallstone-free, normolipidaemic obese subjects had a significantly higher cholesterol saturation than corresponding non obese controls (Figure 4). Cholesterol saturation may increase transiently in obese subjects, during a period of caloric restriction and rapid weight loss, but then frequently decreases after weight reduction and during the maintenance of stable weight[8]. Whiting and Watts[9] recently reported that the gallbladder bile of gallstone-free obese subjects had a longer nucleation time than gallbladder bile from gallstone patients, indicating that factors other than cholesterol supersaturation contribute to the increased risk to gallstones associated with obesity.

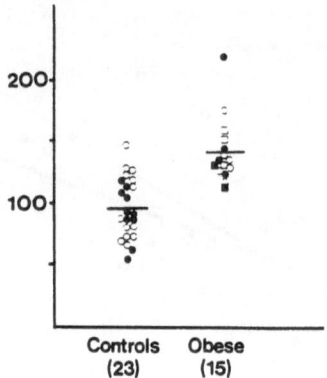

Figure 4 Cholesterol saturation of fasting bile in gallstone-free obese patients and healthy controls[7]. Horizontal bars indicate mean of each group. Open symbols denote females and closed symbols males. Circles denote bile obtained by duodenal intubation and squares gallbladder bile obtained at operation.

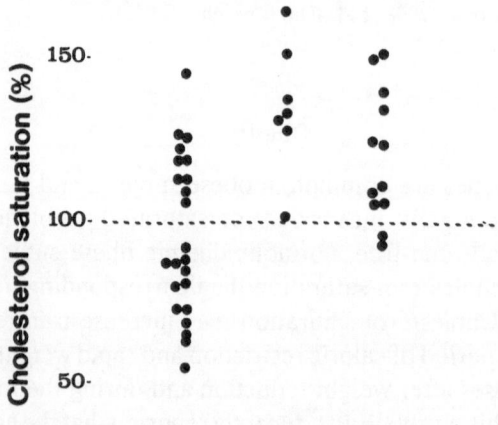

Figure 5 Cholesterol saturation of bile in controls and patients with primary hyper-triglyceridaemia, types IIb and IV, without gallstone disease[18].

102

Hypertriglyceridaemia

Hypertriglyceridaemia is associated with an increased frequency of gallstone disease[10,11], independently of body weight[12-15]. Hypertriglyceridaemia is more common among gallstone patients than in controls[16,17], and is often associated with saturated gallbladder bile[18] (Figure 5). Recent unpublished studies suggest that the genetic basis of the hypertriglyceridaemia may be relevant: patients with familial combined hyperlipidaemia are more likely to have saturated bile than patients with familial hypertriglyceridaemia.

Fibrate Treatment

Treatment with hypolipidaemic drugs may predispose to gallstone forma-

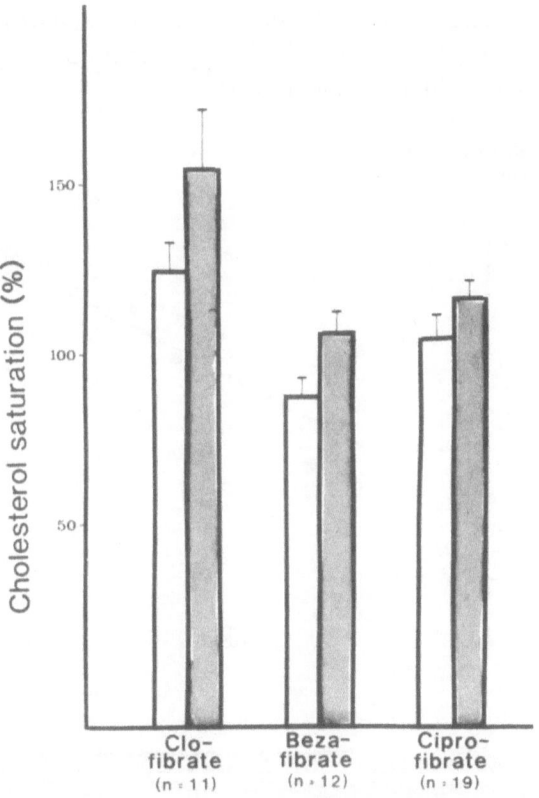

Figure 6 Cholesterol saturation of bile in hyperlipidaemic patients before (open bars) and during (filled bars) treatment with different fibrates. Data combined from refs. 26,30,32

tion[11]. Two large clinical trials with clofibrate, have shown an increased frequency of gallstone disease among users of the drug[19,20]. Clofibrate renders bile supersaturated with cholesterol[21–27] (Figure 6), but does not seem specifically to induce crystal formation[28]. Other fibric acid derivatives[11] such as bezafibrate[29,30] and gemfibrozil[31] seem to have a similar effect in short-term and long-term studies, whilst ciprofibrate in short-term studies, causes an increase in cholesterol saturation which in some patients persists over one year[32].

Oestrogen Treatment

Oestrogen therapy increases the risk of gallstone formation,[20,33,34]. In a recent unpublished study, treatment of elderly men with prostatic cancer with pharmacological doses of oestrogen seemed to induce gallstone formation, whereas orchidectomy did not; new gallstones developed in 5 of 28 patients treated with oestrogen, compared with none of 26 subjected to orchidectomy. In this study, oestrogen increased the cholesterol saturation of bile by about 30%, in accordance with previous studies[23,35,36].

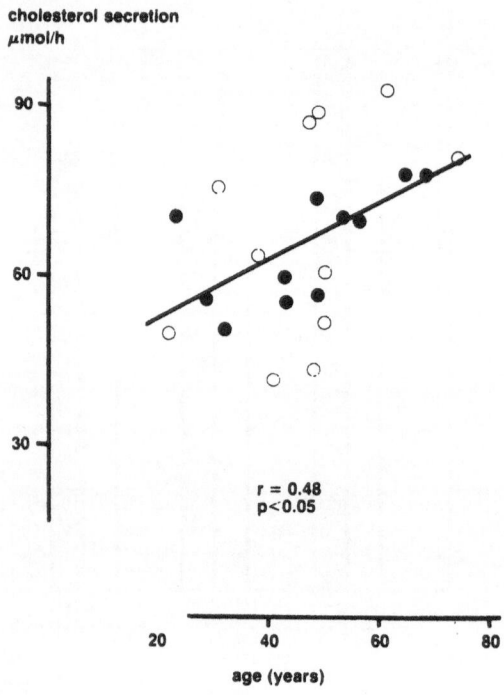

Figure 7 Relation between age and hepatic secretion of cholesterol in 22 healthy individuals[6] (Symbols as in Figure 3).

HEPATIC SECRETION RATES OF BILIARY LIPIDS

In theory, bile may become supersaturated because the liver secretes excessive cholesterol, insufficient bile acids and/or phospholipids, or both[37].

Age

We have studied the secretion of biliary lipids in subjects of different ages. We used the perfusion technique described by Shaffer and Small[38] with a glucose-amino acid mixture as perfusate, but at a higher perfusion rate (5.0 ml per minute) in order to keep the gallbladder contracted. Cholesterol secretion increased with age, whereas bile acid and phospholipid secretion did not (Figure 7)[6]. The degree of cholesterol saturation of bile also correlated positively with the secretion rate of cholesterol. Hypersecretion of cholesterol is evidently very important in the formation of supersaturated bile in this situation.

Obesity and Hypertriglyceridaemia

The hepatic biliary secretion rate of cholesterol is increased in obese subjects with supersaturated bile, whether or not they have gallstones[8,38,39]. We recently found that hypertriglyceridaemic patients with supersaturated bile have a higher cholesterol secretion rate than normolipidaemic controls, but similar bile acid and phospholipid secretion rates.

Treatment with Fibrates and Oestrogen

Fibric acid derivatives also increase cholesterol saturation mainly by increasing biliary output of cholesterol[11], as shown with clofibrate[25] and bezafibrate[29]. We have recently shown that the increase in cholesterol saturation seen in some patients treated with ciprofibrate can be attributed to an increase in cholesterol secretion, with no change in bile acid and phospholipid secretion (Table 1).

Treatment with gemfibrozil increases biliary output of cholesterol but, unlike the other fibrates, also decreases bile acid output[31]. We also compared the secretion rates of biliary lipids in some of our patients with prostatic cancer treated with oestrogen with those of healthy men of the same age. The oestrogen-treated group had significantly higher outputs of cholesterol and phospholipid, but a normal bile acid output.

Table 1 Biliary lipid secretion rates in hyperlipidaemic patients before (B) and during (D) treatment with ciprofibrate[a]. Mean ± SEM.

Patients	Cholesterol secretion (μmol/h)		Bile acid secretion (μmol/h)		Phospholipid secretion (μmol/h)	
	B	D	B	D	B	D
Cholesterol saturation unchanged (n = 3)	94 ± 14	96 ± 26	1357 ± 311	1170 ± 91	196 ± 61	212 ± 59
Cholesterol saturation increased (n = 5)	87 ± 12	120 ± 22[b]	1793 ± 62	1808 ± 255	354 ± 48	398 ± 72

[a] Data from ref. 32
[b] Significantly different compared to pretreatment values, $p < 0.05$

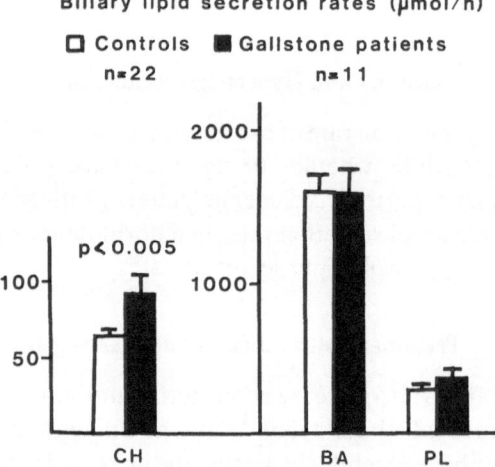

Biliary lipid secretion rates (μmol/h)

☐ Controls ■ Gallstone patients
n = 22   n = 11

Figure 8 Biliary lipid secretion rates in control and in gallstone patients with functioning gallbladders[40].

Gallstone Patients

Gallstone patients have been reported to have a higher cholesterol output than gallstone free controls, with similar bile acid and phospholipid output in Scandinavia[40] (Figure 8), Germany[41] and Chile[42]. Non-obese White Americans with cholesterol gallstones have been reported to have an absolute decrease in bile acid and possibly phospholipid secretion rates, but a normal cholesterol secretion rate[38]. Similar results have been reported from England[39]. It is not clear whether these differences are due to genetic or dietary factors, or to differences in the methods used.

Secretory defects may be primarily genetic in origin, as in the obese Pima Indian females in North America, who develop saturated bile and gallstones at an early age[43,44], associated with increased cholesterol and diminished bile acid secretion[46].

CAUSES OF INCREASED BILIARY CHOLESTEROL SECRETION

Biliary cholesterol is secreted from the liver in non-esterified form (Figure 9). It may be derived from both extrahepatic (diet and lipoprotein) and intrahepatic (synthesis and stored esterified cholesterol) sources. The catabolism of cholesterol to bile acids, and the hepatic secretion of very low density lipoproteins (VLDL) may also influence the amount of cholesterol available for biliary excretion.

Dietary cholesterol is absorbed in the form of chylomicrons which reach the plasma via the lymphatic duct. The chylomicrons are degraded to

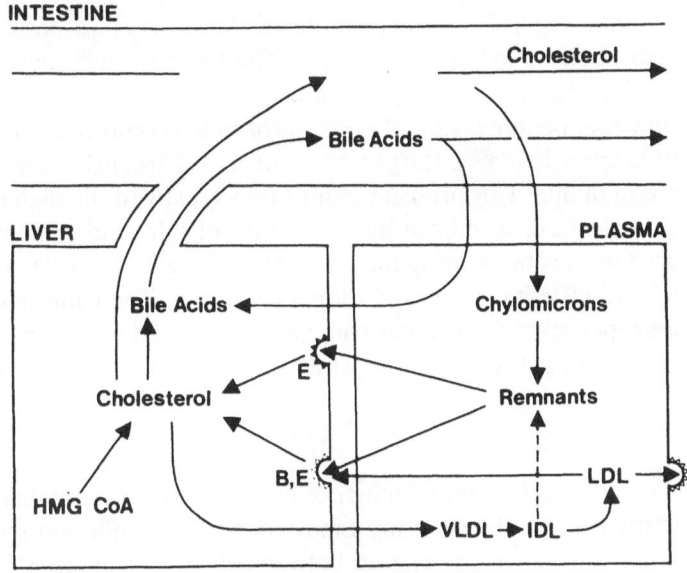

Figure 9 A simplified scheme of cholesterol metabolism in man[45].

chylomicron remnants which are then taken up by the liver, presumably by receptor-mediated endocytosis. VLDL are catabolised to remnant particles called intermediate density lipoproteins (IDL) in a similar way. IDL are removed from the circulation via receptor-mediated uptake in the liver and peripheral tissues or are metabolised to low density lipoproteins (LDL). In man, the liver is a major site of LDL clearance via the LDL (apo-B,E)-receptor. It is now possible to determine the activity of this receptor in liver biopsies obtained at operation. The uptake of LDL from the circulation may also be determined indirectly by studying the plasma clearance of intravenously injected ^{125}I-labelled LDL.

The amount of cholesterol synthesised in the body is greater than the amount derived from the diet, and about half of this synthesis is assumed to occur in the liver in humans. Daily cholesterol turnover can be estimated by laborious cholesterol balance techniques, and the hepatic synthesis of cholesterol may be measured by assaying the activity of the rate-determining enzyme in cholesterol biosythesis,3-hydroxy-3-methylglutaryl coenzyme A(HMG CoA) reductase[47]. The esterification of cholesterol is catalysed by the microsomal enzyme acyl CoA:cholesterol acyl transferase (ACAT)[48], recently characterised in human liver (unpublished work). The rate of cholesterol esterification depends on the accessibility of substrate (cholesterol), and probably also on the expression of ACAT enzymatic activity.

About 30–50% of the daily cholesterol turnover (synthesis + absorption) is catabolised to bile acids in man. This conversion is governed by the rate-limiting microsomal enzyme, cholesterol 7α-hydroxylase[49]. The relatively low rate of conversion of cholesterol to bile acids in man, compared with other animals, leaves a large amount of cholesterol to be secreted as free cholesterol in bile. This probably contributes greatly to the high concentration of cholesterol in human bile. The rate of bile acid synthesis can be measured *in vitro* by assaying the cholesterol 7α-hydroxylase activity[50], and *in vivo* by Lindstedt's isotope dilution technique[51]. The clinical application of these experimental techniques has vastly improved our understanding of the development of supersaturated bile.

Age

We recently investigated the influence of age on bile acid synthesis in healthy gallstone-free subjects using Lindstedt's isotope dilution technique[52], and found a negative correlation between the two (Figure 10). We also demonstrated an inverse relationship between bile acid synthesis and biliary cholesterol saturation, and between bile acid synthesis and cholesterol secretion.

The concentration of LDL cholesterol in man increases with age, and unpublished studies indicate that the rate of LDL catabolism is lower in old than young males. If the main effect of ageing is to decrease the catabolism of cholesterol to bile acids, it may be that the diminished demand for hepatic cholesterol for this purpose results in a down-regulation of LDL-receptor

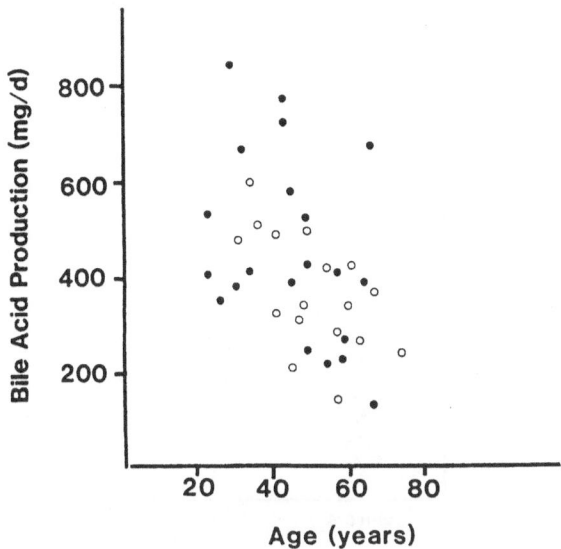

Figure 10 Relation between age and bile acid production rate (measured using Lindstedt's isotope dilution technique) in 38 healthy subjects[52].

activity and thus enhanced secretion of biliary cholesterol. Further work is needed to evaluate this speculation.

Obesity

The excessive output of biliary cholesterol in obese people is probably closely related to over-production of cholesterol, particularly in the liver[8,53,54]. We have found that obese subjects express hepatic HMG coenzyme A reductase activity about twice as high as that of normal weight controls[55] (Figure 11). Obese persons may also display an increased synthesis of bile acids, but lower fractional conversion of cholesterol to bile acids, than non-obese subjects[56].

Hypertriglyceridaemia

The hypersecretion of biliary cholesterol in hypertriglyceridaemia is not explained by a low conversion rate of cholesterol to bile acids. Patients with hypertriglyceridaemia instead have a normal or increased rate of bile acid synthesis[52]. Recent studies indicate that many patients with familial hypertriglyceridaemia have an abnormally high bile acid synthesis[52,57]. It seems more likely that the hypersecretion of biliary cholesterol is due to over-production of cholesterol and lipoproteins in the liver. Most patients with

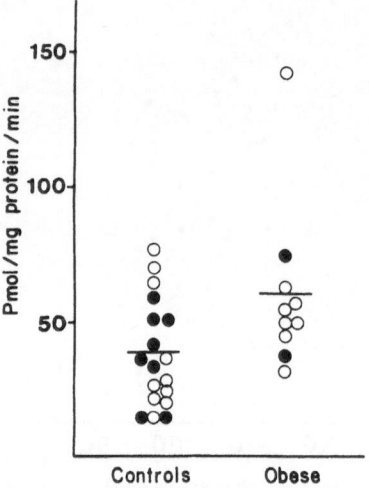

Figure 11 Hepatic microsomal HMG CoA reductase activity in normal weight (< 120% relative body weight) patients with cholesterol gallstones and in obese (> 155% relative body weight) subjects[47] (Symbols as Figure 4).

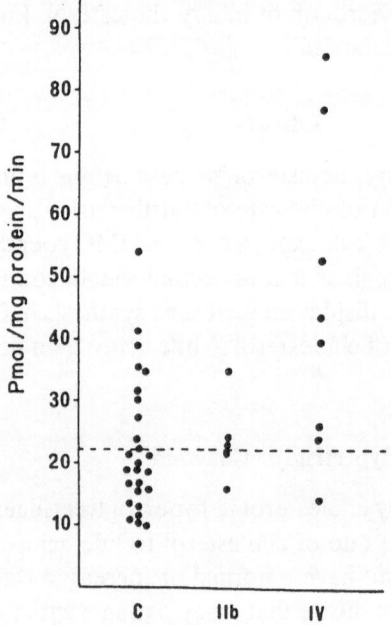

Figure 12 Hepatic microsomal HMG CoA reductase activity in normolipidaemic and hypertriglyceridaemic (types IIb and IV) patients with cholesterol gallstones[58]. The dotted line indicates the mean value of the control group.

110

hypertriglyceridaemia have increased hepatic HMG CoA reductase activity[58] (Figure 12). The hepatic uptake of lipoproteins may also be increased, possibly channelling cholesterol directly into bile. More studies on the different genetic forms of hypertriglyceridaemia are needed to clarify the mechanisms.

Fibrate Treatment

The effects of clofibrate on cholesterol and bile acid metabolism have been extensively investigated[11]. Clofibrate does not consistently influence bile acid synthesis in patients with hypercholesterolaemia[11,22,59], but both clofibrate and ciprofibrate reduce the increased bile acid synthesis seen in many patients with type IV hyperlipidaemia (hypertriglycerid- aemia)[11,22,59,60] (Table 2).

Table 2. Effects of treatment with clofibrate and ciprofibrate on bile acid production in primary hypertriglyceridaemia. Mean ± SEM

	Basal (mg/day) (mg/day)	Treatment
Clofibrate (n = 6)[a]	1379 ± 221	549 ± 97
Ciprofibrate (n = 3)[b]	703 ± 324	318 ± 91

[a] Data from ref. 59
[b] Data from ref. 60

The total faecal output of steroids is generally increased in clofibrate-treated patients[11,22], probably due not to increased synthesis of cholesterol[48] but to mobilisation of cholesterol from peripheral tissues. Kesaniemi and Grundy[61] have studied the effect of gemfibrozil on cholesterol turnover in hyper- lipidaemic patients. They found that the increased excretion of neutral steroids coincided with a decrease in faecal bile acid excretion; there was no change in total steroid excretion. The enhanced biliary secretion of cholesterol during fibrate treatment might therefore be attributable both to a reduction in the catabolism of cholesterol to bile acids and to a recruitment of tissue cholesterol.

Our recent unpublished experiments have shown that fibrates reduce the ACAT activity in rat liver by as much as 50%. We are now studying whether this also occurs in human liver.

Oestrogen Therapy

In an unpublished study, we have shown that pharmacological doses of oestrogen in elderly men with prostatic cancer reduce the LDL cholesterol level in serum by about 40%, and that the relative increment in bile cholesterol correlates with a relative reduction in serum LDL cholesterol. Animal studies have indicated that treatment with oestrogen increases the expression of LDL receptor in rat liver[62,63]. If the catabolism of LDL cholesterol in the human liver increases during oestrogen therapy, the increased in-flow of lipoprotein cholesterol could be attributed to the increased biliary secretion of cholesterol.

SUMMARY

Supersaturated bile is necessary for development of cholesterol gallstones. Gallstone frequency is increased in obesity and hypertriglyceridaemia, during fibrate treatment and oestrogen therapy, and also with increasing age. In all these situations, the enhanced cholesterol saturation appears to be due mainly to an absolute increase in the secretion rate of cholesterol from the liver. A similar defect is observed in patients with overt gallstone disease, at least in the Scandinavian population.

Table 3. Possible main determinants of enhanced secretion rate of biliary cholesterol in man

	Cholesterol synthesis	Bile acid formation	Cholesterol esterification	Lipoprotein uptake
Age		↓		↓
Obesity	↑	↗		↓
Hypertri-glyceridaemia	↑	↗		
Fibrate treatment	→	↘	↓	
Oestrogen therapy				↑

Several factors influence the secretion of cholesterol in bile, the most important being hepatic uptake of lipoprotein cholesterol, endogenous synthesis of cholesterol, catabolism of cholesterol to bile acids, and storage of esterified cholesterol in the liver. There may therefore be several reasons for an increase in the secretion of free cholesterol into bile (Table 3): Increased hepatic synthesis (obesity, hypertriglyceridaemia); decreased catabolism to bile acids (increasing age); reduced cholesterol ester formation (fibrate treatment in rats); and enhanced hepatic uptake of lipoproteins (oestrogen therapy).

Acknowledgements

The authors' work is supported by grants from the Swedish Medical Research Council (03X-4793 and 03X-7137) and from the King Gustaf V and Queen Victoria Foundation. We thank Ms. Inga-Lill Olsson for skilful editorial assistance.

REFERENCES

1. Bennion, L.J. and Grundy, S.M. (1978). Risk factors for the development of cholelithiasis in man. *N. Engl. J. Med.*, 299, 1161–7, 1221–7
2. Oviedo, M.A., Ho, K.J., Biss, K., Soong, S.J., Mikkelson, B. and Taylor, C.B. (1977). Gallbladder bile composition in different ethnic groups. *Arch. Pathol. Lab. Med.*, 101, 208–12
3. Holzbach, R.T., Marsh, M., Olszewski, M. and Holan, K. (1973). Cholesterol solubility in bile: Evidence that supersaturated bile is frequent in healthy man. *J. Clin. Invest*, 52, 1467–79
4. Ahlberg, J., Angelin, B. and Einarsson, K. (1981). Hepatic 3-hydroxy-3-methyl-glutaryl coenzyme A reductase activity and biliary lipid composition in man: Relation to cholesterol gallstone disease and effects of cholic acid and chenodeoxycholic acid treatment. *J. Lipid. Res.*, 22, 410–22
5. Lindström, C.G. (1977). Frequency of gallstone disease in a welldefined Swedish population: A prospective necropsy study in Malmo *Scand. J. Gastroenterol.*, 12, 341–6
6. Einarsson, K., Nilsell, K., Leijd, B. and Angelin, B. (1985). Influence of age on secretion of cholesterol and synthesis of bile acids by the liver. *N. Engl. J. Med.*, 313, 277–82
7. Angelin, B., Einarsson, K., Ewerth, S. and Leijd, B. (1981). Biliary lipid composition in obesity. *Scand. J. Gastroenterol.*, 16, 1015–9
8. Bennion, L.J. and Grundy, S.M. (1975). Effects of obesity and caloric intake on biliary lipid metabolism in man. *J. Clin. Invest.*, 56, 996–1011
9. Whiting, M.J. and Watts, J.McK. (1984). Supersaturated bile from obese patients without gallstones supports cholesterol crystal growth but not nucleation. *Gastroenterology*, 86, 243–8
10. Einarsson, K., Hellström, K. and Kallner, M. (1975). Gallbladder disease in hyperlipoproteinaemia. *Lancet*, 1, 484–7
11. Einarsson, K. and Angelin, B. (1986). Hyperlipoproteinemia, hypolipidemic treatment and gallstone disease. In Grundy, S.M. (ed.) *Bile Acids and Atherosclerosis*, pp. 66–97, (New York: Raven Press)
12. Angelico, M. and the GREPCO Group (1984). Relationships between serum lipids and cholelithiasis: Observations in the GREPCO study. In Capocaccia, L., Ricci, G., Angelico, F., Angelico, M. and Attili, A.F. (eds) *Epidemiology and Prevention of Gallstone Disease*, pp. 77–84 (Lancaster: MTP Press)
13. Angelico, M. and the GREPCO Group (1984). Factors associated with gallstone disease: Observations in the GREPCO study. In Capocaccia, L., Ricci, G., Angelico, F., Angelico, M. and Attili, A.F. (eds) *Epidemiology and Prevention of Gallstone Disease*, pp. 185–192 (Lancaster: MTP Press)
14. Roda, E., for the "Progetto Sirmione". (1984). Factors associated with gallstone disease: Observations in the "Sirmione Study". In Capocaccia, L., Ricci, G., Angelico, F., Angelico, M. and Attili, A.F. (eds) *Epidemiology and Prevention of Gallstone Disease*, pp. 207–9 (Lancaster: MTP Press)
15. Scragg, R.K., Calvert, G.D. and Oliver, J.R. (1984). Plasma lipids and insulin in gallstone disease: A case-control study. *Br. Med. J.*, 289, 523–5
16. Kadziolka, R., Nilsson, S. and Scherstén, T. (1977). Prevalence of hyper-

lipoproteinaemia in men with gallstone disease. *Scand. J. Gastroenterol.,* **12**, 353–5

17. Ahlberg, J. (1979). Serum lipid levels and hyperlipoproteinaemia in gallstone patients. *Acta Chir. Scand.,* **145**, 373–7

18. Ahlberg, J., Angelin, B., Einarsson, K., Hellström, K. and Leijd, B. (1980). Biliary lipid composition in normo- and hyperlipoproteinemia. *Gastroenterology,* **79**, 90–4

19. Cooper, J., Ceizerova, H. and Oliver, M.F. (1975). Clofibrate and gallstones. *Lancet,* **1**, 1083

20. Coronary Drug Project Research Group (1977). Gallbladder disease as a side effect of drugs influencing lipid metabolism. *N. Engl. J. Med.,* **296** 1185–90

21. Thistle, J.L. and Schoenfield, L.J. (1971). Induced alterations in composition of bile of persons having cholelithiasis. *Gastroenterology,* **61**, 488–96

22. Grundy, S.M., Ahrens, E.H., Jr., Salen, G., Schreibman, P.H. and Nestel, P.J. (1972). Mechanisms of action of clofibrate on cholesterol metabolism in patients with hyper-lipidemia. *J. Lipid. Res.,* **13**, 531–51

23. Pertsemlidis, D., Panveliwalla, D. and Ahrens, E.H., Jr. (1974). Effects of clofibrate and of an ostrogen-progestin combination on fasting biliary lipids and cholic acid kinetics in man. *Gastroenterology,* **66**, 565–73

24. Bateson, M.C., Maclean, D. Ross, P.E. and Bouchier, I.A.D. (1978). Clofibrate therapy and gallstone induction. *Dig. Dis.,* **23**, 623–8

25. Grundy, S.M. and Mok, H.Y.I. (1979). Effects of diets and drugs on biliary cholesterol secretion in man. In Fisher, M.M., Goresky, C.A., Shaffer, E.A. and Strasberg, S.M. (eds.) *Gallstones,* pp. 283–98 (New York: Plenum Press)

26. Angelin, B., Einarsson, K. and Leijd, B. (1979). Biliary lipid composition during treat-ment with different hypolipidaemic drugs. *Eur. J. Clin. Invest.,* **9**, 185–90

27. Angelin, B., Einarsson, K. and Leijd, B. (1981). Clofibrate treatment and bile cholesterol saturation: Short-term and long-term effects and influence of combination with chenodeoxycholic acid. *Eur. J. Clin. Invest.,* **11**, 185–9

28. Kesäniemi, Y.A. and Grundy, S.M. (1983). Clofibrate, caloric restriction, supersatura-tion of bile, and cholesterol crystals. *Scand. J. Gastroenterol.,* **18**, 897–902

29. Von Bergmann, K. and Leiss, O. (1984). Effects of short-term treatment with bezafibrate and fenofibrate on biliary lipid metabolism in patients with hyperlipidaemia. *Eur. J. Clin. Invest.,* **14**, 150–4

30. Eriksson, M. and Angelin, B. (1987). Bezefibrate therapy and biliary lipids : effects of short-term and long-term treatment in patients with various forms of hyper-lipoproteinemia. *Eur. J. Clin. Invest.,* **17**, 396–401

31. Leiss, O., von Bergmann, K., Gnasso, A. and Augustin, J. (1985). Effect of gemofibrozil on biliary lipid metabolism in normolipidaemic subjects. *Metabolism,* **34**, 74–82

32. Angelin, B., Einarsson, K. and Leijd, B. (1984). Effects of ciprofibrate treatment on biliary lipids in patients with hyperlipoproteinaemia. *Eur. J. Clin. Invest.,* **14**, 73–8

33. Boston Collaborative Drug Surveillance Program. (1974). Surgically confirmed gallbladder disease, venous thrombo-embolism, and breast tumors in relation to postmenopausal oestrogen therapy. *N. Engl. J. Med.,* **290**, 15–9

34. Stolley, P.D., Tonascia, J.A., Tockman, M.S., Sartwell, P.E., Rutledge, A.H. and Jacobs, M.P. (1975). Thrombosis with low-oestrogen oral contraceptives. *Am. J. Epidemiol.,* **102**, 197–208

35. Bennion, L.J., Ginsberg, R.L., Garnick, M.B. and Bennet, P.H. (1976). Effects of oral contraceptives on the gallbladder bile of normal women. *N. Engl. J. Med.,* **294**, 189–92

36. Andersson, A., James, O.F.W., MacDonald, H.S., Snowball, S. and Taylor, W. (1980). The effects of ethinyloestradiol on biliary lipid composition in young men. *Eur. J. Clin. Invest.,* **10**, 77–80

37. Holzbach, R.T. and Kibe, A. (1985). Pathogenesis of cholesterol gallstones. In Cohen, S. and Soloway, R.D. (eds) *Gallstones,* pp. 73–100, (New York: Churchill Livingstone)

38. Shaffer, E.A. and Small, D.M. (1977). Biliary lipid secretion in cholesterol gallstone dis-ease: The effect of cholecystectomy and obesity. *J. Clin. Invest.,* **59**, 828–40

39. Reuben, A., Maton, P.N., Murphy, G.M. and Dowling, R.H. (1985). Bile lipid secretion in obese and non-obese individuals with and without gallstones. *Clin. Sci.*, **69**, 71–9

40. Nilsell, K., Angelin, B., Liljeqvist, L. and Einarsson, K. (1985). Biliary lipid output and bile acid kinetics in cholesterol gallstone disease: Evidence for an increased hepatic secretion of cholesterol in Swedish patients. *Gastroenterology*, **89**, 287–93

41. Leiss, O. and von Bergmann, K. (1985). Comparison of biliary lipid secretion in non-obese cholesterol gallstone patients with normal, young, male volunteers. *Klin. Wochenschr.*, **63**, 1163–9

42. Valdivieso, V.D., Palma, R., Nervi, F., Covarrubias, C., Severin, C. and Antezana, C. (1979). Secretion of biliary lipids in young Chilean women with cholesterol gallstones. *Gut*, **20**, 997–1000

43. Sampliner, R.E., Bennett, P.H., Commess, L.J., Rose, F.A. and Burch, T.A. (1970). Gallbladder disease in Pima Indians: Demonstration of high prevalence and early onset by cholecystography. *N. Engl. J. Med.*, **283**, 1358–64

44. Bennion, L.J., Knowler, W.C., Mott, D.M., Spagnola, A.M. and Bennett, P.H. (1979). Development of lithogenic bile during puberty in Pima Indians. *N. Engl. J. Med.*, **300**, 873–6

45. Angelin, B. (1984). Regulation of hepatic lipoprotein receptor expression. In Calandra, S., Carulli, N. and Salvioli, G. (eds.) *Liver and Lipid Metabolism*, pp. 187–201 (Amsterdam: Elsevier)

46. Grundy, S.M., Metzger, A.L. and Adler, R.D. (1972). Mechanisms of lithogenic bile formation in American Indian women with cholesterol gallstones. *J. Clin. Invest.*, **51**, 3026–43

47. Angelin, B. and Einarsson, K. (1985). Regulation of HMG CoA reductase in human liver. In Preiss, B. (ed.) *Regulation of HMG CoA Reductase*, pp. 281–320 (New York: Academic Press)

48. Suckling, K.E. and Stange, E.F. (1985). Role of acyl-CoA: cholesterol acyltransferase in cellular cholesterol metabolism. *J. Lipid. Res.*, **26**, 647–71

49. Björkhem, I. (1985). Mechanism of bile acid synthesis in mammalian liver. In Danielsson, H. and Sjövall, J. (eds.) *Sterols and Bile Acids*, pp. 231–278, (Amsterdam: Elsevier Scientific Publishing Company)

50. Einarsson, K., Angelin, B,., Ewerth, S., Nilsell, K. and Björkhem, I. (1986). Bile acid synthesis in man: Assay of hepatic microsomal cholesterol 7 alpha-hydroxylase activity by isotope dilution-mass spectrometry. *J. Lipid. Res.*, **27**, 82–8

51. Lindstedt, S. (1957). The turnover of cholic acid in man. *Acta Physiol. Scand.*, **40**, 1–9

52. Angelin, B. and Einarsson, K. (1986). Bile acids and lipoprotein metabolism. In Grundy, S.M. (ed.) *Bile Acids and Atherosclerosis*, pp. 41–66 (New York: Raven Press)

53. Miettinen, T.A. (1970). Cholesterol production in obesity. *Circulation*, **44**, 842–50

54. Nestel, P.J., Schreibman, P.H. and Ahrens, E.H. Jr. (1973). Cholesterol metabolism in human obesity. *J. Clin. Invest.*, **52**, 2389–97

55. Angelin, B., Backman, L., Einarsson, K., Eriksson, L. and Ewerth, S. (1981). Hepatic cholesterol metabolism in obesity: Activity of microsomal 3-hydroxy-3-methylglutaryl coenzyme A reductase. *J. Lipid. Res.*, **23**, 770–3

56. Leijd, B. (1980). Cholesterol and bile acid metabolism in obesity. *Clin. Sci.*, **59**, 203–6

57. Angelin, B., Hershon, K.S. and Brunzell, J.D. (1987). Bile acid metabolism in hereditary forms of hypertriglyceridemia: Evidence for an increased synthesis rate in monogenic familial hypertriglyceridemia. *Proc. Natl. Acad. Sci. USA.*, **84**, 5434–8

58. Ahlberg, J., Angelin, B., Björkhem, I., Einarsson, K. and Leijd, B. (1979). Hepatic cholesterol metabolism in normo- and hyperlipidemic patients with cholesterol gallstones *J. Lipid. Res.*, **20**, 107–15

59. Einarsson, K., Hellström, K. and Kallner, M. (1973). The effect of clofibrate on the elimination of cholesterol as bile acids in patients with hyperlipoproteinaemia type II and IV. *Eur. J. Clin. Invest.*, **3**, 345–51

60. Angelin, B. (1984). Effects of hypolipidemic treatment on bile acid and cholesterol me-

tabolism in man. In Carlson, L.A. and Olsson, A.G. (eds.) *Treatment of Hyperlipoproteinemia* pp. 121–4 (New York: Raven Press)

61. Kesäniemi, Y.A. and Grundy, S.M. (1984). Influence of gemfibrozil and clofibrate on metabolism of cholesterol and plasma triglycerides in man. *J. Am. Med. Assoc.*, **251**, 2241–6

62. Kovanen, P.T., Brown, M.S. and Goldstein, J.L. (1979). Increased binding of low density lipoprotein to liver membranes from rats treated with 17α-ethinyl estradiol. *J. Biol. Chem.*, **254**, 11367–73

63. Windler, E.E., Kovanen, P.T., Chao, Y.S., Brown, M.S., Havel, R.J. and Goldstein, J.L. (1980). The estradiol-stimulated lipoprotein receptor of rat liver. A binding site that mediates the uptake of rat lipoproteins containing apoproteins B and E. *J. Biol. Chem.*, **255**, 10464–71

8

Pathogenesis of Cholesterol Gallstone Disease: The Physico-chemical Defect

R. T. Holzbach, R.L. Barnhart and J.M. Nader
Department of Gastroenterology and Research Institute
Cleveland Clinic Foundation
9500 Euclid Avenue
Cleveland, OH 44106, USA

INTRODUCTION

About 20 years ago, an era of major advances in clinical and basic research into gallstone pathogenesis began when the principles of physical chemistry were applied to cholesterol solubilisation and transport. The major (experimental) outcome was the reasonably accurate clinical definition of cholesterol saturation and supersaturation. *Supersaturation*, the indispensable prerequisite to cholesterol crystallisation and precipitation, was the first key discovery of this era of advances.

Toward the end of this period came the serendipitous discovery that certain bile salts given orally to humans could reduce cholesterol secretion in bile, and thereby reduce its level of saturation. This led to the first non-surgical treatment of gallstones, by resolubilisation of gallstone cholesterol, resulting often in partial or complete dissolution. The mechanism by which these agents reduce biliary cholesterol, however, still remains unclear. There followed a quest for better insight into the epidemiology and natural history of the clinical disease, and the information gained has had a major impact on therapeutic decision-making.

The next advance came from the investigation of *cholesterol crystal nucleation*, possibly the initial step in gallstone formation. The factors that promote and inhibit cholesterol crystal nucleation, and the balance between them, are almost as important as supersaturation in the pathogenesis of cholesterol gallstones.

The most recent advance has been the description of cholesterol solubility in *vesicles*. Discovery of the role of vesicles in the transport of cholesterol in bile has answered several questions about cholesterol solubility. Aggregation of these vesicles mediated by nucleation-promoting and inhibiting factors may initiate cholesterol crystal nucleation.

This chapter will focus on issues relevant to this latest development, the implications of vesicular transport of cholesterol in bile. There is now general agreement on some points, and controversy on others.

VESICULAR TRANSPORT OF CHOLESTEROL: THE 'NEW' CONCEPT

Many reports appeared from groups working independently and widely distant from one another[1-10], e.g. Israel, New Zealand, Chile, in the last few years. These studies strongly support the concept that vesicles containing phospholipid and cholesterol (in addition to bile salt-lecithin micelles) contribute significantly to the solubilisation and transport of cholesterol in both artificial and native bile. Two groups, using different methods with complementary results, were probably the earliest to identify vesicles in bile[1,2] but they were soon followed by several other groups using a variety of other methods.

The actual amount or proportion of cholesterol solubilised and transported in *in vitro* and *in vivo* solutions varies widely depending primarily upon differences in lipid composition and in the degree of dilution of the solution. For example, variations in the bile salt flow rate have been shown to alter the distribution of cholesterol transport between micelles and vesicles. At low bile salt flow rates, as observed in the fasting state, a greater proportion of cholesterol is transported in vesicles[7]. Vesicles obtained from dilute hepatic bile dissolve upon equilibration with a raised bile salt concentration, so that their contribution to cholesterol solubilisation will appear to diminish[5,11,12]. This suggests that biliary vesicles may be the means by which lipid is secreted by hepatocytes, but the details at present are far from clear. Biliary vesicles about 100 nm diameter (unaggregated small vesicles, USV's) are now widely regarded as an important mode of non-micellar cholesterol transport in both native and artificial systems of supersaturated bile.

Although the idea that vesicles are important in biliary transport of cholesterol seems entirely novel, one may wonder why it did not emerge during the previous decade (approximately 1973–1983). During this period many physico-chemical studies of native and model biles[13-15] were undertaken, both to define better cholesterol saturation and, subsequently (1978–1983), to study the process of cholesterol crystal nucleation in supersaturated systems[16,17]. In retrospect, there seem to be two reasons for the apparent oversight. Firstly, the physical or structural analysis of the solutions and their constituent particles was limited by the resolving power of the light micro-

118

scope (0.5 μm or 5000 Å). Secondly, the equivalent of larger aggregated vesicles were seen in several studies. These precipitates were noted to

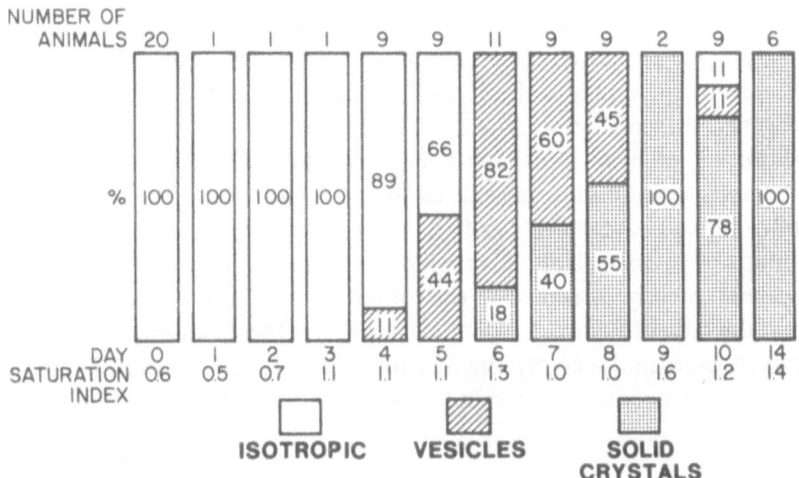

Figure 1 Time-course correlation between biliary cholesterol precipitates observed microscopically and mean saturation indices in gallbladder samples from 87 prairie dogs on a lithogenic diet.

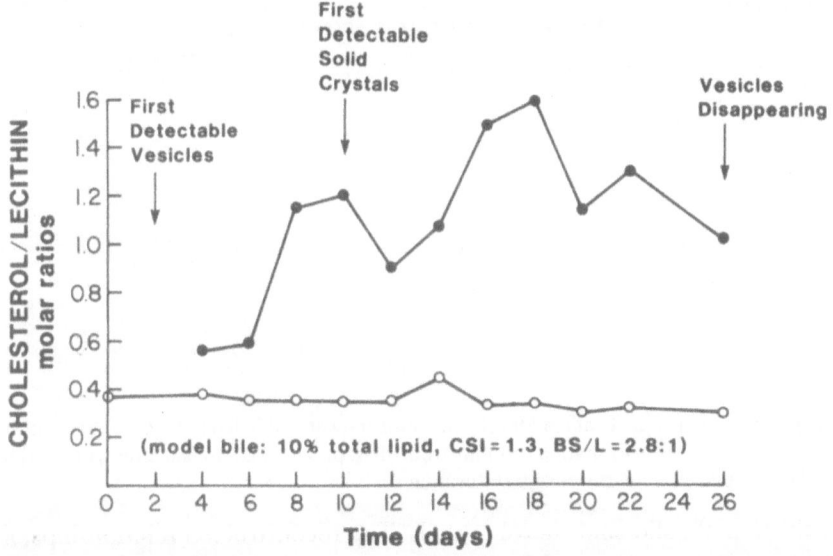

Figure 2 Time-course correlation of cholesterol/lecithin molar ratios for the vesicular phase (filled circles) and micellar phase (open circles) during equilibration from an initially metastably supersaturated isotropic state in a model bile analogue of the indicated composition.

119

precede cholesterol crystallisation both in an animal model of gallstone formation, and in an *in vitro* model bile system moving toward equilibrium from a state of supersaturation[16,18]. In an initial report on these precipitates in human bile they were noted to be associated with cholesterol crystals[13]. The limitation of microscopic resolving power prevented accurate structural assessment of these particles, and obscured their potential significance. They were considered simply to be liquid crystals, based primarily on their birefringence as seen by polarised-light microscopy, and on their lamellar structure as seen by conventional X-ray diffraction. This form of precipitate had been reported earlier in seminal phase-diagram work, but their actual significance had never been clarified. Figures 1 and 2 illustrate in retrospect the interpretive errors from this period and show that the nomenclature can be updated merely by replacing the 'liquid crystals' with 'vesicles'. In particular, the data of Figure 2, replotted in present form, demonstrate a point that was missed until recently: the vesicular phase, but not the micellar phase, demonstrates a considerable increase in cholesterol saturation before

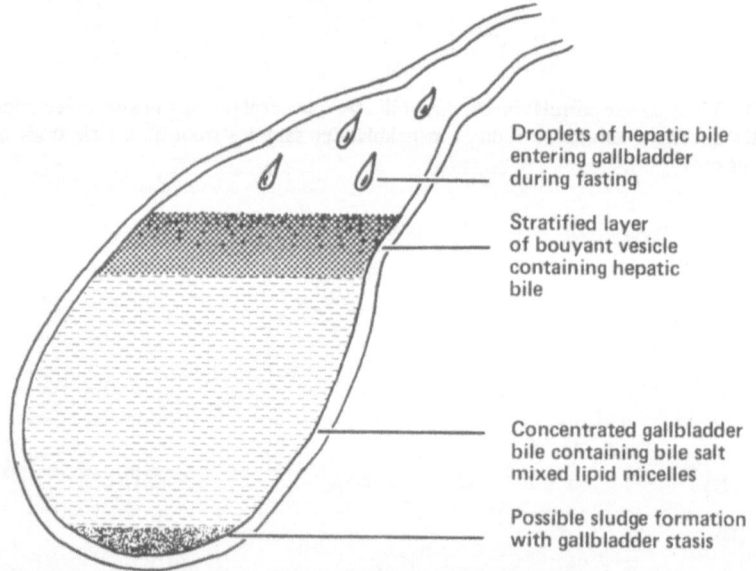

Droplets of hepatic bile entering gallbladder during fasting

Stratified layer of bouyant vesicle containing hepatic bile

Concentrated gallbladder bile containing bile salt mixed lipid micelles

Possible sludge formation with gallbladder stasis

Figure 3   The concept of gallbladder stratification interpreted in light of recent observations on spontaneous vesicle formation resulting from the separate or combined effects of dilution, e.g. hepatic bile, or cholesterol supersaturation.

nucleation of solid cholesterol crystals. The reconstructed relationships, illustrated in Figures 1 and 2, do not, in essence, differ from observations during the past 1–2 years, but are based on a quite different understanding of the process.

Reports from as much as a decade earlier, interpreted in the light of present information, could have led much earlier to the identification of vesicles in bile. The phenomenon referred to as 'stratification,' which began to appear in the surgical literature in the early to mid-1960s, was apparently never taken seriously or clarified[19-21]. Stratification or layering was noted in abnormal gallbladder bile removed at operation and left undisturbed in sealed containers. Denser material invariably settled and the buoyant material floated. Occasionally, the *'creaming-up'* of buoyant opalescent materials in bile was observed *in vitro* (Figure 3)[20]. Inversion of a cylinder

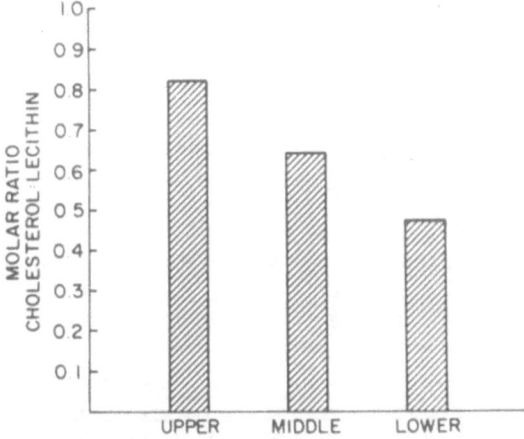

Figure 4 Evidence for cholesterol enrichment in an earlier study of the buoyant stratified upper layer of concentrated human hepatic bile (original data plotted in modified form).

filled with dilute hepatic bile showed reflotation of buoyant material when the solution was allowed to stand[20]. Solute concentrations were higher in the lower dense regions of the fluid, (Figure 4)[20,21] whilst the molar ratio of cholesterol to lecithin was higher in the upper fraction than in the micelles. This suggested the presence in the more dilute upper layer of a cholesterol-carrying 'complex' other than the micelle[20]. The concept of what is today referred to as 'non-micellar' or 'vesicular' transport of cholesterol in bile has probably been around in one form or another for at least 25 years.

Nucleation of Cholesterol Crystals

The belief that cholesterol gallstones must evolve from tiny crystals of cholesterol seems reasonable, but supersaturation of bile with cholesterol *per se* is considered no longer adequate to explain cholelithiasis. it follows, therefore, that factors affecting crystal formation, termed *nucleation*, must be of considerable importance. It is now generally agreed that nucleation, the rate of *de novo* crystal formation, is much more rapid in gallbladder bile from patients with cholesterol gallstones than in gallbladder bile from normal subjects[17,23]. This difference in nucleation time has been shown to separate bile from gallstone patients from normal bile more completely than any other available biochemical or physical criteria. The difference can be explained by the operation of two separate nucleating factors with opposing functions – 'inhibiting' and 'promoting'. These factors can be demonstrated under appropriate conditions but are still uncharacterised[12].

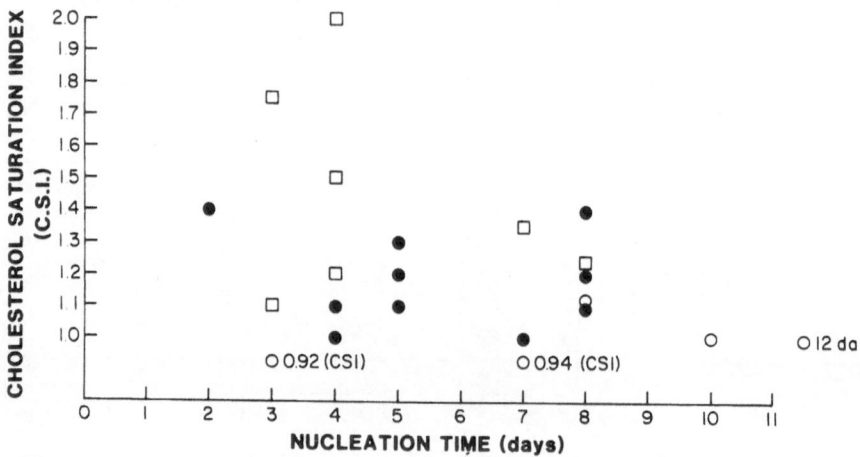

Figure 5 Nucleation times from selected *supersaturated* gallbladder bile samples derived from normal subjects in three studies. (open circles, Holan, K.R. *et al.*[17]; filled circles, Gollish, S.H. *et al.*[23]; open squares, Holzbach, R.T. *et al.*[24]).

The best evidence for the presence of a nucleation-inhibiting agent comes from the prolonged nucleation times observed in 21 *supersaturated* gallbladder bile samples from normal subjects (Figure 5). In another study, a further 7 supersaturated normal gallbladder bile samples were shown to have unspecified nucleation times of over 10 days[24]. This cannot easily be explained on the basis of their lipid composition. An unspecified protein from a crude mixture of bile proteins has been reported to have a similar effect[25], but this observation awaits confirmation. Other evidence suggests that there is a potent nucleation-promoting agent in bile which may also be an unspecified bile protein[26,27]. It is not yet clear whether the inhibiting agent(s) in bile of patients with gallstones is (are) reduced in concentration or even absent, nor whether bile in normal subjects (which surely contains inhibiting agents) also has promoting agents(s) albeit in small quantities. Most important, we do not know whether the disease process itself can be explained by increased secretion of the promoting substance[12]. The co-existence of crystallisation-promoting and inhibiting factors is not unique, but is an ubiquitous biological phenomenon in which small amounts of protein serve as a matrix for crystallisation. This is, for example, the first step in the formation of kidney stones, bone, dental enamel, and possibly in the prevention of ice crystal formation by antifreeze proteins.

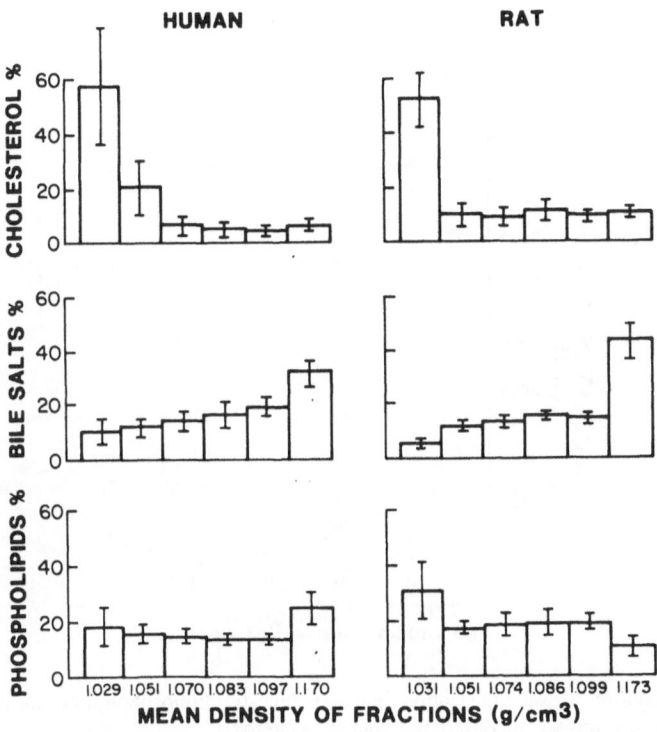

Figure 6 Evidence for the presence of buoyant cholesterol and phospholipid-containing vesicles in human hepatic and rat bile from lipid distributions in continuous density gradients obtained by ultracentrifugation. Fractions of lowest density are on the left and of highest density on the right.

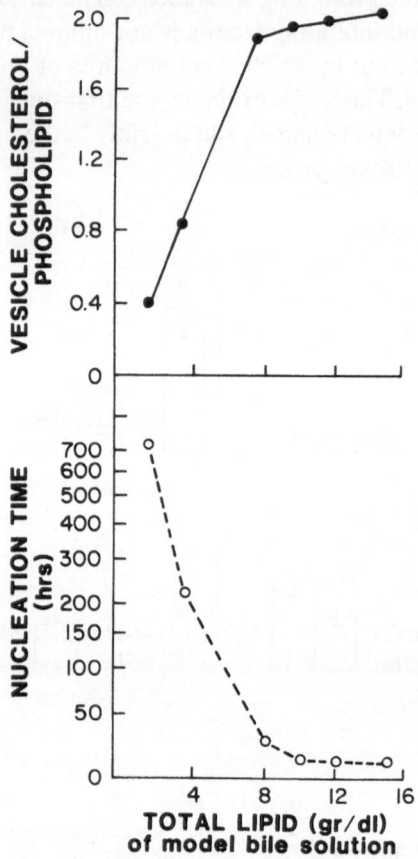

Figure 7 Relation between nucleation time and cholesterol:phospholipid ratios in vesicles as a function of *dilution* from different model bile systems

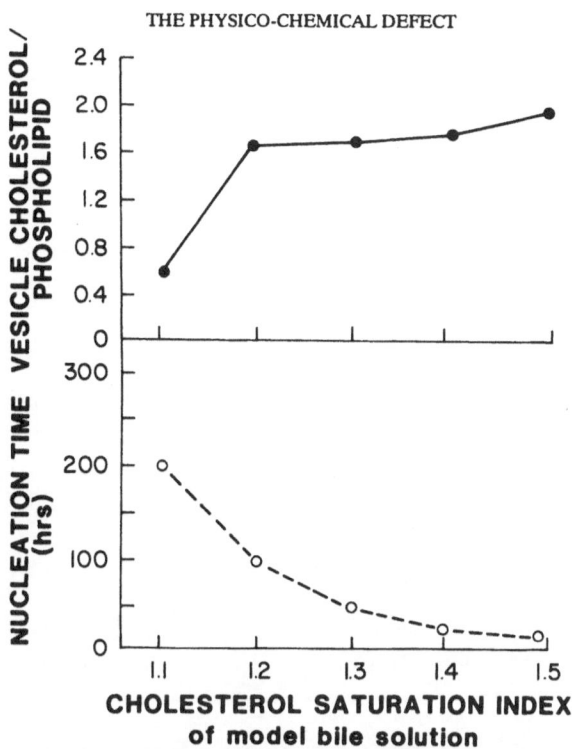

Figure 8   Relation between nucleation time and cholesterol:phospholipid ratios in vesicles as a function of *Cholesterol Saturation Index* in different model bile systems.

Factors Affecting Vesicle Formation and Composition

The presence of vesicles in bile may help to account for the frequently observed, but hitherto unexplained, phenomenon of metastable supersaturation, and the prolonged stability of cholesterol solubilised in supersaturated human bile (Figure 5). For example, hepatic bile, despite marked cholesterol supersaturation, resists cholesterol crystal nucleation[23]. Perhaps crystals are not seen in many supersaturated samples because the samples contain abundant phospholipid vesicles that may transport proportionately more cholesterol than do mixed bile salt lipid micelles. Vesicles in a dilute system, such as in human hepatic bile, rat bile, and in dilute model biles are relatively unsaturated in cholesterol (Figures 6 and 7)[6,10]. This may explain both the stability and the amount of total cholesterol that can be transported in dilute solutions, such as artificial ones or canalicular and hepatic bile. In bile supersaturated with cholesterol, by contrast, individual vesicles are comparatively cholesterol-rich, and the solutions are more prone to nucleation (Figure 8)[28]. An increase in bile salt/phospholipid ratio has also been shown to reduce vesicular stability (Figure 9)[28].

125

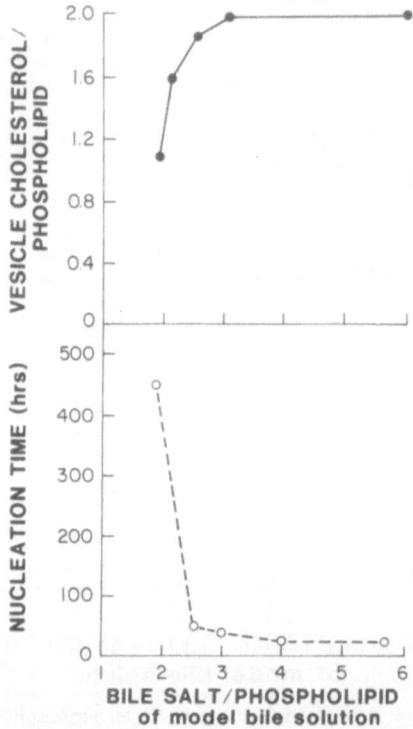

Figure 9 Relation between nucleation time and cholesterol:phospholipid ratios in vesicles as a function of differing *bile salt/phospholipid* molar ratios from different model bile systems.

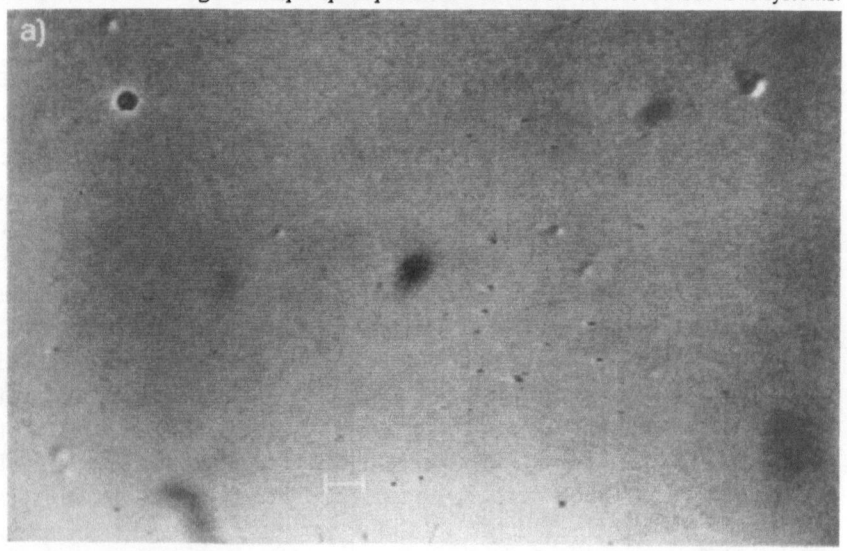

Figure 10 Vesicles as observed by video-enhanced contrast microscopy in normal human gallbladder bile at (a) zero time, and (b) 4 days after zero time (bar – 2500 nm).

Vesicle Aggregation and its Linkage to Nucleation

When observed over several days, vesicles from slowly nucleating super-saturated normal gallbladder bile typically show little *de novo* formation and a comparatively slow rate of vesicle aggregation (Figure 10 a,b). In striking contrast is the rapid rate of both *de novo* vesicle formation and vesicle aggregation observed in bile from gallstone patients (Figure 11a-d)[28]. Super-saturated model bile solutions of appropriate composition can also display, albeit less dramatically, a comparatively rapid aggregation process before crystal nucleation, (Figure 12)[29].

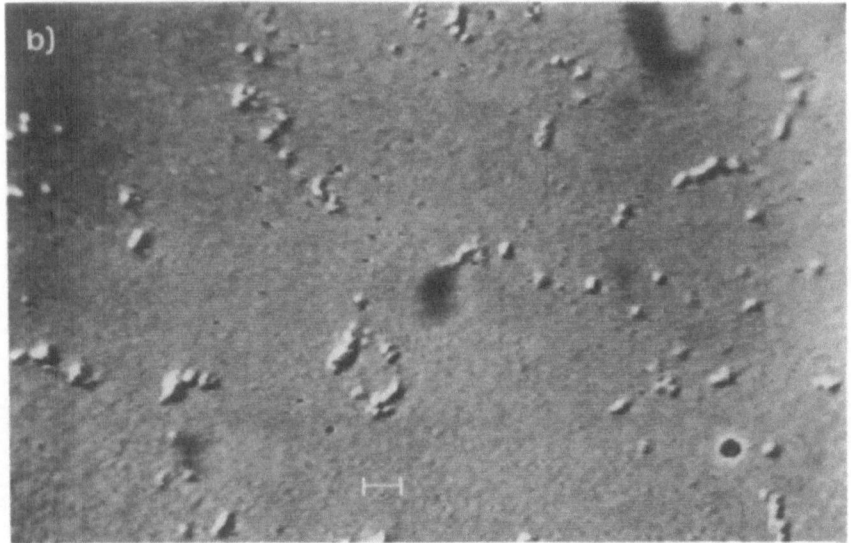

Figure 10(b)

These experiments demonstrate a semiquantitative approach to the assessment of particle dynamics in the nucleation process. Such an approach is clearly limited in quantifying the parallel process in abnormal bile samples because of greater rapidity of nucleation and a broader spectrum of particles and particle aggregates. More recently, a study relating nucleation time to the partitioning of cholesterol to the micellar and non-micellar (vesicular) phases in human bile samples has provided the potential for a more quantitative link (Figure 13). This study showed a strong correlation over time between crystal nucleation and gradual disappearance of the vesicular phase, but no comparable change in the micellar phase. The finding is reminiscent of the reinterpreted data shown in Figure 2, which were published 9 years earlier. All these observations point strongly toward vesicle aggregation as the essential physical phenomenon in cholesterol crystal nucleation.

127

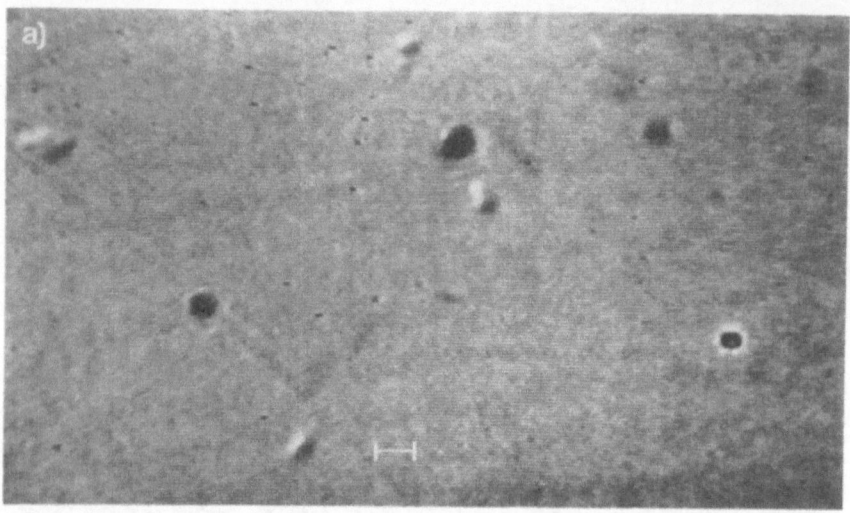

Figure 11(a)

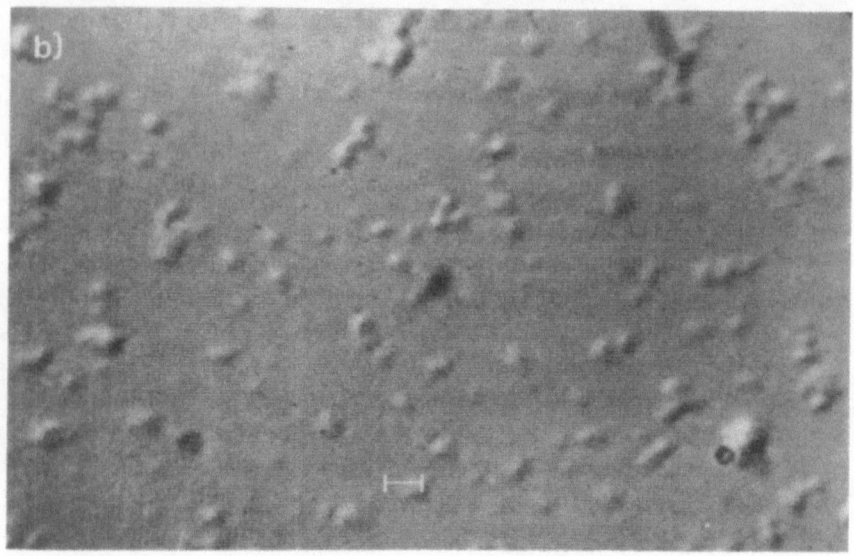

Figure 11(b)

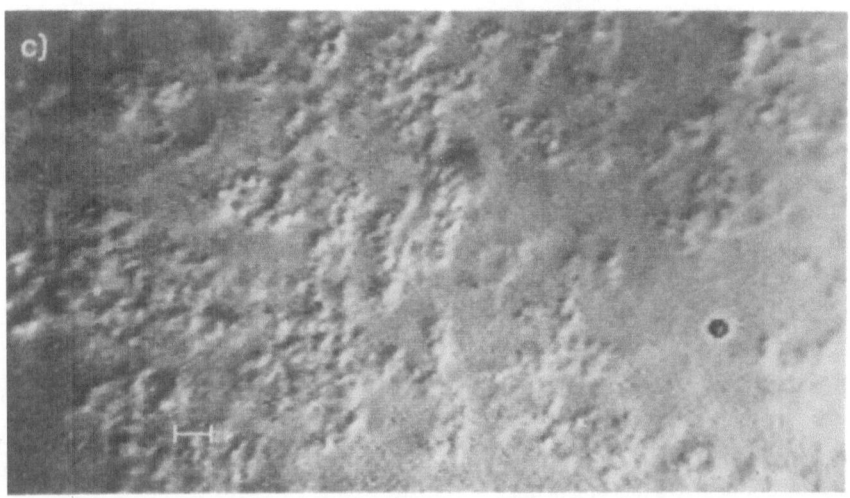

Figure 11(c)

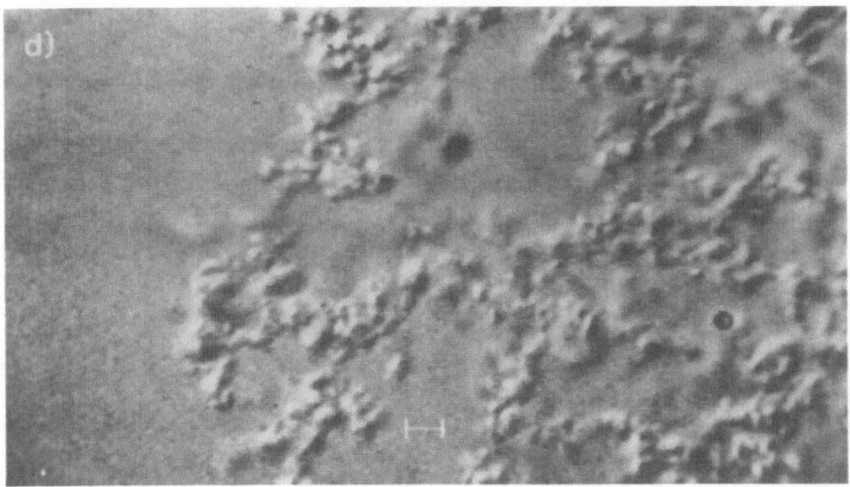

Figure 11(d)

Figure 11 Vesicle formation and rapid aggregation in abnormal human bile: time-lapse video-enhanced contrast microscopy observations at (a) zero time, (b) 2 hours, (c) 4 hours, and (d) 8 hours after zero time (bar – 2500 nm).

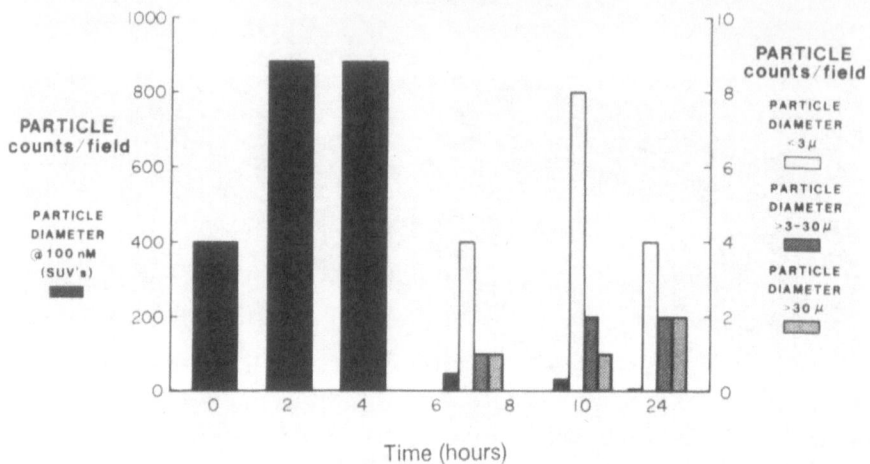

Figure 12 Number of particles observed in supersaturated model bile per video-enhanced microscopy field as a function of time.

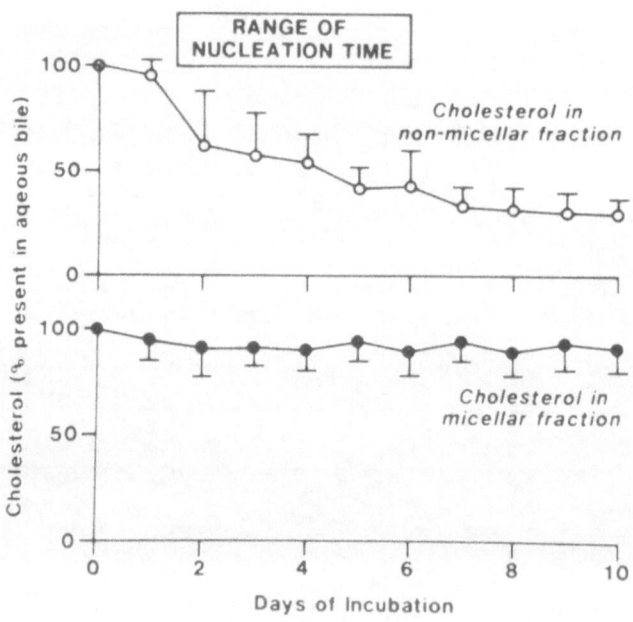

Figure 13 Nucleation time of miceller and non-micellar (vesicular) cholesterol. Results represent mean ± SD of six gallbladder bile samples. Nucleated (crystalline) cholesterol has originated almost exclusively from the non-micellar (vesicular) fraction.

SUMMARY

Vesicular transport of cholesterol in bile is a relatively new and still controversial finding that could be of vital importance regarding cholesterol gallstone formation. The vesicles contain cholesterol and phospholipid and are present together with the classical bile salt–phospholipid–cholesterol micelles. Their main role is probably to supplement micelles as a medium for cholesterol solubilisation in bile. The formation of vesicles is an inherent physicochemical property of bile, since vesicles are present not only in native bile but can be reproduced in model bile solutions. The extent of vesicular transport of cholesterol in bile has an inverse relationship with bile salt concentration, as vesicles tend to increase in quantity in dilute bile systems and disappear in concentrated ones. It is now suggested that aggregation of vesicles might be the initiating step in cholesterol crystal nucleation, an event which is thought to precede cholesterol gallstone formation.

Acknowledgements

This work was supported in part by funds from NIH Research Grant AM-17562 and by funds from the Cleveland Clinic Foundation. Ten figures have been reproduced in original or modified form from the following references by permission from the following copyright owners (including publishers and authors): Figure 1 from Ref. 18 (C.V. Mosby Co.), Figure 2 from Ref. 16 (Elsevier Science Publishing Co., Inc.) Figures 3 and 4 from Ref 22 (Williams & Wilkins), Figure 6 from Ref 10 (Williams & Wilkins), Figures 7–9 in modified form from Ref. 28 (*J. Lipid Res.*), Figure 12 from Ref. 29 (MTP Press), and Figure 13 from Ref 9 (American Physiological Society). The authors gratefully acknowledge the important participation of Ms. Janet Zahn in the manuscript preparation.

REFERENCES

1. Sömjen, G.J. and Gilat, T. (1983). A non-micellar mode of cholesterol transport in human bile. *FEBS Lett.*, **61**, 988
2. Mazer, N.A. and Carey, M.C. (1983). Quasi-elastic light- scattering studies of aqueous biliary lipid systems. Cholesterol solubilisation and precipitation in model bile solutions. *Biochemistry*, **22**, 426
3. Mazer, N.A., Schurtenberger, P., Carey, M.C., Preisig, R., Weigand, K. and Känzig, W. (1984). Quasi-elastic light scattering studies of native hepatic bile from the dog: comparison with aggregative behaviour of model biliary lipid systems. *Biochemistry*, **23**, 1994
4. Pattinson, N.R. (1985). Solubilisation of cholesterol in human bile. *FEBS Lett.*, **181**, 339
5. Sömjen, G.J. and Gilat, T. (1985). Contribution of vesicular and micellar carriers to cholesterol transport in human bile. *J. Lipid Res.*, **26**, 699
6. Kibe, A., Dudley, M.A., Halpern, Z., Lynn, M.P., Breuer, A.C. and Holzbach, R.T. (1985). Factors affecting cholesterol monohydrate crystal nucleation time in model systems of supersaturated bile. *J. Lipid Res.*, **26**, 1102

7.	Pattinson, N.R. and Chapman, B.A. (1986). Distribution of biliary cholesterol between mixed micelles and non-micelles in relation to fasting and feeding in humans. *Gastroenterology*, **91**, 697

8.	Sömjen, G.J., Merikovsky, Y., Lelkes, P. and Gilat, T. (1986). Cholesterol-phospholipid vesicles in human bile: an ultrastructural study. *Biochim. Biophys. Acta*, **879**, 14

9.	Lee, S.P., Park, H.Z., Madani, J. and Kaler, E.W. (1987). Partial characterisation of a non-micellar system of cholesterol solubilisation in bile. *Am. J. Physiol.*, **252**, G374

10.	Ulloa, N., Garrido, J. and Nervi, F. (1987). Ultracentrifugal isolation of vesicular carriers of biliary cholesterol in native human and rat bile. *Hepatology*, **7**, 235

11.	Sömjen, G.J. and Gilat, T. (1986). Changing concepts of cholesterol solubility in bile. *Gastroenterology*, **91**, 772

12.	Holzbach, R.T. (1986). Recent progress in understanding cholesterol crystal nucleation as a precursor to human gallstone formation. *Hepatology*, **6**, 1403

13.	Olszewski, M.F., Holzbach, R.T., Saupe, A. and Brown, G.H. (1973). Liquid crystals in human bile. *Nature*, **242**, 336

14.	Holzbach, R.T., Marsh, M., Olszewski, M., Hermann, R.E., Cooperman, A.M. and Claffey, W.J. (1973). Cholesterol solubility in bile: evidence that supersaturated bile is frequent in healthy man. *J. Clin. Invest.*, **52**, 1467

15.	Carey, M.C. and Small, D.M. (1978). The physical chemistry of cholesterol solubility in bile. *J. Clin. Invest.*, **61**, 988

16.	Holzbach, R.T. and Corbusier, C. (1978). Liquid crystals and cholesterol nucleation during equilibration in supersaturated bile analogs. *Biochim. Biophys. Acta*, **528**, 436

17.	Holan, K.R., Holzbach, R.T., Hermann, R.E., Cooperman, A.M. and Claffey, W.J. (1979). Nucleation time: a key factor in the pathogenesis of cholesterol gallstone disease. *Gastroenterology*, **77**, 611

18.	Holzbach, R.T., Corbusier, C., Marsh, M. and Naito, H.K. (1976). The process of cholesterol cholelithiasis induced by diet in the prairie dog: a physicochemical characterisation. *J. Lab. Clin. Med.*, **87**, 987

19.	Tera, H. (1960). Stratification of human gallbladder bile in vivo. *Acta Chir. Scand.*, **256**, 1

20.	Thureborn, E. (1966). On the stratification of human bile and its importance for the solubility for cholesterol. *Gastroenterology*, **50**, 775

21.	Nakayama, F. and van der Linden, W. (1975). Stratification of bile in the gallbladder and gallstone formation. *Surg. Gynecol. Obstet.*, **141**, 587

22.	Holzbach, R.T. (1984). Effects of gallbladder function on human bile: compositional and structural changes. *Hepatology*, **4**, 57s

23.	Gollish, S.H., Burnstein, J.M., Ilson, R.G., Petrunka, C.N. and Strasberg, S.M. (1983). Nucleation of cholesterol monohydrate crystals from hepatic and gallbladder bile of patients with cholesterol gallstones. *Gut*, **24**, 836

24.	Whiting, M.J. and Watts, J. McK. (1984). Supersaturated bile from obese patients without gallstones supports cholesterol crystal growth but not nucleation. *Gastroenterology*, **86**, 243

25.	Holzbach, R.T., Kibe, A., Thiel, E., Howell, J.H., Marsh, M. and Hermann, R.E. (1984). Biliary proteins. Unique inhibitors of cholesterol crystal nucleation in human gallbladder bile. *J. Clin. Invest.*, **73**, 35

26.	Burnstein, M.J., Ilson, R.G., Petrunka, C.N., Taylor, R.D. and Strasberg, S.M. (1983). Evidence for a potent nucleating factor in the gallbladder bile of patients with cholesterol gallstones. *Gastroenterology*, **85**, 801

27.	Gallinger, S., Taylor, R.D., Harvey, P.R.C., Petrunka, C.N. and Strasberg, S.M. (1985). The effects of mucous glycoprotein on nucleation time of human bile. *Gastroenterology*, **89**, 648

28.	Halpern, Z., Dudley, M.A., Kibe, A., Lynn, M.P., Breuer, A.C. and Holzbach, R.T. (1986). Rapid vesicle formation and aggregation in abnormal human bile. A time-lapse video-enhanced contrast microscopy study. *Gastroenterology*, **90**, 875

29. Holzbach, R.T., Halpern, Z., Dudley, M.A., Lynn, M.P. and Breuer, A.C. (1987). Biliary vesicle aggregation and cholesterol crystal nucleation: evidence for a coupled rationship. In Paumgartner, G., Stiehl, A. and Gerok, W. (eds). *Bile Acids and the Liver*, pp. 301-316 (Lancaster: MTP Press)

9

Pathogenesis of Cholesterol Gallstone Disease: The Motility Defect

I. C. Forgacs
Department of Gastroenterology
King's College Hospital
Denmark Hill
London SE5 9RS, UK

INTRODUCTION

The recent and very considerable expansion in our understanding of the physico-chemical factors leading to cholesterol gallstone formation has, to some extent, diverted attention from the part played by the gallbladder itself in the pathogenesis of gallstones. It was not, however, always thus. An early theory of gallstone formation which emerged in the late 19th century suggested that it was material from the gallbladder wall itself that was the focus for stone formation. A few years earlier, the simple concept that stasis of gallbladder contents might contribute to the development of gallstones was formulated. The historical development of the role of the gallbladder in gallstone pathogenesis is discussed by LaMorte et al.[1] in a valuable but outdated review.

Early attempts to study gallbladder motor function and so test the 'stasis' theory of gallbladder stone formation in man were hindered by the lack of safe, accurate and reproducible techniques for its measurement. In the present decade, however, the advent of both real-time ultrasound and nuclear medicine techniques has enabled frequent and precise observations of changes in gallbladder motility to be made.

In this chapter the pioneering studies of gallbladder motility using oral cholecystography and duodenal intubation will be discussed, before turning to the results of the various studies using ultrasound and radionuclide scanning. The discussion will be predominantly restricted to studies in man but important results from work in experimental animals will be mentioned, particularly with respect to models of gallstone formation.

135

GALLBLADDER EMPTYING AND GALLSTONES

Oral Cholecystography

Until 10 years ago, cholecystography had been the only technique available for studying the size and contraction of the human gallbladder *in vivo*. Several factors limit the usefulness of this technique. Firstly, it involves exposure to radiation which is especially important if frequent observations are to be made. The hazards of radiation were not fully appreciated in the earliest studies of changes in gallbladder emptying using oral cholecystography – three of which were carried out in pregnant women[2-4]. Secondly, successful oral cholecystography relies on intestinal absorption, hepatic uptake and biliary excretion of the contrast material and may fail to give satisfactory opacification of the gallbladder if any of these are abnormal. The technique also requires that the contrast material enters the gallbladder to be concentrated there, so that gallbladder disease itself may preclude satisfactory cholecystographic images. Thirdly, quantitative assessment of gallbladder function requires a calculation of the volume of the gallbladder from its two-dimensional image on X-ray[5,6]. Some of the studies in which such calculations have been made appear to overestimate true gallbladder volume

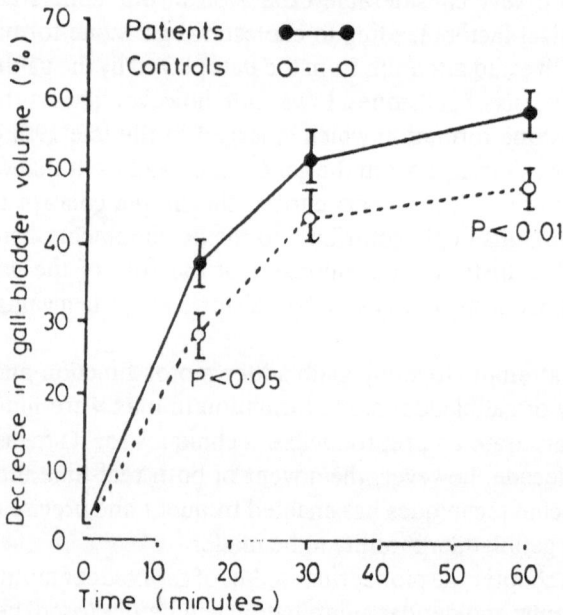

Figure 1 Mean percentage decrease in gallbladder volume, calculated from oral cholecystogram X-rays, at 15, 30 and 60 minutes following a Lundh meal (given at 0 min) in 34 patients with radiolucent gallstones and 34 matched control subjects (reproduced from reference 8 with permission).

considerably[7,8] by comparison with recent more sensitive techniques.

In a study which followed 21 patients in whom initial oral cholecystography had showed no evidence of gallstones, van der Linden[9] categorised

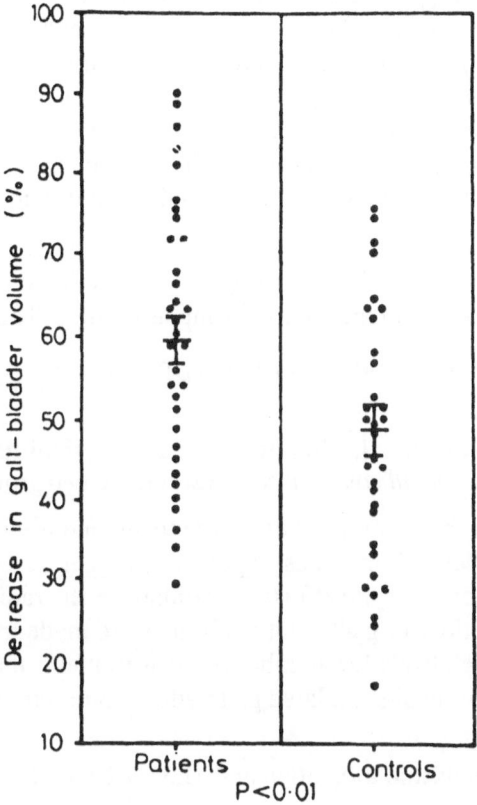

Figure 2 Cumulative percentage decrease in gallbladder volume, calculated from oral cholecystogram X-rays at 60 minutes following a Lundh meal, in 34 patients with radiolucent gallstones and 34 matched control subjects. Individual data points, means ±SEM are shown (reproduced from reference 8 with permission).

the patterns of egg yolk meal-stimulated gallbladder contraction and identified two groups of patients: 12 with 'sluggish' contraction and nine with 'vigorous' contraction. When oral cholecystography was repeated 13–14 years after the initial examination, 7 of 12 in the 'sluggish' group but only one of the nine in the 'vigorous' group had developed gallstones. This study used an unvalidated method for estimating gallbladder volume, employed subjective criteria to select patients and made no attempt to match patients in the two study groups. Nevertheless, despite these drawbacks, this study is an important pioneering landmark.

Maudgal et al.[8] studied serial oral cholecystographic X-rays taken at

0, 15, 30 and 60 minutes after a Lundh meal in 34 patients with radiolucent gallstones and 34 control subjects matched for age, sex and body weight. Gallbladder emptying was quantitated by expressing the calculated gallbladder volume[5] at each postprandial time interval as a percentage of fasting gallbladder volume. Mean cumulative gallbladder emptying was significantly greater in the gallstone patients at 15 minutes and 60 minutes after the Lundh meal (but not at 30 minutes) (Figure 1). However, if the individual data for cumulative percentage emptying are studied (Figure 2) a number of points emerge that handicap interpretation of this and many subsequent comparisons of gallbladder contraction in gallstone patients and control populations:

(1)   The wide range of gallbladder emptying *within* the study groups, which seems as marked in the control group as in the gallstone group.

(2)   The considerable overlap of emptying patterns *between* individuals in the two study groups.

(3)   The relatively small, although statistically significant, difference noted when *overall comparisons* between the two groups are made.

Apart from these considerations, the technique used in this study to calculate gallbladder volume does appear to exaggerate true gallbladder volume. Furthermore, despite efforts to standardise the radiological image, only three observations of gallbladder volume were made in the post-prandial hour. Such a relatively low number of measurements may introduce an error, particularly if meal-stimulated gallbladder contractions is not linear.

Duodenal Intubation and Marker Recovery

In order to study continuously the storage and emptying of the gallbladder, van Bėrge Henegouwen and Hofmann developed a duodenal perfusion technique[10]. A continuous intravenous (IV) infusion of indocyanine green (ICG) was given. ICG is a marker which undergoes hepatic extraction and excretion into bile, but is not reabsorbed in the intestine. Using steady-state IV infusion of ICG with simultaneous naso-duodenal aspiration, the difference between ICG infused and ICG recovered from the duodenum represents either net storage (duodenal recovery < IV input) or emptying (duodenal recovery > IV input) of the gallbladder.

Comparison of nocturnal gallbladder storage and emptying patterns between gallstone patients and matched control subjects showed that over half of the night-time secretion of bile by-passed the gallbladder in both groups. No abnormalities of nocturnal gallbladder motor function were seen in the patients with gallstones.

Mok *et al.*[11] used a similar technique but measured duodenal recovery of 'endogenous' bilirubin as a marker of biliary secretion, obviating the need for an 'exogenous 'infusate. They obtained a similar pattern of results to van Berge Henegouwen and Hofmann: about half of the total bile acid pool was stored overnight in the gallbladder both in control subjects and in patients with radiolucent gallstones.

Duodenal intubation techniques are, however, somewhat indirect; they reflect only net changes in gallbladder motor function and give no information about gallbladder size or the extent of its emptying. Furthermore the intraduodenal tube might itself disturb gastrointestinal physiology.

Radionuclide Studies of Gallbladder Contraction

The development of radionuclide techniques enabled Englert and Chiu[12] to measure external radioactivity over the gallbladder after oral administration of ^{131}I-labelled iopanoic acid. Their limited ability either to image continuously or to adjust for activity in the liver and intestine, and the use of a beta-emitting isotope, limited the usefulness of this method. However with the emergence of modern gamma cameras, sophisticated computer techniques and more suitable radionuclides, in particular ^{99m}Tc-HIDA, the methods of nuclear medicine have been successfully applied to the study of gallbladder motor function[13].

Protocol for ^{99m}Tc-HIDA Scanning

The schematic illustration of the protocol for quantitative ^{99m}Tc-HIDA radionuclide scanning used in the studies of Forgacs *et al.*[14] is shown above

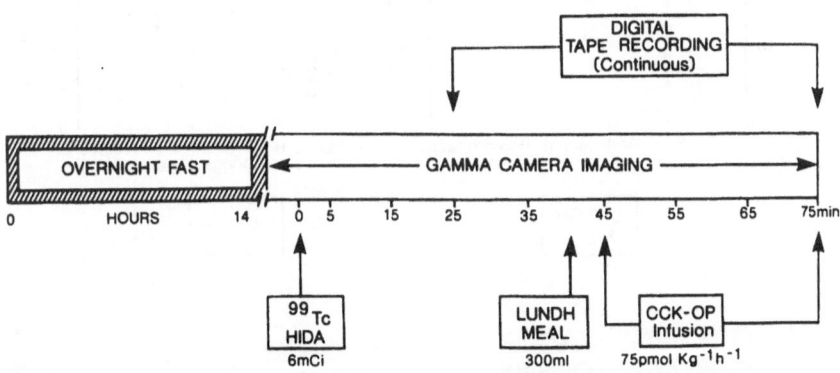

Figure 3 Scheme of protocol for quantitative ^{99m}Tc-HIDA radionuclide studies of gallbladder contraction in response to either a Lundh meal (at min 40) or a CCK-OP infusion (min 45 – min 75) (reproduced from reference 14 with permission).

in Figure 3. After a 12–14 hour fast, patients were given an IV bolus injection of ^{99m}Tc-HIDA and studied when activity over the gallbladder region had reached maximum or near-maximum (usually after 40–45 minutes). Patients were then given *either* a 30 minute infusion of CCK-octapeptide (CCK-OP, dose: 75 pmol kg^{-1} h^{-1}), *or* a Lundh meal. The t$_{1/2}$ of the exponential decline in counts over the gallbladder region (corrected for background and decay) was used as the index of gallbladder contraction.

Results

The t$_{1/2}$ values for gallbladder emptying in control subjects and patients with gallstones are shown in Figure 4. Following the Lundh meal, t$_{1/2}$ in control subjects was 10.2 (SEM: 1.5) min. Prolonged t$_{1/2}$ values were seen both in patients with radiolucent stones : 21.7 (3.1) and radio-opaque stones : 26.7 (3.1). Similar results were seen with the CCK-OP stimulus.

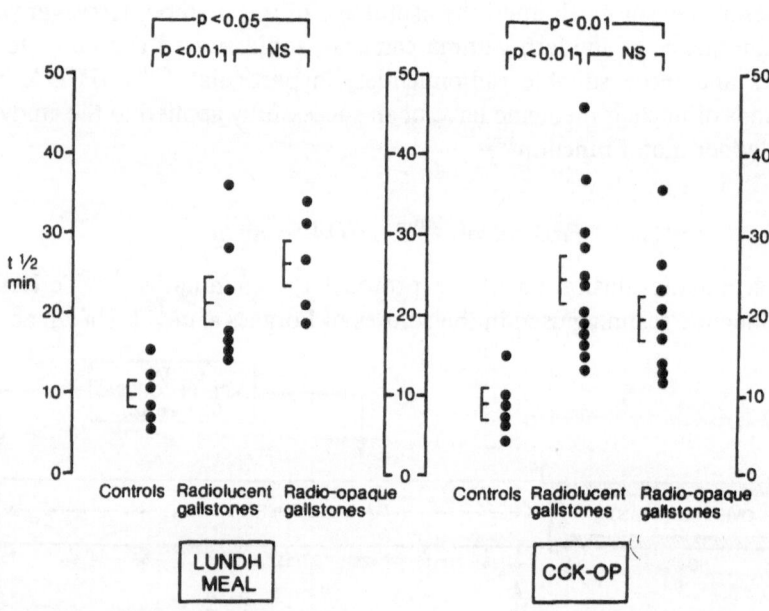

Figure 4 Gallbladder emptying (t$_{1/2}$) in control subjects and patients with radiolucent or radio-opaque stones given either a Lundh meal or CCK-OP stimulus. Individual data points, mean ± SEM are shown (reproduced from reference 14 with permission).

Related Radionuclide Studies in Patients with Gallstones

Fisher *et al.*[15] studied meal-stimulated gallbladder emptying by ^{99m}Tc-HIDA scanning in 15 patients with gallstones (of whom at least 10 had radiolucent stones) and 15 control subjects. Gallbladder emptying at 15 minute intervals was calculated from the gallbladder counts expressed as a percentage of the maximum count before administration of the meal. The % gallbladder emptying was less in patients with gallstones at each time interval for the 2-hour study period following the meal (Figure 5).

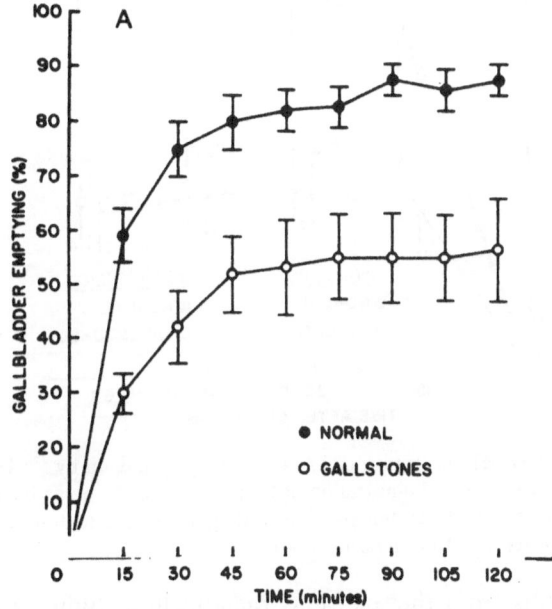

Figure 5 Mean (± SEM) percentage gallbladder emptying judged by ^{99m}Tc-HIDA scanning at 15 min intervals following a liquid (Meriten/Lipomul) meal in 15 patients with gallstones and 15 control subjects (reproduced from reference 15 with permission).

Gallbladder emptying was also studied following administration of CCK-OP either by IV bolus injection (0.04 µg kg^{-1}) or by IV infusion (5 ng kg^{-1} min^{-1} in normal subjects and 10 patients with gallstones. The results of these studies are shown in Figure 6. In contrast to the results seen following the liquid meal (Figure 5) and the results of Forgacs *et al.* (Figure 4) gallbladder emptying following CCK-OP was the same in the patients with gallstones and the control subjects.

In a preliminary study[16], Shaffer *et al.* reported impaired gallbladder emptying following a 30-minute CCK-OP (9.2 ng kg^{-1} h^{-1}) infusion in six gallstone patients. They have now studied 26 gallstone patients and 41 normal subjects[17]. As in the studies discussed above[14-16], they found an exponential decline in counts over the gallbladder region and a significantly longer $t_{1/2}$ in patients with gallstones. They also, however, identified two groups of gallstone patients: those with normal gallbladder emptying ($t_{1/2}$ < 19.1 min) and those with impaired emptying ($t_{1/2}$ > 19.1 min).

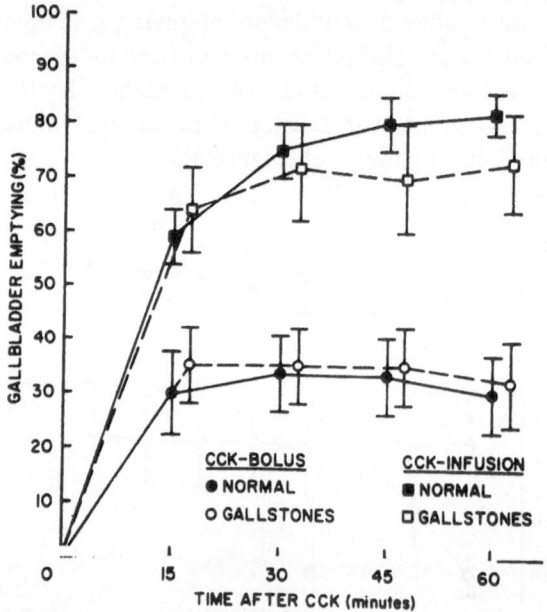

Figure 6 Mean (± SEM) percentage gallbladder emptying judged by ^{99m}Tc-HIDA scanning at 15 min intervals after administration of CCK-OP either by bolus injection or by infusion (for dosage, see text) in ten patients with gallstones and ten control subjects (reproduced from reference 15 with permission).

The results from these various radionuclide studies are discussed below in conjunction with the results of ultrasound studies.

Real-time Ultrasound Studies of Gallbladder Emptying

The earlier technique of examining the gallbladder by grey-scale ultrasonography has been superseded by high-resolution, real-time scanners. A preliminary report suggested that the ability of such scanners to take rapid serial images of the gallbladder would enable its kinetics to be assessed quantitatively[18]. An elegant method of calculating gallbladder volume has been described and fully validated[19], and this technique has enabled several groups to study patterns of gallbladder contraction by making frequent real-time measurements of gallbladder volume over prolonged periods of time.

Protocol for Ultrasound Studies

Patients were studied after an over-night fast. Two measurements of fasting gallbladder volume were made and then serial measurements of volume were recorded at five minute intervals following either a Lundh meal or a 30-minute CCK-OP infusion (75 pmol kg^{-1} h^{-1}). Gallbladder contraction was expressed as the delta volume (ΔV), the difference between the fasting volume and, when the meal stimulus was given, the smallest volume observed in the 2-hour post-prandial period. When the CCK-OP infusion was used, ΔV represented the difference between the fasting volume and the volume remaining at the end of the 30-minute infusion.

Results

Fasting gallbladder volumes were similar in patients with radiolucent gallstones and control subjects (data not shown), but after the meal mean ΔV was less in the seven patients with gallstones than in the control subjects: (9.1 ± 1.5) vs. 14.8 ± 0.9 ml, mean $\pm$ SEM. A similar pattern of results were seen with the CCK-OP infusion (Figure 7).

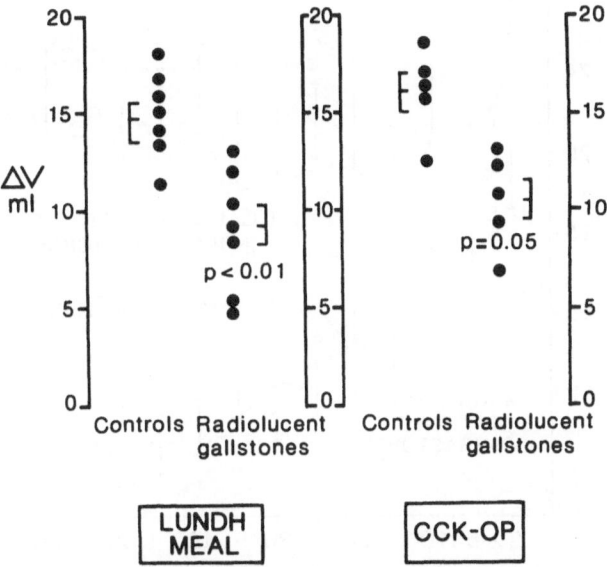

Figure 7 Difference between fasting and post-stimulus gallbladder volumes (ΔV) measured by real-time ultrasound in control subjects and patients with radiolucent gallstones, given either a Lundh meal or CCK-OP infusion. Individual data points and mean $\pm$ SEM are shown (reproduced from reference 14 with permission).

Related Ultrasound Studies in Patients with Gallstones

In an earlier study with a similar design, Thompson et al. took serial ultrasonographic measurements of absolute gallbladder volume at frequent intervals after a fatty meal (Lipomul) in 12 control subjects and 24 patients with gallstones[20]. Gallbladder emptying patterns in the patients with gallstones fell into three groups (Figure 8): four patients had dilated, non-contractile gallbladders, 14 had emptying indistinguishable from normal and six patients had non-dilated gallbladders but showed only slight contraction in response to the meal.

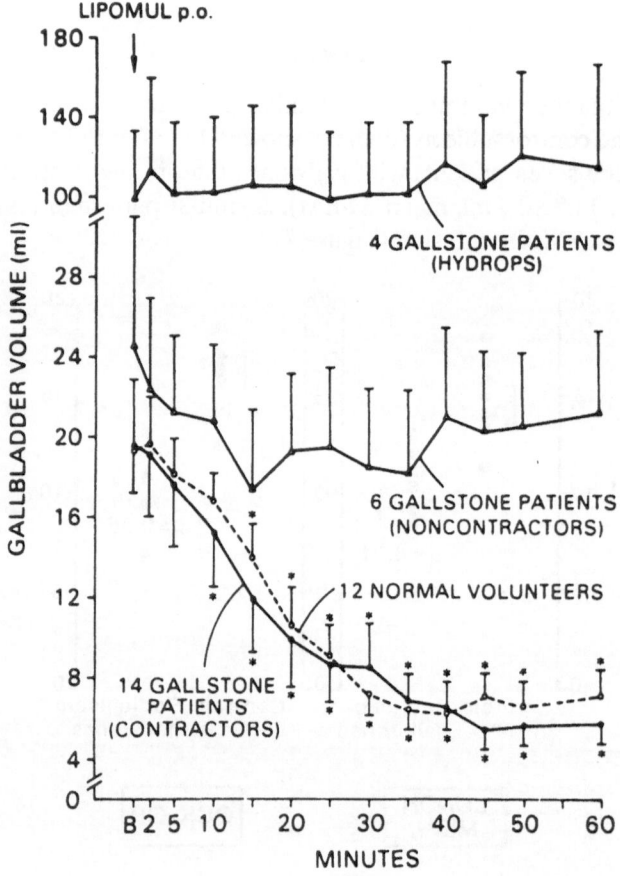

Figure 8 Serial measurements of gallbladder volume by real-time ultrasound in response to a liquid meal (Lipomul) in 24 patients with gallstones and 12 control subjects. Means ± SEM for each group and sub-group are shown. Figures marked with an asterisk indicate a significant decrease from fasting volume at 0 min (reproduced from reference 20 with permission).

THE IMPORTANCE OF THE STIMULUS TO GALLBLADDER CONTRACTION

Meal Stimuli

In each study where a meal stimulus was used, the meal was predominantly fatty and consisted of an emulsion rich in long-chain triglyceride (LCT). LCT-rich meals are known to be a powerful stimulus to gallbladder contraction, probably by acting as a potent secretagogue for CCK[21]. Despite the potency of the stimulus, the resulting CCK release and gallbladder contraction may be no greater than are produced by a standard breakfast[22] (eggs, toast, marmalade and orange juice) and, in that sense, such fatty meals may be deemed 'physiological'. Plasma CCK release has been measured in two of the above studies. In one study, Lundh-meal stimulated CCK release was normal in patients with gallstones[23], while in the other, Lipomul-stimulated CCK release was either normal or reduced[20].

If the reduced gallbladder contraction of patients with gallstones is *not* associated with impaired CCK-release, then a 'physiological' infusion of CCK-OP should give a degree of gallbladder contraction comparable to that produced by a meal. One of the above studies showed such a pattern[14], but not the other[15]. Were the CCK-OP infusions 'physiological'?

CCK-OP Stimuli

Two studies have attempted to define the physiological dose of CCK-OP. Walsh *et al.*[24] infused CCK-OP in stepwise increments of 16, 43 and 98 pmol $kg^{-1} h^{-1}$. These resulted in mean increments of plasma CCK (ΔCCK) of 6.5, 20 and 30 pmol l^{-1} respectively. A plasma CCK-OP concentration of 7–8 pmol l^{-1} produced an output of pancreatic amylase that was one-half of the maximal observed amylase response. A physiological meal produced a much lower CCK-OP suggesting that CCK-OP was not solely responsible for this physiological response.

Maton *et al.* infused doses of CCK-OP of 1,5,20 and 50 pmol $kg^{-1} h^{-1}$ which gave mean plasma CCK concentrations of 0 (undetectable), 6.6, 13.3 and 26.9 pmol l^{-1} respectively[25]. The highest infusion rate produced plasma CCK levels and gallbladder contraction similar to those found after a meal.

The postprandial levels of circulating CCK are still ill defined, and it is not clear which the major biologically-active molecular forms in plasma are. This makes the studies of gallbladder response to CCK-OP infusion very difficult to interpret. Certainly the dose that Fisher *et al.*[15] used is clearly supra-physiological, and this may explain why they found a normal gallbladder response to CCK-OP in gallstone patients. We should, however, be cautious in imparting physiological significance to any of these studies in

145

which CCK was given in this present climate of uncertainty.

CAN TWO POPULATIONS OF GALLSTONE PATIENTS BE DISTINGUISHED?

Both Thompson et al.[20] and Pomeranz and Shaffer[17] were able to divide their gallstone patients into one sub-group that showed a normal pattern of gallbladder contraction, and another with reduced contraction. All studies, however, include some patients with normal gallbladder emptying. It is not yet clear whether the division of patients into groups with 'normal' and 'abnormal' contraction represents distinct pathophysiological entities or is merely arbitrary.

MECHANISM OF REDUCED GALLBLADDER CONTRACTION

There are several possible explanations for the slower and less complete gallbladder emptying in gallstone disease.

The presence of stones in the gallbladder might mechanically impede contraction. Although several of the above studies do not provide data on stone size, in the largest study[14] only two of the 40 patients had stones that occupied > 15% of the cholecystographic gallbladder area. Such a purely mechanical inhibitory effect from the stones seems unlikely[26].

The presence of gallstones might be associated with chronic inflammation of the gallbladder wall with corresponding reduction in its contractility. Histological studies of gallbladders removed for apparently uncomplicated cholelithiasis often show chronic cholecystitis, with abnormalities in the muscle coats and particularly the mucosa, although these changes are often mild[27]. Most of the patients with gallstones in the contractility studies had radiologically functioning gallbladders, but this implies only that the cystic duct was patent and that the gallbladder concentrated the contrast material and expelled it in response to a fatty meal. Radiological 'function' is a crude guide to motor function and patients with chronic cholecystitis may show normal 'function'. No study has compared gallbladder contraction using the recent sensitive techniques with the degree of pathological change in the gallbladder wall. Such a study might clarify the role of chronic cholecystitis in impaired gallbladder contraction. This mechanism seems likely to be important, since the data from CCK-OP infusions and plasma CCK levels suggest an end-organ (gallbladder) lack of responsiveness to a normal contractile stimulus.

Is Impaired Contraction a Primary Phenomenon?

The third and most intriguing of the possibilities is that impaired motor function might be a primary phenomenon, antedating gallstone formation. This speculation receives some support from the work of van der Linden[9] and from a study by Brugge *et al.*[28]. The latter investigated 36 patients with symptoms suggestive of biliary tract disease who all had normal gallbladders by both oral cholecystography and ultrasound. Sixteen of these patients had cholesterol crystals in samples of bile-rich duodenal fluid, while the remaining 20 did not. The 16 patients with cholesterol crystals showed markedly reduced gallbladder emptying measured by radionuclide scanning CCK infusion.

Both these studies raise the possibility that abnormal gallbladder contraction might precede, rather than result from, gallstone formation. This idea receives further support from animal studies.

GALLBLADDER CONTRACTION IN ANIMAL MODELS OF GALLSTONE FORMATION

Prairie dogs form gallstones when fed a cholesterol-enriched diet, and this animal model has been widely used to study lithogenesis. Using a surgical technique, Doty *et al.* measured gallbladder emptying directly through indwelling gallbladder cannulas, and found (see Figure 9) that gallbladder emptying was significantly reduced as cholesterol crystals formed within

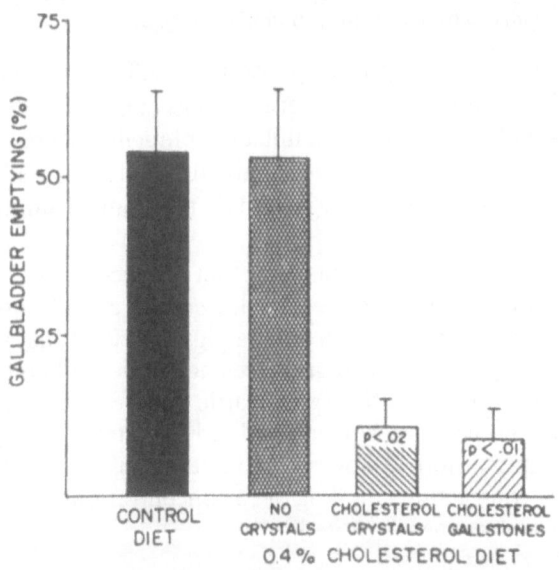

Figure 9 Mean ($\pm$SEM) percentage gallbladder emptying in groups of prairie dogs fed a control or cholesterol-enriched diet, who failed to develop, or did develop, cholesterol crystals or gallstones – for methodology, see text (reproduced from reference 29 with permission).

147

gallbladder bile[29].

Reduced gallbladder contractility, measured *in vitro* as the isometric tension generated in gallbladder wall muscle, was also seen in a study of the ground squirrel which, like the prairie dog, develops crystals and then gallstones on a high-cholesterol diet[30]. Lower wall tension was seen when the lithogenic index of the bile had increased but before cholesterol crystals had formed.

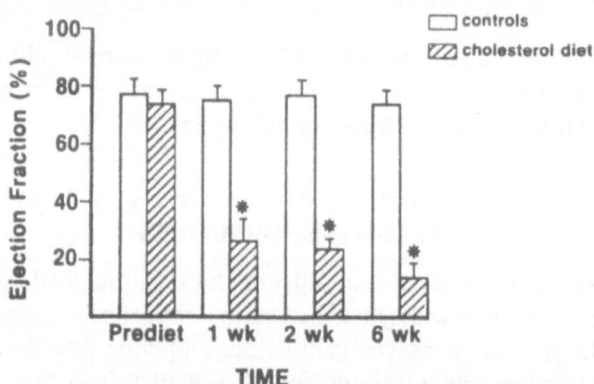

Figure 10 Mean (± SEM) gallbladder emptying (ejection fraction) in response to CCK-33 infusion in prairie dogs fed a control diet and at 1,2 and 6 weeks after feeding on a cholesterol-enriched diet (reproduced from reference 30 with permission).

Gallbladder emptying in response to a CCK infusion has been examined by radionuclide scanning in prairie dogs at 0, 1, 2 and 6 weeks after starting a high-cholesterol diet[31]. Gallbladder emptying decreased after only one week of the lithogenic diet (see Figure 10), and remained significantly lower throughout the 6-week study period than in control animals fed a normal diet.

The mechanism by which a lithogenic diet produces these changes in advance of stone formation is not resolved. Feeding a high cholesterol diet caused gallbladder enlargement in guinea pigs, an effect that was inhibited by indomethacin – suggesting that a prostaglandin-mediated mechanism might be involved[32]. Li *et al.* showed in prairie dogs fed a lithogenic diet that the gallbladder smooth muscle developed reduced stress in response to calcium-induced contraction[33]. However no alterations in membrane excitation, excitation–contraction coupling or in concentrations of the contractile proteins, actin or myosin were noted.

EFFECT OF BILE ACID TREATMENT ON
GALLBLADDER EMPTYING

A potentially important collateral benefit from bile acid treatment for gallstones is that the frequency and severity of biliary colic falls within a few weeks of starting treatment – an effect seen in some[34–36], but not all[37], studies of bile acid therapy.

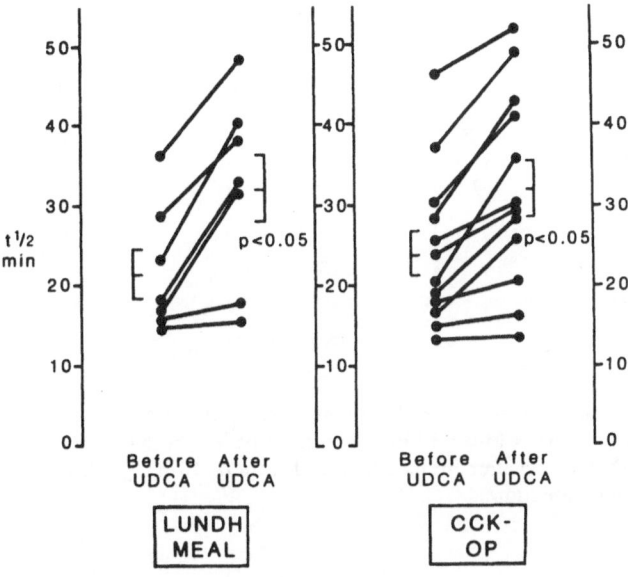

Figure 11 Effect of one month's treatment with ursodeoxycholic acid (8–10 mg kg^{-1} day^{-1}) on the t$_{1/2}$ of gallbladder emptying in patients with radiolucent gallstones given a Lundh meal or CCK-OP stimulus. Individual data points, means ±SEM are shown (reproduced from reference 14 with permission).

Forgacs *et al.* speculated that the reason biliary pain might be reduced during bile acid treatment could be that gallstone patients experience a reduction in gallbladder contraction leading to less forceful expulsion of small stones or other debris into the biliary tree[14]. They measured gallbladder emptying by radionuclide scanning (Figure 11) and by ultrasound before and again after, one months treatment with ursodeoxycholic acid (8–10 mg kg^{-1} day^{-1}). Gallbladder emptying was slower (increased t$_{1/2}$) and less complete (reduced ΔV) during ursotherapy.

Fasting and Lundh-meal stimulated plasma CCK levels (Figure 12) in the patients with gallstones were indistinguishable from normal both before and after bile acid treatment. A direct inhibitory effect from the bile acid treatment on the gallbladder therefore seems likely. Intraduodenal perfusion of sodium taurocholate has been found to inhibit biliary secretion in

149

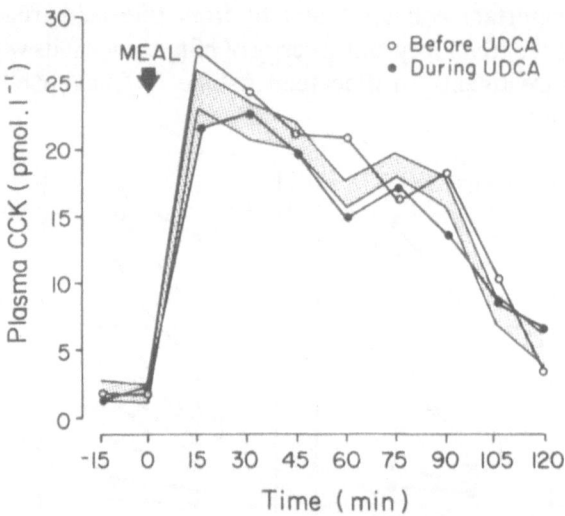

Figure 12 Fasting and 2-hour post-Lundh-meal stimulated plasma CCK levels in six control subjects (shaded zone = Mean ±SEM), and seven patients with radiolucent gallstones who were studied before and after one month's ursotherapy (8–10 mg kg^{-1} day^{-1}). Mean values for gallstone patients are shown.

man[38] but the mechanism for this is not known.

SUMMARY

A consistent pattern emerges from the results of radionuclide and ultrasound studies of gallbladder contraction in patients with radiolucent gallstones. Despite some variations in study design, patient groups, stimuli to gallbladder contraction and expression of emptying, gallstone patients clearly show impaired *meal-stimulated* gallbladder contraction. The results of gallbladder contraction in patients given the CCK-OP infusion are not, however, uniform – perhaps because of the different doses used in the various studies.

   It is not yet clear why patients with gallstones have reduced gallbladder contraction, although experimental evidence is now emerging that this abnormality may antedate and predispose to gallstone formation. The ability to study gallbladder emptying accurately and safely with ultrasound means that it should now be possible to study prospectively patterns of gallbladder contraction in man. Such prospective studies in high-risk groups should determine whether decreased gallbladder emptying is indeed a precursor, rather than an accompaniment, of gallstone disease.

Bile acid therapy inhibits gallbladder emptying. This may be of importance in the management of patients who have had their gallstones fragmented by extracorporeal shock wave lithotripsy. Adjuvant bile acid therapy may speed dissolution of gallstone fragments but may hinder expulsion of such fragments[40].

Those of us who study gallbladder motor function have long been used to playing second fiddle to the bile acid chemists. At last we are now moving towards centre-stage.

Acknowledgements

I wish to thank Mrs. Alison C Roberts for typing the manuscript; Professor Hermon Dowling and other former colleagues at Guy's Hospital for their help, advice, encouragement and practical support in enabling some of the foregoing studies to be carried out; Gipharmex SpA and Roussel Pharmaceuticals Ltd for financial support.

REFERENCES

1. LaMorte, W., Schoetz, D., Birkitt, D. and Williams, L. (1979). The role of the gallbladder in the pathogenesis of cholesterol gallstones. *Gastroenterology*, 77, 580–92.
2. Mann, F.C. and Higgins, G.M. (1927). Effect of pregnancy on the emptying of the gallbladder. A preliminary report. *Arch. Surg.*, 15, 552–9.
3. Levyn, L., Beck, E.C. and Aaron, A.H. (1933). Further cholecystographic studies in the late months of pregnancy. *Am. J. Roetgenol.*, 30, 774–8.
4. Gerdes, M.M. and Boyden, E.A. (1938). The rate of emptying of the human gallbladder in pregnancy. *Surg. Gynaecol. Obstet.*, 66, 145–56.
5. Silva, G. (1949). A simple method for computing the volume of the human gallbladder. *Radiology*, 52, 904–12.
6. Edholm, P. (1960). Gallbladder evacuation in the normal male induced by cholecystokinin. *Acta Radiol.*, 53, 257–65.
7. Inberg, M.V. and Vuorio, M. (1969). Human gallbladder function after selective gastric and total abdominal vagotomy. *Acta Chir. Scand.*, 135, 625–33.
8. Maudgal, D.P., Kupfer, R.M., Zentler-Munro, P.L. and Northfield, T.C. (1980). Postprandial gallbladder emptying in patients with gallstones. *Br. Med. J.*, 280, 141–3.
9. van der Linden, W. (1974). Emptying of the human gallbladder and predisposition to gallstone formation. *Tidjschr. Gastroenterol.*, 17, 121–8.
10. van Berge Henegouwen, G. and Hofmann, A.F. (1978). Nocturnal gallbladder storage and emptying in gallstone patients and healthy subjects. *Gastroenterology*, 75, 879–85.
11. Mok, H.Y.I., von Bergmann, K. and Grundy, S.M. (1980). Kinetics of the enterohepatic circulation during fasting: biliary lipid secretion and gallbladder storage. *Gastroenterology*, 78, 1023–33.
12. Englert, Jr. E. and Chiu, V.S. (1966). Quantitation of human biliary evacuation with a radioisotope technique. *Gastroenterology*, 50, 506–18.
13. Spellman, S.J, Shaffer, E.A. and Rosenthall, L. (1979). Gallbladder emptying in response to cholecystokinin. A cholescintigraphic study. *Gastroenterology*, 77, 115–20.
14. Forgacs, I.C., Maisey, M.N., Murphy, G.M. and Dowling, R.H. (1984). Influence of gallstones and ursodeoxycholic acid therapy on gallbladder emptying. *Gastroenterology*,

87, 299–307.

15. Fisher, R.S., Stelzer, F., Rock, E. and Malmud, L.S. (1982). Abnormal gallbladder emptying in patients with gallstones. *Dig. Dis. Sci.*, **27**, 1019–24.

16. Shaffer, E.A., McOrmond, P. and Duggan, H. (1980). Quantitative cholescintigraphy : assessment of gallbladder filling and emptying and duodeno-gastric reflux. *Gastroenterology*, **79**, 899–906.

17. Pomeranz, I.S. and Shaffer, E.A. (1985). Abnormal gallbladder emptying in a subgroup of patients with gallstones. *Gastroenterology*, **88**, 787–91.

18. Palframan, A. and Meire, H.B. (1979). Real-time ultrasound. A new method for studying gallbladder kinetics. *Br. J. Radiol.*, **52**, 801–3.

19. Everson, G.T., Braverman, D.Z., Johnson, M.L. and Kern, Jr. F. (1980). A critical evaluation of real-time ultrasonography for the study of gallbladder volume and contraction. *Gastroenterology*, **79**, 40–6.

20. Thompson, J.C., Fried, G.M., Ogden, W.D., Fagan, C.J., Inoue, K., Wiener, I. and Watson, L.C. (1982). Correlation between release of cholecystokinin and contraction of the gallbladder in patients with gallstones. *Ann. Surg.*, **195**, 670–5.

21. Isaacs, P.E.T., Ladas, S., Forgacs, I.C., Dowling, R.H., Ellam, S.V., Adrian, T.E. and Bloom, S.R. (1987). Comparison of effects of ingested medium – and long-chain triglyceride on gallbladder volume and release of other gut peptides. *Dig. Dis. Sci.*, **32**, 481–6.

22. Forgacs, I.C., Isaacs, P.E.T., Ladas, S., Murphy, G.M. and Dowling, R.H. (1983). Meal composition influences plasma immunoreactive cholecystokinin (IR-CCK) levels and gallbladder (GB) contraction. *Gastroenterology*, **84**, 1157 (Abstract).

23. Forgacs, I.C., Murphy, G.M. and Dowling, R.H. (1985). Gallbladder contraction and plasma immunoreactive CCK in gallbladder and intestinal disease. In Paumgartner G., Stiehl A., Gerok W. (eds). Enterohepatic Circulation of Bile Acids and Sterol Metabolism, pp. 147–153 (Lancaster: MTP Press).

24. Walsh, J.H., Lamers, C.B., Valenzuela, J.E. (1982). Cholecystokinin-like-immunoreactivity in human plasma. *Gastroenterology*, **82**, 438–44.

25. Maton, P.N., Selden, A.C., Fitzpatrick, M.L. and Chadwick, V.S. (1984). Infusion of cholecystokinin octapeptide in man : relationship between plasma cholecystokinin concentrations and gallbladder emptying rates. *Eur. J. Clin. Invest.*, **14**, 37–41.

26. Pomeranz, I.S., Davison, J.S. and Shaffer, E.A. (1985). The effects of prosthetic gallstones on gallbladder function and bile composition. *J. Surg. Res.*, **41**, 47–52.

27. Edlund, Y. and Zettergren, L. (1959). Histopathology of the gallbladder in gallstone disease related to clinical data. *Acta Chir. Scand.*, **116**, 450–60.

28. Brugge, W.R., Brand, D.L., Atkins, H.L., Lane, B.P. and Abel, W.G. (1986). Gallbladder dyskinesia in chronic acalculous cholecystitis. *Dig. Dis. Sci.*, **31**, 461–7.

29. Doty, J.E., Pitt, H.A., Kuchenbecker, S.L. and Den Besten, L. (1983). Impaired gallbladder emptying before gallstone formation in the prairie dog. *Gastroenterology*, **85**, 168–74.

30. Fridhandler, T.M., Davison, J.S. and Shaffer, E.A. (1983). Defective gallbladder contractility in the ground squirrel and prairie dog during the early stages of cholesterol gallstone formation. *Gastroenterology*, **85**, 830–6.

31. Pellegrini, C.A., Ryan, T., Broderick, W., and Way, L.W. (1986). Gallbladder filling and emptying during cholesterol gallstone formation in the prairie dog. A cholescintigraphic study. *Gastroenterology*, **90**, 143–9.

32. Brotschi, E.A., LaMorte, W.W. and Williams, Jr. L.F. (1986). Effect of dietary cholesterol and indomethacin on cholelithiasis and gallbladder motility in guinea pig. *Dig. Dis. Sci.*, **29**, 1050–6.

33. Li, Y.F., Weisbrodt, N.M., Moody, F.G., Coelho, J.C. and Gouma, D.J. (1987). Calcium-induced contraction and contractile protein content of gallbladder smooth muscle after high-cholesterol feeding of prairie dogs. *Gastroenterology*, **92**, 746–50.

34. Maton, P.N., Iser, J.H., Reuben, A., Saxton, H.M., Murphy, G.M. and Dowling, R.H.

(1982). Outcome of chenodeoxycholic acid treatment in 125 patients with radiolucent gallstones: factors influencing efficacy, withdrawal, symptoms and side-effects and post-dissolution recurrence. *Medicine (Baltimore)*, **61**, 86–97.

35. Iwamura, K. (1980). Clinical studies on cheno- and ursodeoxycholic acid treatment for gallstone dissolution. *Hepato-gastroenterology*, **27**, 26–34.

36. Meredith, T.J., Williams, G.V., Maton, P.N., Murphy, G.M., Saxton, H.M. and Dowling, R.H. (1982). Retrospective comparison of 'cheno' and 'urso' in the medical treatment of gallstones. *Gut*, **23**, 382–9.

37. Schoenfield, L.J., Lachin, J.M. The Steering Committee and the National Cooperative Gallstone Study Group (1981). The National Cooperative Gallstone Study. A controlled trial of efficacy and safety. *Ann. Intern. Med.*, **95**, 257–82.

38. Bjornsson, O.G., Maton, P.N., Fletcher, D.R., Chadwick, V.S. (1982). Effects of duodenal perfusion with sodium taurocholate on biliary and pancreatic secretion in man. *Eur. J. Clin. Invest.*, **12**, 97–105.

39. Sylwestrowicz, T., Logan, K., Kloiber, R. and Shaffer, E. (1987). Effect of bile acid therapy and gallstone dissolution on gallbladder motility. *Gastroenterology*, **92**, 1784 (Abstract).

40. Forgacs, I.C. (1987). Shock news for gallstones. *Br. Med. J.*, **295**, 737–8.

SECTION C
GALLSTONE
PREVENTION

10
Gallstone Prevention: Clues from Epidemiology

K.W. Heaton
University Department of Medicine
Bristol Royal Infirmary
Bristol BS2 8HW, UK

INTRODUCTION

In this chapter I first consider the evidence that the prevalence of gallstones in a population is not immutable, a proposition which implies that gallstones are preventable. I then look at the scope for prevention in terms of modifiable risk factors, and in terms of those eating and drinking habits which have been linked with gallstones themselves or with lithogenic bile.

EPIDEMIOLOGY

Geographical Variations in Prevalence

Accurate data for national prevalence and incidence are not available for any country. This is because gallstones rarely lead to death; indeed, most are symptomless and are never diagnosed. In theory, the data could be obtained by a nation-wide programme of abdominal ultrasonography or cholecystography in random samples of the population, but it is unlikely that the money and manpower for such a vast project will ever be available.

Autopsy surveys suffer from selection bias but can at least give a rough idea of prevalence in the cities where they are carried out. Such surveys have shown that, even after standardisation for age and sex, there are big differences between different countries (Figure 1)[1-16]. Overall, it seems that gallstones are commoner in Northern than in Southern Europe and that they are rare in sub-Saharal Africa.

The special propensity of America Indian women to gallstones has been documented (by cholecystography) in both the USA[17] and Canada[18].

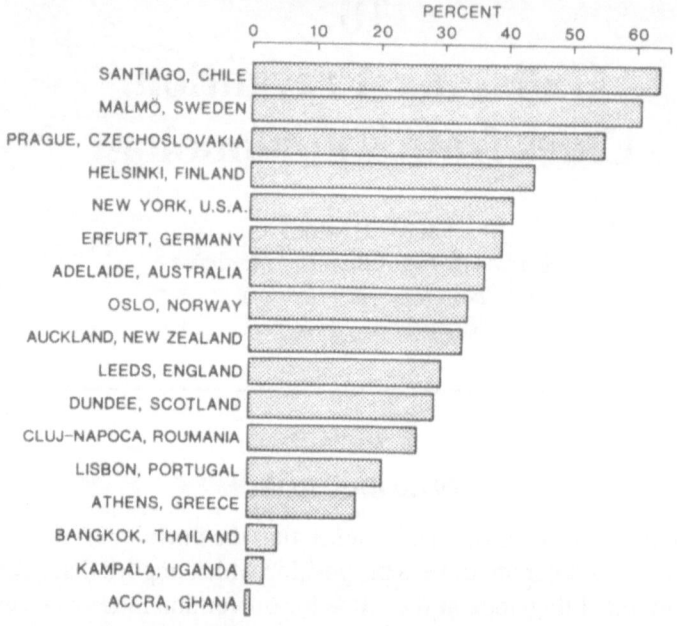

Figure 1   Prevalence of gallstones at autopsy in women aged 70–79 in 17 different countries. The data are taken from reports published since 1951.

These geographical and ethnic variations may in part be due to differences in genetic susceptibility, but this cannot be said of the differences between urban and rural populations or of the changes in prevalence with migration or with time.

Urban-Rural and Social Class Differences

The few reports available suggest that urban–rural and social class differences do exist in developing countries. In Japan in the late 1950s cholesterol stones were found at autopsy much more often in people from the cities than in people from the country[19,20]. In Indian railway workers gallstones were 13–22 times more likely to be diagnosed in the wealthier executive class than in the labouring classes although, it was claimed, medical facilities were comprehensive for all classes[21]. In contrast, ultrasonographic surveys in a developed country, Italy, have shown gallstones to be just as common in a rural area as in the city[22].

Changes in Prevalence with Migration

Documentation is scanty but suggestive. The admission of an Italian to hospital in the 1960s was three times more likely to be due to gallstones if he or she lived in Melbourne than if he or she lived in Italy itself (4.8% vs 1.5%)[23]. Hospital admission for cholelithiasis in Philadelphia is just as common in the black population as in the white[24]. This implies a big increase in gallstone incidence in the blacks, since gallstones are rare in West Africa where the US blacks originated.

Studies of this sort are subject to biases of several kinds but, taken at face value, they suggest that when they were done people were more likely to form gallstones in the environment of the USA and Australia than in those of West Africa and Italy.

Temporal Changes

Repeated surveys of gallstone prevalence in the same place over a period of time are few, but there are enough to suggest a rise in prevalence during this century, at least in Westernised countries. In the Romanian city of Cluj-Napoca the prevalence of gallstones at autopsy was several-fold higher in 1973–82 than it had been 100 years previously (Table 1), even after standardisation for age and sex[11]. Less confidence can be attached to non-standardised data, but such data do suggest that in seven European countries the mean autopsy prevalence of gallstones between 1870 and 1939 was 10.5%, whereas in six European countries between 1940 and 1973 it was 18.5%[25]. The unstandardised autopsy prevalence of gallstones in Tokyo more than doubled from 1949 to 1964 – a period of rapid Westernisation[26]. Similar increases were noted when pre- and post-World War 2 autopsy surveys from England, Sweden and USA were compared[27].

Table 1 Autopsy prevalence of gallstones in Romanian women of different ages in 1873–82 and 1973–82[11]

| | Age (years) | | | | | | |
	20–29	30–39	40–49	50–59	60–69	70–79	80–89
1873–82	1/110	1/89	0/77	1/68	2/23	1/18	1/8
	(0.9%)	(1.1%)	(0)	(1.5%)	(6.0%)	(5.5%)	(12.5%)
1973–82	0/83	6/105	15/255	65/435	121/638	131/498	32/14
	(0)	(5.7%)	(5.9%)	(14.9%)	(19.0%)	(26.3%)	(21.6%)

During and just after the War there was a drop in the standardised autopsy prevalence of gallstones in Essen, Germany[28]. Many believe, anecdotally, that this occurred all over Europe.

Descriptive epidemiology thus, for all its defects, suggests consistently that environmental factors characteristic of modern Western civilisation and urbanisation may be responsible for most gallstones, or at least for most cholesterol rich gallstones.

One group of people in our civilisation seems to have a lower than expected prevalence of gallstones – vegetarians. Only 12% of 130 vegetarian women aged 40–69 had gallstones on ultrasonography, compared with 25% of 632 meat-eating women in the same age group[29]. This is, perhaps, the most direct evidence for environmental factors to date, but it gives little clue to the nature of these factors since there are many life-style and dietary differences between vegetarians and omnivores.

MODIFIABLE PERSONAL RISK FACTORS

Associations between the risk of gallstones and personal characteristics have been sought from autopsy data, from studies of symptomatic patients and, most convincingly, from studies of asymptomatic cases discovered in screening surveys of the general population. All these studies use much the same approach, namely, to look for differences between people with gallstones and people who are stone-free (case control studies). Unmodifiable risk factors such as age and female sex are first established, and then controlled in the search for other factors. Nowadays this is usually done by the statistical technique of multiple regression analysis (multivariate analysis). The case-control approach can be used to look for differences in life-style, such as eating and drinking habits, and this has been done with increasing sophistication in recent years.

Most of the published case-control studies suffer from inadequate sample size or various types of selection bias which confound the results[30]. Scragg has calculated that as many as 200 cases and the same number of controls may be needed for a study to have a reasonable chance of showing dietary differences of the order of 10%, but the exact number depends on how much dietary intakes vary within the population[30]. Small studies are liable to yield false negative results, that is, to fail to reveal a genuine difference. Selection bias is also liable to manufacture non-existent differences, that is, false positive results.

Studies of asymptomatic cases picked up by population screening should yield the most reliable data, and so I shall pay particular attention to such studies. The older literature has been ably summarised by Pixley[27] and especially by Scragg[30,31].

160

Obesity

Obesity was recognised as a risk factor for gallstones in the nineteenth century, and has been extensively documented[31,32]. Nevertheless, there are people in whom this seems not to be true. In the case of Pima Indians[17] and Italian countrywomen[22], the lack of difference in obesity between gallstone cases and controls can be explained by their universal obesity. However, it is less easy to explain why, in some studies where the sexes have been analysed separately, men have shown no association between gallstones and obesity[31] or why, when women over the age of 50 were analysed separately from younger women, they too showed little or no association[33]. Scragg attempts to explain these findings by postulating 'a role for reproductive or hormonal factors, or both, in the association between obesity and gallstones'[31] but another factor may be the relative rarity of slimness in older women. Certainly, overnutrition has endocrine and sexual effects. The fatter a woman is the more likely she is to have had an early menarche[34] and the earlier she had her menarche the more likely she is to have gallstones[35]. Does this simply mean that overnutrition causes gallstones, or that increased exposure to endogenous oestrogens causes gallstones, or both?

Obesity is generally believed to raise the risk of gallstones by increasing the biliary secretion of cholesterol leading to supersaturated bile[36]. Supersaturated bile is a feature of fat men as well as of fat women[37] so that the failure of fat men to be prone to gallstones still needs explaining. Perhaps fat men are less likely than fat women to have other prerequisites for gallstone formation such as gallbladder stasis or crystal nucleating factors. It is possible too that it is not obesity itself which promotes supersaturated bile and gallstones, but an associated metabolic abnormality such as hyperinsulinaemia.

Does thinness protect against gallstones? The GREPCO study of office workers in Rome suggested that it does, at least in women, by showing that body mass index and the risk of gallstones were correlated across the whole range of body mass indices[38] (Figure 2).

Obesity is preventable and reversible. In theory, therefore, many gallstones are preventable by control of body weight, at least in women. Shedding of excess body fat reduces cholesterol secretion into bile[36], but does not necessarily result in normalisation of the cholesterol saturation index except with total starvation[39,40]. This discouraging fact is unexplained, but again suggests that it is not obesity *per se* which leads to gallstones but an associated metabolic abnormality.

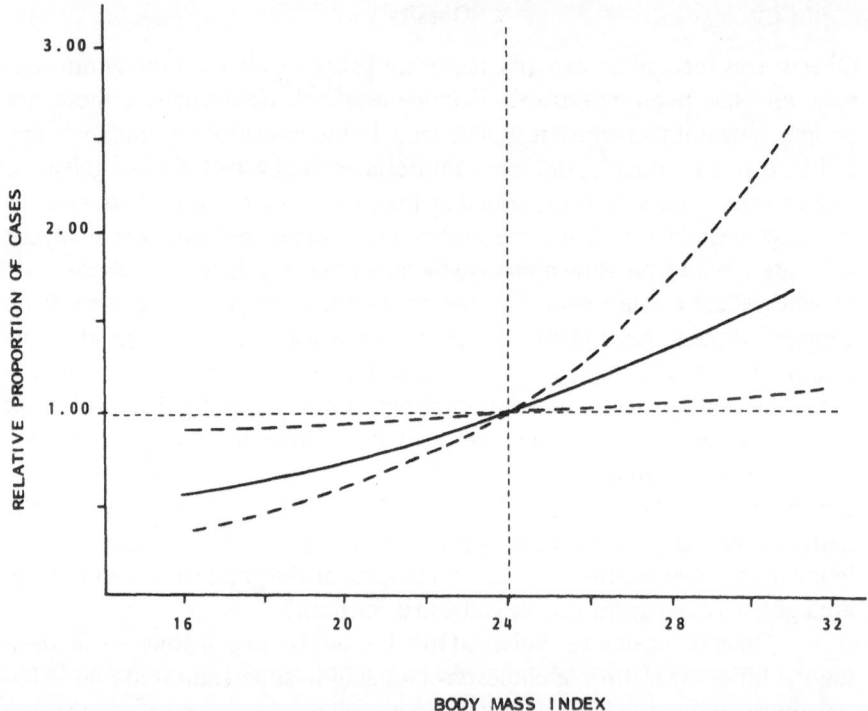

Figure 2 Correlation between body mass index and the relative risk of gallstones in women in the GREPCO study[38]. The data are derived from a multiple logistic analysis including 19 independent variables. Dotted lines indicate 95% confidence limits.

Raised Plasma Triglycerides

An association between gallstones and fasting hypertriglyceridaemia has been demonstrated in several ways. Patients with fasting hypertriglyceridaemia have been shown to have a high prevalence of gallstones[41,42] probably even when they are not overweight (at least in men)[42]. Conversely, patients with gallstones have an increased prevalence of hypertriglyceridaemia[43], and their mean plasma triglyceride levels are increased compared with stone-free controls[43-45]. The latter finding has been confirmed in asymptomatic cases of gallstones discovered by ultrasound screening of the general population[38,46] and, in patients aged under 50, in a large case-control study[47].

The association has a biochemical explanation. Nearly all patients with hypertriglyceridaemia have supersaturated gallbladder bile, even if they are slim[48]. There is a positive correlation between the fasting plasma triglyceride concentration and the cholesterol saturation index of gallbladder bile even in normolipidaemic subjects[49,50] (though not necessarily in patients with gallstones[51]). This association is probably due to a relationship between plasma concentration of triglyceride (or its carrier protein, very low density lipoprotein), and the biliary secretion of cholesterol. Cholesterol synthesis rises with the plasma triglyceride concentration[52] (as does bile acid synthesis but, presumably, not enough to prevent a fall in the bile acid : cholesterol ratio in bile[53]).

The association between gallstones and plasma triglyceride concentration is closer than that between gallstones and body weight, and is independent of it; it holds for men as well as women. The cholesterol saturation of bile correlates more consistently with plasma triglyceride levels than with body mass index.

Hypertriglyceridaemia is preventable and reversible. Much of it is associated with obesity but some is not. A high intake of saturated fat may raise plasma triglycerides[54] but there is no evidence linking saturated fat with gallstones apart from their contribution to calorie intake[31]. A high carbohydrate intake is the dietary factor most widely recognised to raise plasma triglycerides. It is necessary to distinguish between different forms of carbohydrates: a large intake of rapidly absorbed forms of starch and sugar certainly raises the plasma triglyceride level[55,56], but a high intake of slowly digested starch, as in whole grains and pulses, does not[55,57]. Prevention of hypertriglyceridaemia requires control of weight, avoidance of rapidly absorbed carbohydrate, and moderation in alcohol intake.

Other Blood Lipids

Most studies have found no relationship between plasma *total cholesterol* and gallstones[31], but recent epidemiological surveys suggest that an increased plasma cholesterol actually decreases the risk of gallstones[38,47]. This fits with the observation that clofibrate (which lowers plasma total cholesterol) increases the risk of gallstones[58], and with the disputed suggestion that a diet supplemented with polyunsaturated fatty acids has the same effect[59,60].

Three epidemiological studies suggest that the risk of gallstones varies inversely with plasma total *HDL cholesterol* [47,61,62] and one does not[46]. In healthy subjects there is an inverse relationship between biliary cholesterol saturation and plasma HDL cholesterol[49,63] or HDL$_3$ cholesterol[50], which suggests that the relationship is a real one (though it was not found in a study of gallstone patients)[51]. The relationship may, on the other hand, reflect the strong association between plasma triglycerides and gallstones since plasma triglycerides and HDL cholesterol are inversely correlated.

A low plasma HDL cholesterol is to some extent preventable and reversible by changes in life-style. Physical exercise, regular use of alcohol and avoidance of smoking and of refined or added sugars each raise plasma HDL cholesterol[64,65].

High Plasma Insulin

The Adelaide case-control study showed a raised fasting plasma insulin concentration to be a risk factor for gallstones[47] independent of obesity and plasma triglycerides. Not much is known of life-style factors affecting the fasting plasma insulin, but it can be increased by overfeeding and, in some people, by a high intake of refined or added sucrose[66].

DIETARY HABITS

Nutritional epidemiology is an inexact science fraught with pitfalls[67]. Nevertheless, with large samples and careful use of well-designed food frequency questionnaires, it is possible to obtain valid information about some nutrients and some eating habits. Negative findings are hard to interpret as they could be due to the imprecision of dietetic methods.

Sugar Intake

The Adelaide case-control study[33] was large (267 patients) and meticulous, and deserves most attention even though it concerned only symptomatic gallstones. Its most consistent finding was that an increased intake of refined or added sugars in drinks and sweets increased the risk of gallstones in both sexes, under and over the age of 50. Calculating energy intake from questionnaires is somewhat hazardous, but a high energy intake (like obesity) appeared to be a risk factor in younger women in Adelaide. Drinking alcohol had a consistent protective effect, even at low intakes.

Three other case-control studies, all from Italy, have looked at sugar intake. One found higher sugar intakes in the gallstone patients[68], but the other two did not[69,70]. All three studies can be criticised, the first for being based on symptomatic cases, and the others for their small size (60 and 64 subjects respectively). With respect to sugar, therefore, 2 studies with 427 mainly symptomatic cases found sugar to be a risk factor, and 2 studies with 124 asymptomatic cases failed to do so. These negative studies also failed to find a protective effect of alcohol, although this effect is well documented[31] and explained[63].

A high sugar intake increases several risk factors for gallstones. It inflates energy intake and promotes weight gain[65], raises plasma triglycerides and lowers plasma HDL cholesterol[56,65], and raises fasting plasma insulin levels, at least in some people[66]. Most if not all of these risk factors probably operate by raising the cholesterol saturation of bile. It is therefore surprising that, after 6 weeks on high and low sugar diets, there is no difference in the saturation index of bile[65]. Perhaps sugar's *modus operandi* is slow.

Dietary fibre has an opposite position. The experimental evidence that it is protective is quite good: a high intake of fibre, in the form of wheat bran supplements, lowers the cholesterol saturation of bile[71]. The epidemiological evidence is, however, rather weak. The second largest case-control study[68] found patients with gallstones to have a slightly reduced intake of fibre, but the largest one found dietary fibre to be protective only on multiple regression analysis and when certain assumptions were made[33]. The two GREPCO studies found an inverse relationship between the frequency of vegetable consumption and the risk of gallstones, but this did not reach statistical significance (possibly because of small sample size)[69,70]. The lower prevalence of gallstones in vegetarians[29] does not necessarily favour a protective effect of dietary fibre since many vegetarians limit their intake of refined sugars. The great heterogeneity of dietary fibre, the problems of defining and measuring it, the lack of population data on fibre intake and, especially, the uncertainty of interpreting these measurements[72], all mean that it will not be easy to unravel the role of fibre in protecting against gallstones. The best way forward may be to look at slowly digested and absorbed carbohydrate foods (which tend to be rich in intact fibre) rather than at fibre itself.

Fasting seems an improbable risk factor as its opposite, overnutrition, is certainly one. But fasting in the short term increases the cholesterol saturation of gallbladder bile[73] and, in the longer term, the gallbladder stasis attendant on fasting can lead to sludge in the gallbladder and eventually stones[74,75]. Younger women with gallstones are more prone to skip breakfast than controls[76], so that their mean overnight fast was two hours longer. In the first GREPCO study, women with gallstones had fewer snacks between meals than stone-free subjects[69]. If fasting is a risk factor it is, presumably, operative only in overnourished people.

Other Preventable Risk Factors

Oral contraceptive usage seems to accelerate the development of gallstones in some users, especially younger women[31]. Similarly, pregnancy increases gallstone risk only in younger women[31]; this seems to apply to pregnancies which end in abortion as well as to those which go to full term[35].

165

SUMMARY

Overnutrition and habitual consumption of rapidly absorbed carbohydrate, especially sugars, explain many of the reversible risk factors for cholesterol-rich gallstones, including obesity, hypertriglyceridaemia, low plasma HDL cholesterol and high plasma insulin. This nutritional hypothesis is also consistent with geographical and historical variations in the prevalence of gallstones which suggest that gallstones are a disease of modern Western civilisation. However, other factors must exist to explain the formation of gallstones in some slim people, even in some slim vegetarians, and also their occurrence in older people. Promising areas for future investigation are the frequency and duration of fasting episodes[77] and, perhaps, large bowel function in relation to deoxycholic acid metabolism[78,79]. A moderate intake of alcohol seems to have a protective effect.

The author suggests that people who wish to avoid gallstones should limit their intake of energy and especially of readily absorbed carbohydrate, so as to remain slim, should eat enough dietary fibre to avoid constipation, should take breakfast, and should if they like it drink a little alcohol.

References

1. Marinovic, I., Guerra, C. and Larach, G. (1972). Incidencia de litiasis biliar en material de autopsias y analisis de composicion de los calculos. *Revista Méd. Chile*, **100**, 1320–7

2. Záhor, Z., Sternby, N.H., Kagan, A., Uemera, K., Vanecek, R. and Vichert, A.M. (1974). Frequency of cholelithiasis in Prague and Malmö. An autopsy study. *Scand. J. Gastroenterol.*, **9**, 3–7

3. Domellöf, L., Lowenfels, A.B. and Sipponen, P. (1984). Prevalence of gallstones in Finland: an autopsy study in the Helsinki area. *Scand. J. Gastroenterol.*, **19**, 761–4

4. Newman, H.F. and Northup, J.D. (1959). The autopsy incidence of gallstones. *Int. Abst. Surg.*, **109**, 1–13

5. Rodewald, H. (1957). Zur Pathologie der Gallenblase. II Mitteilung. Über die Häufigkeit der Gallensteine. *Zentbl. Allg. Path.*, **96**, 300–2

6. Cleland, J.B. (1953). Gallstones in seven thousand post-mortem examinations. *Med. J. Austr.*, **2**, 488–9

7. Torvik, A. and Høivik, B. (1960). Gallstones in an autopsy series. Incidence, complications, and correlations with carcinoma of the gallbladder. *Acta Chir. Scand.*, **120**, 168–74

8. Douss, T.W. and Castleden, W.M. (1973). Gallstones and carcinoma of the large bowel. *N.Z. Med. J.*, **77**, 162–5

9. Watkinson, G. (1967). The autopsy incidence of gallstones in England and Scotland. *Proc 3rd World Congress Gastroenterol, Tokyo*, **4**, 157–62

10. Bateson, M.C. (1984). Gallbladder disease and cholecystectomy rate are independently variable. *Lancet*, **2**, 621–4

11. Acalovschi, M., Dumitrascu, D., Caluser, I. and Ban, A. (1987). Comparative prevalence of gallstone disease at 100–year interval in a large Romanian town, a necropsy study. *Dig. Dis. Sci.*, **32**, 354–7

12. Galvão, H., Menezes, M.L. and Correia, J.P. (1981). The prevalence of gallstones in the Portuguese population: a necrops study. *Ital. J. Gastroenterol.*, **13**, 100–4

13. Kalos, A., Delidou, A., Kordosis, T., Archimandritis, A., Gananis, A. and Angelopoulos,

B. (1977). The incidence of gallstones in Greece; an autopsy study. *Acta Hep-Gastroenterol.*, **24**, 20–3

14. Stitnimankarn, T. (1960). The necroscopy incidence of gallstones in Thailand. *Am. J. Med. Sci.*, **240**, 349–52

15. Owor, R. (1964). Gallstones in the autopsy population at Mulago Hospital, Kampala. *E. Afr. Med. J.*, **41**, 251–3

16. Edington, G.M. (1957). Observations on hepatic disease in the Gold Coast: with special reference to cirrhosis. *Trans. R. Soc. Trop. Med. Hyg.*, **51**, 48–55

17. Sampliner, R.E., Bennett, P.H., Comess, L.J., Rose, F.A. and Burch, T.A. (1970). Gallbladder disease in Pima Indians. Demonstration of high prevalence and early onset by cholecystography. *N. Engl. J. Med.*, **283**, 1358–64

18. Williams, C.N., Johnston, J.L. and Weldon, K.L.M. (1977). Prevalence of gallstones and gallbladder disease in Canadian Micmac Indian women. *Can. Med. Assoc. J.*, **117**, 758–60

19. Yagi, T. (1960). Some observations on chemical components of gallstones in the Sendai district of Japan. *Tohoku. J. Exp. Med.*, **72**, 117–30

20. Maki, T. (1961). Cholelithiasis in the Japanese. *Arch. Surg.*, **82**, 599–612

21. Malhotra, S.L. (1968). Epidemiological study of cholelithiasis among railroad workers in India with special reference to causation. *Gut*, **9**, 290–5

22. Progetto Distretto Sezze Controllo Comunitario (DISCO), the National Research Council and the Rome Group for Epidemiology and Prevention of Cholelithiasis (GREPCO)(1987). Epidemiology of gallstone disease in Italy: comparison between a rural and urban female population. *Ital. J. Gastroenterol.*, **19**, 129–33

23. Hills, L.L. (1971). Cholelithiasis and immigration. *Med. J. Austr.*, **2**, 94–5

24. Trotman, B.W. and Soloway, R.D. (1973). Influence of age, race or sex on pigment and cholesterol gallstone incidence. *Gastroenterology*, **65**, 573

25. Brett, M. and Barker, D.J.P. (1976). The world distribution of gallstones. *Int. J. Epidemiol.*, **5**, 335–41

26. Kameda, H. (1967). Gallstones, compositions, structural characteristics and geographical distribution. In: *Proc 3rd World Congress Gastroenterol, Tokyo 1966*, **4**, 117–24

27. Pixley, F. (1986). Epidemiology. In: Bateson, M.C. (ed), *Gallstone Disease and its Management*, pp. 1–23. (Lancaster: MTP Press)

28. Balzer, K., Goebell, H., Breuer, N., Ruping, K.W. and Leder, L.D. (1986). Epidemiology of gallstones in a German industrial town (Essen) from 1940–1975. *Digestion*, **33**, 189–97

29. Pixley, F., Wilson, D., McPherson, K. and Mann, J. (1985). Effect of vegetarianism on development of gallstones in women. *Br. Med. J.*, **291**, 11–2

30. Scragg, R.K.R. (1984). Diet, obesity, plasma lipids and insulin in gallstone disease. *PhD Thesis*, University of Adelaide

31. Scragg, R.K.R. (1986). Aetiology of cholesterol gallstones. In: Bateson, MC (ed), *Gallstone Disease and its Management*, pp. 25–55. (Lancaster: MTP Press)

32. Bennion, L.J. and Grundy, S.M. (1978). Risk factors for the development of cholelithiasis in man. *N. Engl. J. Med.*, **299**, 1161–7 and 1221–7

33. Scragg, R.K.R., McMichael, A.J. and Baghurst, P.A. (1984). Diet, alcohol, and relative weight in gallstone disease: a case-control study. *Br. Med. J.*, **288**, 1113–9

34. Garn, S.M., La Velle, M., Rosenberg, K.R. and Hawthorne, V.M. (1986). Maturational timing as a factor in female fatness and obesity. *Am. J. Clin. Nutr.*, **43**, 879–83

35. Jørgensen, T. (1988). Gallstones in a Danish population: fertility period, pregnancies, and exogenous female sex hormones. *Gut*, (In press)

36. Bennion, L.J. and Grundy, S.M. (1975). Effects of obesity and caloric intake on biliary lipid metabolism in man. *J. Clin. Invest.*, **56**, 996–1011

37. Angelin, B., Einarsson, K., Ewerth, S. and Leijd, B. (1981). Biliary lipid composition in obesity. *Scand. J. Gastroenterol.*, **16**, 1015–9

38. Angelico, F. and the GREPCO group (1984). Factors associated with gallstone disease:

observations in the GREPCO study. In: Capocaccia, L., Ricci, G., Angelico, F., Angelico, M. and Attili, A.F. (eds). *Epidemiology and Prevention of Gallstone Disease*, pp.185–92. (Lancaster: MTP Press)

39. Reuben, A., Qureshi, Y., Murphy, G.M. and Dowling, R.H. (1985). Effect of obesity and weight reduction on biliary cholesterol saturation and the response to chenodeoxycholic acid. *Eur. J. Clin. Invest.*, 16, 133–42

40. Schlierf, G., Schellenberg, B., Stiehl, A., Czygan, P. and Oster, P. (1981). Biliary cholesterol saturation and weight reduction – effects of fasting and low calorie diet. *Digestion*, 21, 44–9

41. Einarsson, K., Hellström, K. and Kallner, M. (1975). Gallbladder disease in hyperlipoproteinaemia. *Lancet*, i, 484–7

42. Ahlberg, J., Angelin, B., Einarsson, K., Hellström, K. and Leijd, B. (1979). Prevalence of gallbladder disease in hyperlipoproteinemia. *Dig. Dis. Sci.*, 24, 459–64

43. Kadziolka, R., Nilsson, S. and Schersten, T. (1977). Prevalence of hyperlipoproteinaemia in men with gallstone disease. *Scand. J. Gastroenterol*, 12, 353–5

44. Bell, G.D., Lewis, B., Petrie, A. and Dowling, R.H. (1973). Serum lipids in cholelithiasis: effect of chenodeoxycholic acid therapy. *Br. Med. J.*, 3, 520–3

45. Ahlberg, J. (1979). Serum lipid levels and hyperlipoproteinaemia in gallstone patients. *Acta Chir. Scand.*, 145, 373–7

46. Barbara, L., Sama, L., Labate, A.M.M. *et al.* (1987). A population study on the prevalence of gallstone disease. The Sirmione study. *Hepatology*, 7, 913–7

47. Scragg, R.K.R., Calvert, G.D. and Oliver, J.R. (1984). Plasma lipids and insulin in gallstone disease: a case-control study. *Br. Med. J.* , 289, 521–5

48. Ahlberg, J., Angelin, B., Einarsson, K., Hellström, K. and Leijd, B. (1980). Biliary lipid composition in normo- and hyperlipoproteinaemia. *Gastroenterology*, 79, 90–4

49. Thornton, J.R., Heaton, K.W. and Macfarlane, D.G. (1981). A relation between high-density-lipoprotein cholesterol and bile cholesterol saturation. *Br. Med. J.*, 283, 1352–4

50. Alvaro, D., Angelico, F., Attili, A.F. *et al.* (1986). Plasma lipid lipoproteins and biliary lipid composition in female gallstone patients. *Biomed. Biochem. Acta*, 45, 761–8

51. Marks, J.W., Cleary, P.A. and Albers, J.J. (1984). Lack of correlation between serum lipoproteins and biliary cholesterol saturation in patients with gallstones. *Dig. Dis. Sci.*, 29, 1118–22

52. Sodhi, H.S. and Kudchodkar, B.J. (1973). Correlating metabolism of plasma and tissue cholesterol with that of plasma-lipoproteins. *Lancet*, 1, 513–9

53. Angelin, B. (1977). Cholesterol and bile acid metabolism in normo- and hyperlipoproteinaemia. *Acta Med. Scand.*, Suppl. 610, 1–40

54. Lewis, B. (1976). Influence of diet, energy balance and hormones on serum lipids. In: Lewis, B., *The Hyperlipidaemias. Clinical and Laboratory Practice*, pp.131–80. (Oxford: Blackwell Scientific Publications)

55. Anderson, J.W., Chen, W.-J.L. and Sieling, B. (1980). Hypolipidemic effects of high-carbohydrate, high-fiber diets. *Metabolism*, 29, 551–8

56. Reiser, S., Hallfrisch, J., Michaelis, O.E., Lazar, F.L., Martin, R.E. and Prather, E.S. (1978). Isocaloric exchange of dietary starch and sucrose in humans. I Effects on levels of fasting lipids. *Am. J. Clin. Nutr.*, 32, 1659–69

57. Simpson, H.C.R., Simpson, R.W., Lousley, S., Carter, R.D., Geekie, M., Hockaday, T.D.R. and Mann, J.I. (1981). A high carbohydrate leguminous fibre diet improves all aspects of diabetic control. *Lancet*, i, 1–5

58. Coronary Drug Project Research Group (1977). Gallbladder disease as a side effect of drugs influencing lipid metabolism. *N. Engl. J. Med.*, 296, 1185–90

59. Sturdevant, R.A.L., Pearce, M.L. and Dayton, S. (1973). Increased prevalence of cholelithiasis in men ingesting a serum cholesterol lowering diet. *N. Engl. J. Med.*, 288, 24–7

60. Miettinen, M., Turpeinen, O., Karvonen, M.J., Paavilainen, E. and Elosuo, R. (1976). Prevalence of cholelithiasis in men and women ingesting a serum-cholesterol-lowering

diet. *Ann. Clin. Res.*, **8**, 111–6

61. Angelico, M. and the GREPCO group (1984). Relationship between serum lipids and cholelithiasis: observations in the GREPCO study. In: Capocaccia, L., Ricci, G., Angelico, F., Angelico, M. and Attili, A.F. (eds), *Epidemiology and Prevention of Gallstone Disease*, pp.77–84. (Lancaster: MTP Press)

62. Petitti, D.B., Friedman, G.D. and Klatsky, A.L. (1981). Association of a history of gallbladder disease with a reduced concentration of high-density-lipoprotein cholesterol. *N. Engl. J. Med.*, **304**, 1396–8

63. Thornton, J., Symes, C. and Heaton, K. (1983). Moderate alcohol intake reduces bile cholesterol saturation and raises HDL cholesterol. *Lancet*, **2**, 819–22

64. Stubbe, I., Eskilsson, J. and Nilsson-Ehle, P. (1982). High-density lipoprotein concentrations increase after stopping smoking. *Br. Med. J.*, **284**, 1511–3

65. Werner, D., Emmett, P.M. and Heaton, K.W. (1984). The effects of dietary sucrose on factors influencing cholesterol gallstone formation. *Gut*, **25**, 269–74

66. Reiser, S., Handler, H.B., Gardner, L.B., Hallfrisch, J.G., Michaelis, O.E. and Prather, E.S. (1979). Isocaloric exchange of dietary starch and sucrose in humans. II Effect on fasting blood insulin, glucose, and glucagon and on insulin and glucose response to a sucrose load. *Am. J. Clin. Nutr.*, **32**, 2206–16

67. Willett, W. (1987). Nutritional epidemiology: issues and challenges. *Int. J. Epidemiol.*, **16**, 312–7

68. Alessandrini, A., Fusco, M.A., Gatti, E. and Rossi, P.A. (1982). Dietary fibres and cholesterol gallstones: a case control study. *Ital. J. Gastroenterol.*, **14**, 156–8

69. Attili, A.F. and the GREPCO group (1984). Dietary habits and cholelithiasis. In: Capocaccia, L., Ricci, G., Angelico, F., Angelico, M. and Attili, A.F. (eds), *Epidemiology and Prevention of Gallstone Disease*, pp. 175–81. (Lancaster: MTP Press)

70. Attili, A.F. and the Rome Group for the Epidemiology and Prevention of Cholelithiasis (GREPCO) (1987). Diet and gallstones: result of an epidemiologic study performed in male civil servants. In: Barbara, L., Bianchi Porro, G., Cheli, R. and Lipkin, M. (eds), *Nutrition in Gastrointestinal Disease*, pp. 225–31. (New York: Raven Press)

71. Heaton, K.W. (1987). Effect of dietary fiber on biliary lipids. In: Barbara, L., Bianchi Porro, G., Cheli, R. and Lipkin, M. (eds), *Nutrition in Gastrointestinal Disease*, pp. 213–22. (New York: Raven Press)

72. Eastwood, M.A. (1986). What does the measurement of dietary fibre mean? *Lancet*, **1**, 1487–8

73. Bloch, H.M., Thornton, J.R. and Heaton, K.W. (1980). Effects of fasting on the composition of gallbladder bile. *Gut*, **21**, 1087–9

74. Messing, B., Bories, C., Kunstlinger, F. and Bernier, J.J. (1983). Does total parenteral nutrition induce gallbladder sludge formation and lithiasis? *Gastroenterology*, **84**, 1012–9

75. Bolondi, L., Gaiani, S., Testa, S. and Labo, G. (1985). Gallbladder sludge formation during prolonged fasting after gastrointestinal tract surgery. *Gut*, **26**, 734–8

76. Capron, J.P., Delamarre, J., Herve, M.A., Dupas, J.L., Poulain, P. and Descombes, P. (1981). Meal frequency and duration of overnight fast: a role in gallstone formation? *Br. Med. J.*, **283**, 1435

77. Bouchier, I.A.D. (1987). Nutrition and gallstone disease. In: Barbara, L., Bianchi Porro, G., Cheli, R. and Lipkin, M. (eds), *Nutrition in Gastrointestinal Disease*, pp. 205–12. (New York: Raven Press)

78. Marcus, S.N. and Heaton, K.W. (1986). Intestinal transit, deoxycholic acid and the cholesterol saturation of bile – three inter-related factors. *Gut*, **27**, 550–8

79. Marcus, S.N. and Heaton, K.W. (1988). Deoxycholic acid and the pathogenesis of gallstones. *Gut*, **29**, 522–33

11
Gallstone Prevention: Post-dissolution Trials

K.A. Hood
Gastroenterology Unit
UMDS of Guy's and St Thomas' Hospitals
Guy's Campus
London SE1 9RT, UK

INTRODUCTION

Oral bile acids have been in use for several years for the dissolution of cholesterol-rich gallstones. During this time, much information has been gained about patients treated in this manner – their response to treatment, the difficulty of confirming complete gallstone dissolution, and then, after treatment is withdrawn, the rebound increase in biliary cholesterol saturation and the recurrence of stones.

It is probable that many factors are involved in recurrence:-

(1) Cholesterol supersaturation is considered a prerequisite for the initial development of cholesterol-rich gallstones. Following withdrawal of treatment, most patients develop supersaturated bile again within 4 weeks[1-3]. Not all such patients develop recurrent gallstones, however; resaturation is a poor predictor of recurrence, and this suggests that other mechanisms must also be involved.

(2) Abnormal nucleation. There is good evidence that a nucleation defect contributes to the pathogenesis of primary gallstones. It is, unfortunately, impracticable to obtain samples of gallbladder bile for such studies from patients who have become stone free, so that little is known about nucleating factors in gallstone recurrence.

(3) Abnormal gallbladder motor function. Gallbladder emptying is impaired in patients with gallstones[4-7], but it is not known whether the stones are the cause or the effect of this abnormality. Recent reports[8] indicate that gallbladder motor function does not improve after stone dissolution.

Studies of patients who have achieved complete gallstone dissolution show that stones recur in 30–50%[9-12] within 5 years of treatment withdrawal. Several post-dissolution trials have tried to identify suitable methods of keeping the gallbladder free of stones. Such prophylactic treatment should be safe and free of unwanted effects, convenient to take and reasonably cheap. Prophylactic treatments have so far been directed towards reducing the cholesterol saturation of bile, using either low-dose bile acid treatment or dietary modification.

Some gallstone recurrences, particularly those occurring within a few months of treatment withdrawal, are probably really regrowth of dissolved stone fragments undetected at the time complete dissolution was diagnosed.

(4)   Diagnosis of complete gallstone dissolution. Complete dissolution must be established before treatment is withdrawn. Traditionally, this has involved two consecutive normal oral cholecystograms, but in recent years ultrasound scanning has been more widely used. The sensitivity of this technique in detecting small gallstones has increased as equipment and radiological skills have developed. The reporting in 1982[13,14] of a significant number of patients said to have complete stone dissolution on the basis of cholecystography who had small stones on an ultrasound examination has drawn attention to the possible inaccuracy of diagnosing gallstone dissolution. Jazrawi et al.[15] confirmed these findings by establishing the presence of such stones at cholecystectomy.

POST-DISSOLUTION TRIALS

The American National Co-Operative Gallstone Study[17]

After the large American multicentre trial on the safety and efficacy of dissolution therapy using chenodeoxycholic acid (CDCA) (NCGSG), patients with complete dissolution were entered into a post-dissolution study[17]. 53 patients were randomised in double-blind fashion to receive either CDCA 375 mg/day or placebo, and followed for a maximum of 41/2 years. The cumulative recurrence rate was reported after 31/2 years because only seven patients continued follow up after this time. The overall recurrence rate by life table analysis was 27%, with 23.9% in the treated group and 28.5% in the placebo group. The authors concluded that CDCA 375 mg/day did not prevent recurrence. No factors capable of predicting recurrence could be identified in this study.

Perez Aguilar[18]

A group from Valencia studied 31 patients in whom complete dissolution had been confirmed by ultrasound and/or cholecystogram. The patients were randomised into three groups A, B and C. Group A received no treatment, and no medical follow up other than an ultrasound examination after 4–8 years. Patients in group B received 'low-dose' CDCA (250 mg/day) and those in group C 'medium-dose' ursodeoxycholic acid (UDCA) (300 mg/day). Groups B and C were followed with 6 monthly ultrasound scans for 18 months.

	GROUP A No treatment	GROUP B CDCA (250mg/day)	GROUP C UDCA (300mg/day)
NUMBER OF PATIENTS	10	12	9
NUMBER OF RECURRENCES	6	3	0

Figure 1 Perez Aguilar *et al.* Distribution of patients and gallstone recurrences between treatment groups.

The results are summarised in Figure 1. 60% of the untreated patients developed recurrent gallstones, compared with 25% of those receiving low-dose CDCA and none of those taking medium-dose UDCA.

The much longer period of follow-up in the untreated patients may, in part, explain their greater recurrence rate. The doses of the two bile acids are not comparable in terms of their pharmacological effects, making it difficult to draw any conclusions regarding their relative efficacy in prophylaxis. Nevertheless, this study suggests that UDCA may be effective in preventing recurrence.

Villanova[19]

Investigators from Italy recently reported a follow up study of 96 cases of complete dissolution in 86 patients (10 patients having had recurrence and re-dissolution). Complete dissolution was established by two consecutive cholecystograms and/or ultrasound scans. The patients were followed for up to 12 years with annual ultrasound scans or cholecystograms – a potential source of error in view of the well documented discrepancies between these two techniques. Patients were allocated to post-dissolution treatment with

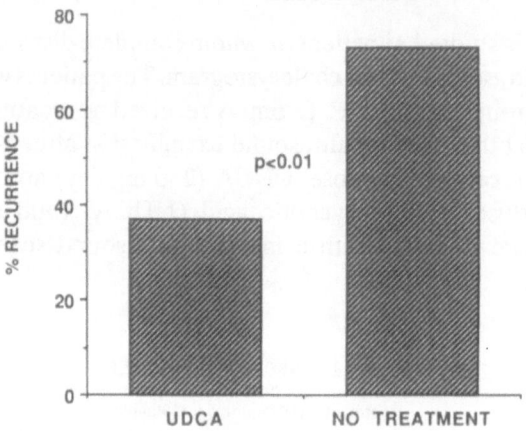

Figure 2 Villanova *et al*. Cumulative gallstone recurrence by life table analysis at 12 years in the UDCA-treated compared with the untreated group.

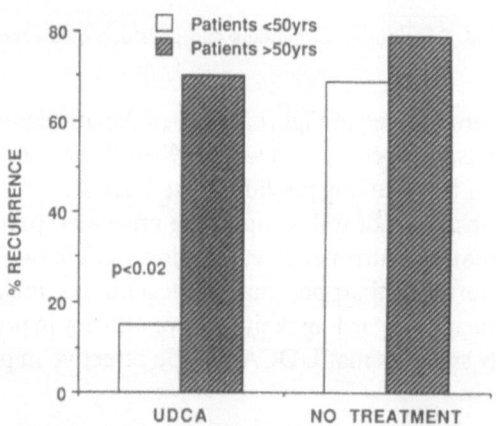

Figure 3 Effect of age on gallstone recurrence (Villanova *et al.*). Cumulative recurrence by life table analysis at 12 years in treated and untreated patients according to age group.

UDCA 300 mg/day on 36 occasions and to no treatment on 60 occasions not in a randomised fashion. The overall cumulative recurrence rate by life table analysis was 12.5% after 1 year, reaching a plateau of 64% by the ninth year (total follow up 12 years). Gallstone recurrence in the treated group was significantly ($p < 0.01$) lower than that seen in the untreated group (Figure 2).

Retrospective sub-group analysis suggested that the benefit of UDCA was confined to the few younger patients (arbitrarily defined as those under 50 years of age) (Figure 3). This apparent age difference is difficult to explain, and was not seen in the British–Belgian post-dissolution trial.

The Italian study identified an interesting predictive factor: patients who initially had a solitary gallstone had a significantly lower recurrence rate than did those presenting with multiple stones (33% vs 71% by life table analysis at 12 years). The British–Belgian study suggested a similar trend but there were too few subjects presenting with a solitary stone to allow statistical comparison.

Tint, Salen and Chazen[20]

An American study by Tint and colleagues, whilst not a true post-dissolution trial with regular follow-up, provides certain information about gallstone recurrence. 33 patients who had had complete gallstone dissolution (method of confirmation not stated) were reviewed by ultrasound or oral cholecystogram and by interview. 21 of these patients had recurrence within 7 years. Of the 12 patients who remained gallstone free (after varying lengths of follow-up), five had received UDCA (90–300 mg/day) since dissolution.

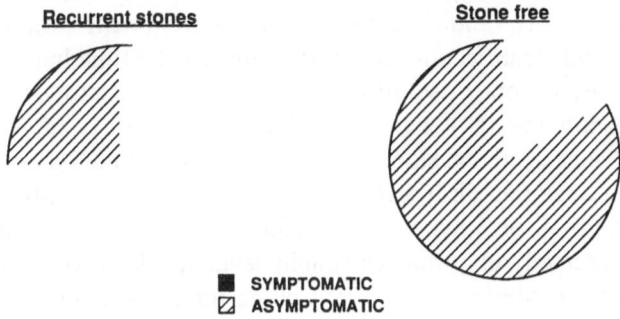

Figure 4 Proportion of patients with recurrent symptons at follow up: patients with gallstone recurrence compared with patients continuing stone free (Tint *et al.*).

Most of those patients reported biliary and dyspeptic symptoms, far more than those who were stone free (Figure 4). In other studies most of the recurrences were asymptomatic at the time of diagnosis.

THE BRITISH–BELGIAN GALLSTONE STUDY GROUP POST-DISSOLUTION TRIAL is the most ambitious study so far performed. It has been reported only in abstract, and is reported here in some detail:

Aims

This post-dissolution study was a prospective, multicentre, randomised trial aimed to compare the safety and efficacy of

(i)   low-dose (3 mg/kg/day) UDCA given at bedtime,

(ii)   placebo (given in a double-blind fashion with UDCA) and

(iii)   a diet high in fibre (30 g/day) and low in refined carbohydrates (15 g/day)

in preventing gallstone recurrence. The trial was initially for 2 years, later extended to 5 years. It aimed to gain information about timing and frequency of recurrence, and how commonly this is associated with symptoms. It also compared the efficacy of oral cholecystography and ultrasonography in the detection of recurrent stones, and tried to identify risk factors which might predict recurrence.

Protocol

All patients had complete gallstone dissolution confirmed by two successive oral cholecystograms, and by ultrasonography in all except four patients. Both ultrasonography and cholecystography preceded trial entry by not more than 6 weeks. Patients were randomised to one of the treatment groups from a central office after stratification for obesity, and for the time between confirmed complete gallstone dissolution and entry to the trial (stone free interval). The reason for the latter was that early reports of gallstone recurrence[9,10] suggested that stones recurred within the first 2 years of stopping treatment or not at all. It was considered that those patients who had remained stone free for 2 years or more since treatment withdrawal might represent a 'protected' sub-group who might never develop recurrent stones.

Patients attended an out-patient clinic for clinical review every 3 months, for ultrasound scan every 6 months and for oral cholecystography every year. Whenever recurrence was diagnosed on ultrasound, cholecystography was performed soon after. In the event of a discrepancy between the results obtained with ultrasonography and cholecystography, the decision was based on the results of oral cholecystography. Patients sensitive to contrast media were diagnosed by two successive positive ultrasound examinations.

Patient Study Group

93 patients were randomised to the three treatment groups (73 women and 20 men aged 20–85 years). The maximum duration of follow up was 5 years.

11 patients withdrew before their first 6 monthly ultrasound scan, due to unrelated death in one patient, intolerance to treatment in four patients and default in six patients. These patients were similar in all respects to those remaining. Approximately equal numbers of patients remained in each treatment group.

Results

A total of 21 recurrences was detected, all within 3 1/2 years of randomisation, and all but two asymptomatic. Cumulative recurrence rate by life table analysis was 34% after 3 1/2 years and rose higher thereafter. Four recurrences occurred in the UDCA-treated group, six in the placebo group and eleven in the diet group, corresponding to 21%, 27% and 46% respectively at 3 1/2 years by life table analysis. There were no significant differences between recurrence rate in the placebo group and either of the two treatment groups.

Ultrasound Compared with Oral Cholecystogram

Ultrasonography detected recurrent stones more frequently and earlier than did oral cholecystography. Two recurrences were diagnosed by cholecystography, but not by ultrasound, while five recurrences were detected by ultrasonography alone. Where both techniques were in agreement, recurrence was seen earlier by ultrasound than by oral cholecystogram in two thirds of cases and simultaneously only in one third.

These observations highlight the difficulty of using different imaging techniques in this type of study.

Factors Influencing Gallstone Recurrence

Many factors were assessed as possible predictors of recurrence, but most were not shown to influence the outcome. Pre-treatment gallstone size and type of bile acid dissolution therapy had no effect on recurrence. Gallstone recurrence was less common in patients who had had single stones than in those who had had multiple stones, but this did not reach statistical significance. The patients' age and the presence of obesity appeared unimportant. In the women, history of pregnancy either in the past or since dissolution therapy, menopausal status and the ingestion of oestrogen containing preparations were not shown to influence recurrence.

Recurrence seemed more common in men than in women, although the number of men with recurrent stones was too small to permit statistical comparison.

Because of recent work[22,23] showing that non-steroidal antiflammatory drug (NSAID) ingestion may influence the development of gallstones in experimental animals fed a lithogenic diet, a retrospective analysis of patient's consumption of aspirin and NSAIDs was undertaken by questionnaire, to which 71 patients have so far replied. Few patients took these drugs on a regular basis and none of these suffered gallstone recurrence. Although this is a small group, it suggests that aspirin and NSAIDs may influence gallstone recurrence.

The interval between confirmed gallstone dissolution and treatment withdrawal, and entry to the trial varied from one to 80 months, with a median of 9 months. When patients with stone free intervals on either side of this median were compared, recurrence appeared significantly less frequent in those who had already been stone free for at least 9 months. It appears that even this relatively short time interval defines a 'low risk' subgroup.

SUMMARY

Up to 50% of patients who achieve complete gallstone dissolution develop recurrent stones within 5 years of treatment withdrawal. Few patients have been followed up beyond 5 years, so that the plateau in recurrence rate usually reported at this time cannot be substantiated. Longer trials are needed. Most recurrent gallstones are asymptomatic at the time of diagnosis.

Comparison between different post-dissolution studies is hindered by the different study designs, particularly the admission criteria and the manner and duration of follow-up. It would be desirable in future studies to use the same imaging techniques throughout – to establish complete gallstone dissolution at the outset, and in diagnosing recurrence. There are well documented discrepancies between different techniques.

Post-dissolution studies should begin from the time of treatment withdrawal, as the British–Belgian study showed that those who had remained stone-free even for nine months without treatment were at lower-risk of recurrence.

Low dose UDCA[18,19,21] probably reduces, but does not prevent, gallstone recurrence. A high-fibre low refined carbohydrate diet does not prevent recurrence. Younger patients may benefit more than older patients from post-dissolution treatment with UDCA.

Few variables predictive of gallstone recurrence have been identified. Solitary stones, once dissolved, seem to recur less commonly than multiple stones.

It is probable that recurrence will be seen to the same extent in those patients treated by extracorporeal shock wave lithotripsy or by contact dissolution using solvent infusion into the gallbladder as has been documented in those treated with oral bile acids.

Patients whose stones have been dissolved constitute a group with an approximately 50% risk of developing gallstones. Comparison between those who do develop recurrent stones and those who do not may ultimately provide information about the pathogenesis of gallstone disease.

Acknowledgement

The author gratefully acknowledges the contributions of Professor R.H. Dowling and Doctors David Ruppin and Dermot Gleeson, and wishes to thank Mrs Ann Hollington for secretarial assistance.

REFERENCES

1. Mok, H.Y.I., Bell, G.D. and Dowling, R.H. (1974). Effects of different doses of chenodeoxycholic acid on bile lipid composition and on frequency of side-effects in patients with gallstones. *Lancet*, 2, 253–7.
2. Thistle, J.L., Yu, P.Y.S., Hofmann, A.F. and Ott, B.J. (1974). Prompt return of bile to supersaturated state followed by gallstone recurrence after discontinuance of chenodeoxycholic acid therapy. *Gastroenterology*, 66, 789 (Abstr).
3. Iser, J.H., Murphy, G.M. and Dowling, R.H. (1979). Speed of change in biliary lipids and bile acids with chenodeoxycholic acid – is intermittent therapy feasible? *Gut*, 18, 7–15.
4. Forgacs, I.C., Murphy, G.M. and Dowling, R.H. (1984). Gallbladder contraction and plasma immuno reactive CCK in gallbladder and intestinal disease. In: Paumgartner, G., Stiehl, A. and Gerok, W. (eds.) *Enterohepatic Circulation of Bile Acids and Sterol Metabolism*. pp. 147–53 (Lancaster: MTP Press).
5. Forgacs, I.C., Maisey, M.N., Murphy, G.M. and Dowling, R.H. (1984). Influence of gallstones and UDCA therapy on gallbladder emptying. *Gastroenterology*, 87, 299–307.
6. Fisher, R.S., Stelzer, F., Rock, E. and Malmud, L.S. (1982). Abnormal gallbladder emptying in patients with gallstones, *Dig. Dis. Sci.*, 27, 1019–24.
7. Pomeranz, I.S. and Shaffer, E.A. (1985). Abnormal gallbladder emptying in a sub group of patients with gallstones. *Gastroenterology*, 88, 787–91.
8. Sylwestrowicz, T., Logan, K., Kloiber, R. and Shaffer, E. (1987). Effect of bile acid therapy and gallstone dissolution on gallbladder motility. *Gastroenterology*, 92, 1784 (Abstr).
9. Ruppin, D.C. and Dowling, R.H. (1982). Is recurrence inevitable after gallstone dissolution by bile acid treatment? *Lancet*, 1, 181–5.
10. Thistle, J.L. (1981). Medical management of gallstones; *Prac. Gastroenterol.*, 5, 351–6.
11. O'Donnell, L. and Heaton, K.W. (1986). Success and failure in the medical treatment of gallstones. *Gut*, 27, A1234, (Abstr).
12. Lanzini, A., Jazrawi, R.P., Kupfer, D.M., Maudgal, D.P., Joseph, A.E.A. and Northfield, T.C. (1986). Gallstone recurrence after medical dissolution – an overestimated threat? *J. Hepatol.*, 3, 241–6.
13. Somerville, K.W., Rose, D.H., Bell, G.D., Ellis, W.R. and Knapp, D.R. (1982). Gallstone dissolution and recurrence: are we being misled? *Br. Med. J.*, 284, 1295–7.
14. Shapero, T.F., Rosen, I.E., Wilson, S.R. and Fisher, M.M. (1982). Discrepancy between ultrasound and oral cholecystography in the assessment of gallstone dissolution. *Hepatology*, 2, 587–90.
15. Jazrawi, R.P., Joseph, A.E.A., Wilson, A.G. and Northfield, T.C. (1984). Comparison of cholecystography and ultrasonography for detection of gallstones. *Gut*, 25, A561 (Abstr).

16. Gleeson, D. and Ruppin, D.C. and the British Gallstone Study Group. (1985). Discrepancies between cholecystography and ultrasonography in the detection of recurrent gallstones. *J. Hepatol.*, **1**, 597–607.

17. Marks, J.W., Lan, S.P., The Steering Committee and the National Cooperative Gallstone Study Group. (1984). Low-dose Chenodiol to prevent gallstone recurrence after dissolution therapy. *Ann. Intern. Med.*, **100**, 376–81.

18. Perez Aguilar, F., Breto, M., Alfonso, V., Martinez-Silvestre, M. and Berenguer, J. (1985). Gallstone recurrence following cessation of dissolving treatment and during prophylactic administration of either low-dose chenodeoxycholic acid (CDCA) or medium-dose ursodeoxycholic acid (UDCA). *J. Hepatol.*, **1**, S305 (Abstr).

19. Villanova, N., Bazzoli, F., Frabboni, R., Mazzella, G., Morselli Labate, A.M., Barbara, L. and Roda, E. (1987). Gallstone recurrence after successful oral bile acid treatment: a follow up study and evaluation of long-term post-dissolution treatment. *Gastroenterology*, **92**, 1789 (Abstr).

20. Tint, G.S., Salen, G. and Chazen, D. (1987). Symptomatic gallstones are likely to reoccur after dissolution with ursodeoxycholic acid (UDCA) but this may be prevented by low-dose UDCA. *Gastroenterology*, **92**, 1787 (Abstr).

21. Hood, K.A., Gleeson, D., Ruppin, D.C., Dowling, R.H. and the BBGSG. (1987). The British-Belgian Gallstone Study Group's post-dissolution trial. *Gut*, **28**, A1359 (Abstr).

22. Lee, S.P., Carey, M.C. and Lamont, J.T. (1981). Aspirin prevention of cholesterol gallstone formation in prairie dogs. *Science*, **211**, 1429–30.

23. Lamont, J.T., Turner, B.S., Dibenedetto, D., Handin, R. and Schafer, A.I. (1983). Arachidonic acid stimulates mucin secretion in prairie dog gallbladder. *Am. J. Physiol.*, **245**, 992–8.

SECTION D
NON-SURGICAL TREATMENT OF GALLSTONES

12
Non-Surgical Treatment: of Gallstones Cheno- versus Ursodeoxycholic Acid

L. Barbara, F. Bazzoli and E. Roda
Istituto di Clinica Medica e Gastroenterologia,
Università di Bologna, Italy

INTRODUCTION

Chenodeoxycholic acid (cheno) and ursodeoxycholic acid (urso) are the two agents now available for the oral dissolution of cholesterol gallstones.

The rationale for using oral bile acids to dissolve gallstones is, essentially, to reduce the ratio of cholesterol to bile acids plus phospholipids in bile. Although this method was first conceived by Johnston and Nakayama in 1957[1], it was not until 1972 that the Mayo Group reported the first dissolution in man, using chenodeoxycholic acid[2]. In 1975, Makino reported gallstone dissolution using ursodeoxycholic acid, a bile acid which had been used in Japan for decades as a cholagogue[3]. In 1982, we published a study comparing cheno and urso for gallstone dissolution[4].

In this chapter, we summarise the effects of cheno and urso on cholesterol and bile acid metabolism, and we focus on the clinical aspects of their use and on the place oral bile acid treatment in managing gallstone disease.

PHARMACOLOGY

After ingestion, cheno and urso are rapidly and efficiently absorbed in the terminal ileum, transported in the portal blood to the liver, and then rapidly extracted, conjugated and resecreted into bile[5]. The concentrations of cheno and urso which are present in the systemic circulation are therefore much lower than those in the enterohepatic circulation. This is crucial, as their efficacy is related to biliary and not to serum concentrations.

MECHANISM OF ACTION

Both cheno and urso lower the lithogenic index of bile by reducing biliary cholesterol output, but they do this by different mechanisms. Urso, in acute bile acid pool replacement studies[6], probably reduces cholesterol secretion by virtue of its limited capacity for transporting cholesterol in micellar form through the canalicular membrane. It also seems to reduce the intestinal absorption of cholesterol and to enhance bile acid synthesis[7], thus promoting a normal or negative cholesterol balance despite diminished biliary cholesterol secretion. Cheno, in chronic administration only, probably reduces cholesterol secretion by inhibiting cholesterol synthesis[8,9]; intestinal absorption[10] is not modified. The different cholesterol solubilising capacity of the two bile acids also contributes to the different mechanism of dissolution: cheno solubilises cholesterol in micelles, but urso also transports cholesterol in liquid crystals[11].

CLINICAL EFFECTS

The two agents have similar overall efficacy, achieving complete dissolution in about 40% of conventionally selected patients. Cheno, in the optimal dose (15/mg/day), induces troublesome diarrhoea in about 40% of patients. This unwanted effect is usually temporary, but discourages patients and is a major cause of drop outs. Cheno also induces hypertransaminasaemia and increases serum LDL-cholesterol[4,12]. Urso is free of unwanted effects and seems to dissolve gallstones faster than cheno[4]. For these reasons we believe that the problem now is no longer choosing between cheno and urso, but rather defining the reasons for the relatively low efficacy of oral bile acid therapy.

There are three major limitations to oral gallstone dissolution: its efficacy only in small radiolucent gallstones in functioning gallbladders, the occurrence of calcification during treatment, and the tendency for gallstones to recur after dissolution.

The first point applies equally to urso and cheno. Calcification during treatment, which precludes further dissolution, was initially observed only during urso treatment, due to the formation of calcium-glycoursodeoxycholate; it was suggested that the administration of tauroursodeoxycholic acid could prevent it. In recent studies[14], however, we have shown gallstone calcification during both cheno and urso treatment which was not avoided by giving tauroursodeoxycholic acid simultaneously. We found no factors predicting gallstone calcification, except that it seemed more common in older patients. Our results, together with reports of calcification during placebo administration[12], suggest that calcification may simply be part of the natural history of gallstone disease rather than an unwanted effect of oral bile acid treatment.

In a recent long-term study[15] we evaluated the effect of continuous treatment with low-dose urso, and factors predicting gallstone recurrence. The cumulative gallstone recurrence rate was 12.5% in the first year, rising to 61% by the eleventh year. Urso 300 mg/day significantly reduced the frequency of gallstone recurrence, by comparison with no treatment, only in patients aged under 50. Recurrence was significantly more common in patients who presented with multiple stones than in those with solitary stones. No other factors could be identified.

SUMMARY

Cheno and urso are the two alternative bile acids available for gallstone dissolution. They both lower cholesterol saturation in bile by reducing cholesterol output. Although they have similar overall efficacy in dissolving gallstones, urso is preferred because it has no side-effects (diarrhoea, hypertransaminasaemia and increased serum LDL-cholesterol) and because it induces faster dissolution especially for small gallstones. The limitations to dissolution therapy include the need to select small radiolucent stones in functioning gallbladders; the occurrence of calcification during treatment (especially on urso); and the high recurrence rate following successful gallstone dissolution.

REFERENCES

1. Johnston, C.G. and Nakayama, F. (1957). Solubility of cholesterol and gallstones in metabolic material. *Arch. Surg.*, **75**, 436
2. Danzinger, R.G., Hofmann, A.F. and Shoenfield, L.J. (1972). Dissolution of cholesterol gallstones by chenodeoxycholic acid. *N. Engl. J. Med.*, **286**, 1
3. Makino, I. and Shginozaky, K. (1975). Dissolution of cholesterol gallstones by ursodeoxycholic acid. *Jap. J. Gastroenterol.*, **72**, 690
4. Roda, E., Bazzoli, F. and Labate, A.M.M. *et al.* (1982). Ursodeoxycholic acid vs chenodeoxycholic acid as cholesterol dissolving agents: a comparative randomised study. *Hepatology*, **2**, 804
5. van Berge Henegouwen, G.P. and Hofmann, A.F. (1977). Pharmacology of chenodeoxycholic acid: II Absorption and Metabolism. *Gastroenterology*, **73**, 300
6. Sama, C., La Russo, N.F. and Lopez del Pino, V. *et al.* (1982). Effects of bile acids administration on biliary lipid secretion in healthy volunteers. *Gastroenterology*, **82**, 515
7. Hardison, W.G.M. and Grundy, S.M. (1984). Effect of ursodeoxycholic acid and its taurine conjugate on bile acid synthesis and cholesterol absorption. *Gastroenterology*, **87**, 130
8. Coyne, M.J., Bonorris, G.G. and Goldstein, L.I. *et al.* (1976). Effect of chenodeoxycholic acid and phenobarbital on the rate limiting enzymes of hepatic cholesterol and bile acid synthesis in patients with gallstones. *J. Lab. Clin. Med.*, **87**, 281
9. Ahlberg, J., Angelin, B. and Einarsson, K. (1981). Hepatic 3-hydroxy-3-methylglutaril Coenzyme A reductase activity and biliary lipid composition in man: relation to cholesterol gallstone disease and effects of cholic and chenodeoxycholic acid treatment. *J. Lipid. Res.*, **22** 410
10. Einarsson, K. and Grundy, S.M. (1980). Effects of feeding cholic acid and

chenodeoxycholic acid on cholesterol absorption and hepatic secretion of biliary lipid in man. *J. Lipid. Res.*, **21**, 23

11. Salvioli, G., Igimi, H. and Carey, M.C. (1983). Cholesterol gallstone dissolution in bile. Dissolution kinetics of crystalline cholesterol monohydrate by conjugated cheno- deoxycholate-lecithin and conjugated ursodeoxycholate-lecithin mixtures: dissolution phase equilibria and dissolution mechanisms. *J. Lipid. Res.*, **24**, 701

12. Shoenfield, L.J. and Lachin, J.M. (1981). The Steering Committee and The National Cooperative Gallstone Study Group. Chenodiol (chenodeoxycholic acid) for dissolu- tion of gallstones: The National Cooperative Gallstone Study. *Ann. Intern. Med.*, **95**, 257

13. Frabboni, R., Bazzoli, F. and Mazzella, G. *et al.* (1985). Acquired gallstone calcification during cholelitholytic treatment with chenodeoxycholic, ursodeoxycholic and taurour- sodeoxycholic acids. *Hepatology*, **5**, 1004

14. Villanova, N., Bazzoli, F., Frabboni, R. *et al.* (1987). Gallstone recurrence after success- ful oral bile acid treatment: a follow up study and evaluation of postdissolution treat- ment. *Gastroenterolgy*, **92**, 1789

13

Non-Surgical Treatment
of Gallstones:
Cheno- plus Ursodeoxycholic Acid

M. Podda, M. Zuin and P.M. Battezzati
Istituto di Medicina Interna
Milan University
Italy

INTRODUCTION

Oral therapy for gallstones has, some say, induced more disillution than dissolution[1,2]; others are less pessimistic[3]. Few patients with gallstones fulfill the criteria for successful treatment[4] and many are disappointed by the limited efficacy of dissolution therapy, or discouraged by its adverse effects, duration and cost.

The increasing use of abdominal ultrasonography, by detecting stones earlier, might make more patients eligible for litholytic therapy, but a recent epidemiological study suggests that the increase will be small[5]. New oral litholytic drugs will probably increase efficacy and safety, and reduce the duration and costs of treatment in patients suitable for dissolution therapy[6]. At present, however, these objectives could be pursued by a more rational use of the litholytic bile acids already available – cheno and urso. One approach is to administer cheno and urso together. The combination of the different properties of each bile acid should allow a lower dosage, and thus reduce cost and toxicity.

In this chapter we shall review the mechanism of action of cheno and urso and then show how giving both together enhance efficacy and reduces cost.

RATIONALE FOR CHENO PLUS URSO

Several reviews on this topic have been recently published[7,8] and a detailed discussion is beyond the scope of this chapter.

Table 1 shows the physico-chemical and metabolic properties of cheno and urso and emphasises how different, but in some respects complementary, they are.

Table 1 Differences in physico-chemical and metabolic properties of cheno and urso

	Cheno	Urso
Detergent capacity	↑↑	↑
Cholesterol solubilisation in micelles	↑↑	↑
Cholesterol solubilisation in liquid crystals	o	↑↑
Cholesterol secretion	↓	↓↓
Bile acid synthesis	↓↓	(↑)
Cholesterol absorption	o	↓

The most important advantage of combined therapy is the possibility of exploiting the two mechanisms of cholesterol solubilisation. Uro has, in fact, lower capacity to solubilise cholesterol into micelles than cheno, but only urso also dissolves cholesterol by forming liquid crystals[9]. The combination therefore allows the formation of a mesophase[10] and its subsequent dispersion into mixed micelles, whilst unsaturated micelles still collide with the surface of the stone and solubilise cholesterol from it. Each drug exerts different but possibly complementary effects on cholesterol metabolism which has a key role in dissolution[7,8].

Urso reduces biliary cholesterol secretion much more than cheno does[11,12], but it does not reduce *de novo* synthesis of bile acids from cholesterol – indeed, it may even increase it[11,12].

Cheno may be associated with transient hypertransaminasaemia[13,14], whilst urso prevents liver injury induced by mono- and dihydroxy bile acids both *in vitro* and *in vivo* [15-18]. Table 2 shows the other unwanted effects of urso and cheno alone, which may be reduced or even eliminated by combined therapy.

Table 2 Advantages and disadvantages of treatment with cheno and urso

	Cheno	Urso
Gallstone calcification	±	+
Hypertransaminaemia	+	o
Diarrhoea	+	o
Plasma triglycerides	↓	o
Plasma LDL-cholesterol	↑	o
Cost of treatment	+	+ +

CHANGES IN BILIARY LIPIDS WITH CHENO PLUS URSO

We[19] and others[20] have compared the effects of a combination of equimolar cheno and urso (5–8 mg/kg of each) with those of each bile acid alone in the same total dose (10–15 mg/kg) on biliary lipid composition after 6–12 weeks of treatment within the same patients. In both studies, the molar percentage of cholesterol in bile was significantly lower on urso alone and on the combination than on cheno alone. When, however, the capacity to solubilise cholesterol into micelles was calculated, taking into account the percentage of urso in bile, using the correction factor of Carey[21], cholesterol saturation fell more on cheno plus urso than on either bile acid alone (Figure 1).

Table 3 Biliary lipids and biliary bile acid composition before and during treatment with urso (10 mg/kg) and cheno plus urso (5 mg/kg of each)

	URSO (n = 21)		CHENO + URSO (n = 24)	
	Before[o]	During	Before	During
Bile acids (molar %)	70.5 ± 6.6	73.3 ± 7.0	68.5 ± 8.6	69.3 ± 7.1
Cholesterol (molar %)	9.8 ± 2.5	5.4 ± 1.9*	9.5 ± 2.2	5.2 ± 1.7*
Phospholipids (molar) %)	19.7 ± 4.7	21.3 ± 6.0	22.2 ± 7.1	25.4 ± 6.5
Urso (%)	1.1 ± 1.3		43.2 ± 8.7*	0.8 ± 0.6
Cheno (%)	31.7 ± 7.2	23.7 ± 6.5*	31.1 ± 8.4	49.4 ± 6.2**
Deoxycholic acid (%)	29.5 ± 9.0	15.6 ± 5.6*	20.9 ± 8.9	7.4 ± 2.0**
Lithocholic acid (%)	3.2 ± 1.5	3.3 ± 1.6	3.2 ± 1.9	3.8 ± 1.7
Cholic acid (%)	34.4 ± 6.4	14.1 ± 5.4*	35.0 ± 8.7	9.4 ± 2.8**

[o]means ± SD
*   p < 0.01 vs initial values by analysis of variance
**   p < 0.01 urso vs cheno + urso, by analysis of covariance

Uncontrolled studies have recently shown changes in biliary lipids with the combination at a total dose of about 15 mg/kg[22].

In conclusion, the combination induces those changes in biliary lipid composition (a marked decrease in biliary cholesterol saturation and a high proportion of litholytic bile acids) which most favour the rapid removal of cholesterol from gallstones.

CLINICAL EFFICACY OF CHENO PLUS URSO

Only preliminary or uncrontrolled studies have been reported on the efficacy of the cheno plus urso combination for gallstone dissolution.

Roehrkasse et al.[22] treated 16 patients with about 6.5 mg/kg urso and 7.5 mg/kg cheno for an average of 19 months. They reported a response rate of 60% at 1 year, with one complete and eight partial dissolutions. Longer periods of treatment gave further improvements and no side effects were noted. Thistle *et al.*[23] treated 10 patients with 5 mg/kg urso plus 10 mg/kg cheno for 24 months and claimed 'more effective stone dissolution' than with urso alone (10 mg/kg) or urso (10 mg/kg) plus taurine (2 g/day).

Czygan[24] has reported, in preliminary form, the results of three prospective controlled trials involving a total of 159 patients. In each trial the dissolution rate was significantly higher in patients treated with urso (5–8 mg/kg) plus cheno (5–10 mg/kg) than in those treated with urso (10–12.4 mg/kg) alone. Total dissolution rates with the combination were 53%, 80% and 58% in the three studies, compared with 33%, 40% and 40% respectively with urso alone. Czygan claimed[24] that the efficacy of the combination may be further enhanced by the administration of the entire dose at bedtime, rather than in three divided doses with meals.

Kawamoto *et al.*[25] compared the efficacy of different proportions of urso and cheno in combination. They found that increasing the proportion of urso from 33% to 50% and 66% (with a total dose of bile acid of about 10 mg/kg) increased dissolution rates from 29% to 48% and 72% respectively.

We have recently compared the efficacy of an equimolar combination of cheno (5 mg/kg) plus urso (5 mg/kg) with urso (10 mg/kg) alone in a total of 120 patients with radiolucent gallstones less than 15 mm in diameter (Table 4), mostly diagnosed at a screening ultrasonography. Patients were stratified into two groups according to the diameter of their largest stone before randomisation. Cholecystography and ultrasonography were repeated after 6, 12 and 24 months of treatment. At 6 months we found a significantly higher complete dissolution rate in patients with smaller stones treated with the combination (52%) than in those treated with urso alone (24%).

Table 4 Characteristics of patients at enrolment

	URSO (n = 60)	CHENO + URSO (n = 60)	TOTAL (n = 120)
Men (n)	20	19	39
Women (n)	40	41	81
Age (years, mean ± SD)	46 ± 11	48 ± 11	47 ± 11
Weight (kg, mean ± SD)	64 ± 6	65 ± 7	65 ± 7
With stones ≤ 5 mm (n)	25	25	50
With single stones (n)	19	18	37
With floating stones (n)	27	29	56

The complete plus partial dissolution rate also showed the combination to be more efficacious (68% vs 48% at 6 months). After longer treatment we found even higher dissolution rates with the combination, but the improvement over urso alone became smaller and non-significant. As expected, we found lower dissolution rates in the patients with larger stones, the difference between the two treatments being significant only for partial dissolution at 6 months (51% vs 26%).

The combination of urso plus cheno, unlike urso alone[26] does not seem to promote calcification of radiolucent gallstones. Czygan found no calcification during combination therapy[24], whilst we found acquired calcification in 7 of the 60 patients treated with urso alone and only in one of the 60 treated with the combination.

CLINICAL SAFETY

The cheno plus urso combination has been well tolerated[19,20,22-24] in all studies so far reported. About 10% of patients noted occasional diarrhoea during the first weeks of treatment but none needed to interrupt treatment.

Roehrkasse *et al.*[22] reported no change in liver function tests, particularly transaminase, whilst we found that on the combination transaminases rose above twice the upper limit of normal only transiently in a few patients.

Serum levels of triglycerides, total and HDL cholesterol do not change during the combination treatment[21,22].

IS THE COMBINATION THE BEST CHOICE?

Efficacy

The clinical trial data so far reported and our recent contolled study have demonstrated that the combined administration of cheno plus urso can achieve high dissolution rates. Comparative studies would have to be very large to demonstrate that the combination is clearly better than either bile acid alone in achieving complete dissolution, after prolonged treatment – the most relevant and objective outcome measurement for cholelitholytic therapy. We and others[24] have, however, already found the combination to achieve higher response rates (partial plus complete dissolutions, or complete dissolution of small stones) after short periods of treatment. This suggests that the combination of cheno with urso dissolves stones more quickly than urso alone, just as urso alone dissolves stones more rapidly than cheno alone[27,28] so that the it may be the best choice for rapid dissolution. The combination has therefore been chosen as adjuvant treatment in extracorporeal shock wave lithotripsy[29].

A different proportion of urso, or a higher total dose of bile acid, could prove more effective than the equimolar combination of 10 mg/kg we used, whilst the administration of the entire dose at bedtime would probably further enhance efficacy.

Stone calcification

The calcification of stones during treatment may greatly hinder complete stone dissolution. It was acquired by 12% of patients on urso alone in our study, an incidence similar to that reported in other trials[26]. It has been attributed mainly to the high concentration of poorly soluble glyco-conjugates of urso in bile during treatment with urso[30], though during treatment with cheno alone, calcification has also been demonstrated[31,32].

Why the incidence appears to be lower on the combination regimen is not known. It might be because on the combination the concentration of poorly soluble glycourso conjugates in bile is lower, or the proportion of other soluble conjugates is higher, or both. It might be because the proportion of unconjugated urso in bile is lower, as this has been suggested to increase the amount of bicarbonate and free calcium ions[33], thus leading to the deposition of calcium carbonate on the stone surface.

Safety

The unwanted effects of cheno[13,14] have decreased its popularity, whilst the good tolerability and safety of urso has been widely confirmed in many trials[34]. The combined regimen also seems to be well tolerated despite the presence of cheno. This is not surprising, since the toxicity and unwanted effects of cheno are dose-related[13] and the dose used in the combination is lower than that associated with significant unwanted effects. The administration of cheno with urso probably also avoids toxicity, as several experimental models have shown for bile acid-induced liver injury[15-17].

Cost

Both cheno and urso are relatively expensive but, as a raw material, urso costs about twice as much as cheno, from which it is derived. In Italy, a branded cheno is now 3-4 times cheaper than urso, but this does not vitiate its major unwanted effects. The cost of the combination is therefore most relevantly compared with that of urso alone. In Italy, the combination we used costs 30% less than urso alone. The same may not be true in other countries, or if the combination is marketed as a single formulation.

SUMMARY

The administration of cheno with urso combines the different actions of each bile acid in dissolving gallstones. It achieves a greater reduction in cholesterol saturation of bile than does either bile acid alone and, in the few clinical trials so far reported, greater clinical efficacy in dissolution treatment. The combination also avoids the unwanted effects of cheno, and appears to cause stone calcification less often than urso. It is likely to prove the treatment of choice for oral gallstone dissolution therapy.

REFERENCES

1. Dissolving hopes for gallstone dissolution (Editorial) (1981). *Lancet*, **2**, 905–6
2. Isselbacher, K.J. (1981). Chenodiol for gallstones: dissolution or disillusion? (Editorial). *Ann. Intern. Med.*, **95**, 377–9
3. Palmer, R.H. and Carey, M.C. (1982). An optimistic view of the National Cooperative Gallstone Study. *N. Engl. J. Med.*, **306**, 1171–4
4. Northfield, T.C. and Maudgal, D.P. (1986). Oral medical therapy. In: Bateson, M.C. (ed.), *Gallstone Disease and its Management*, pp. 203–27. (Lancaster: MTP Press)
5. Barbara, L., Sama, C., Morselli Labate A.M. *et al.* (1987). A Population study on the prevalence of gallstone disease: the Sirmione study. *Hepatology*, **7**, 913–7
6. Fromm, H. (1986). Gallstone dissolution therapy. Current status and future prospects. *Gastroenterology*, **91**, 1560–7
7. Fromm, H. (1984). Gallstone dissolution and the cholesterol-bile acid-lipoprotein axis. Propitious effect of ursodeoxycholic acid. *Gastroenterology*, **87**, 229–33
8. Tint, G.S., Salen, G. and Shefer, S. (1986). Effect of ursodeoxycholic acid and chenodeoxycholic acid on cholesterol and bile acid metabolism. *Gastroenterology*, **90**, 1007–18
9. Salvioli, G., Igimi, H. and Carey, M.C. (1983). Cholesterol gallstone dissolution in bile. Dissolution kinetics of crystalline cholesterol monohydrate by conjugated chenodeoxycholate-lecithin mixtures: dissimilar phase equilibria and dissolution mechanism. *J. Lipid Res.*, **24**, 701–20
10. Corrigan, O.I., Su, C.C., Higuchi, W.I. and Hofmann, A.F. (1980). Mesophase formation during cholesterol dissolution in ursodeoxycholate-lecithin solutions: new mechanism for gallstone dissolution in humans. *J. Pharm. Sci.*, **69**, 869–71
11. von Bergmann, K., Epple-Gutsfeld, M. and Leiss, O. (1984). Differences in the effects of chenodeoxycholic and ursodeoxycholic acids in biliary lipid secretion and bile acid synthesis in patients with gallstones. *Gastroenterology*, **87**, 136–43
12. Nilsell, K., Angelin, B., Leijd, B. and Einarsson, K. (1983). Comparative effect of ursodeoxycholic acid and chenodeoxycholic acid on bile acid kinetics and biliary lipid secretion in man. Evidence for different modes of action on bile acid synthesis. *Gastroenterology*, **85**, 1248–56
13. Mok, H.Y.I., Bell, G.D. and Dowling, R.H. (1974). Effect of different doses of chenodeoxycholic acid on bile lipid composition and on frequency of side effects in patients with gallstones. *Lancet*, **2**, 253–7
14. Thistle, J.L., Hofmann, A.F., Ott, B.J. and Stephens, D.H. (1978). Chenotherapy for gallstone dissolution: I. Efficacy and safety. *J. Am. Med. Assoc.*, **239**, 1041–6
15. Miyai, K., Toyota, N., Jones, H.M. and Gochman, N. (1982). Protective effect of ursodeoxycholic acid against cholestatic and hepatotoxic effects of lithocholic acid (Abstr.). *Hepatology*, **2**, 705
16. Krol, T., Kitamura, T., Miyai, K. and Hardison, W. (1983). Tauroursodeoxycholate reduces dictular proliferation in bile duct-ligated hamsters (Abstr.). *Hepatology*, **3**, 881
17. Tanikawa, K., Kawahara, T., Kumashiro, R. *et al.* (1986). Effects of bile acids on the cultured hepatocyte and Kupffer cell (Abstr.). *Hepatology*, **6**, 779
18. Poupon, R., Chretien, Y., Poupon, R.E. *et al.* (1987). Is ursodeoxycholic acid an effective treatment for primary biliary cirrhosis? *Lancet*, **1**, 834–6
19. Podda, M., Zuin, M., Dioguardi, M.L., Festorazzi, S. and Dioguardi, N. (1982). A combination of chenodeoxycholic acid and ursodeoxycholic acid is more effective than

either alone in reducing biliary cholesterol saturation. *Hepatology*, **2**, 334–9

20. Stiehl, A., Raedsch, R., Czygan, P., Gotz, R., Manner, C.H. and Walker, S. (1980). Effects of biliary bile acid composition on biliary cholesterol saturation in gallstone patients treated with chenodeoxycholic acid and/or ursodeoxycholic acid. *Gastoenterology*, **79**, 1192–8

21. Carey, M.C. and Ko, G. (1979). The importance of total lipid concentration in determining cholesterol solubility in bile and the development of critical tables for calculating 'percent cholesterol saturation' with a correction factor for ursodeoxycholic-rich bile. In: Paumgartner, G., Stiehl, A. and Gerok, W. (eds.), *Biological Effects of Bile Acids*, pp. 299–308. (Lancaster: MTP Press).

22. Roehrkasse, R., Fromm, H., Malavolti, M., Tunuguntla, A.K. and Ceryak, S. (1986). Gallstone dissolution treatment with a combination of chenodeoxycholic and ursodeoxycholic acids. Studies of safety, efficacy and effects on bile lithogenicity, bile acid pool and serum lipids. *Dig. Dis. Sci*, **31**, 1032–40

23. Thistle, J.L. (1987). Dissolution of gallstones using ursodeoxycholic acid with or without chenodeoxycholic acid or taurine. In: Paumgartner, G., Stiehl, A. and Gerok, W. (eds.), *Biological Effects of Bile Acids*, pp. 353–4. (Lancaster: MTP Press).

24. Czygan, P (1987). Efficacy of combined ursodeoxycholic and chenodeoxycholic acid treatment. In: Paumgartner, G., Stiehl, A. and Gerok, W. (eds.), *Biological Effects of Bile Acids*, pp. 343–4. (Lancaster: MTP Press).

25. Kawamoto, T., Horiuchi, I., Hino, F., Okahashi, M. and Kajiyama, G. (1984). Combination treatment with different doses of urso (U)- and chenodeoxycholic acid (C) in patients with cholesterol gallstones (Abstr.). In: *Proceedings of the VIII International Bile Acid Meeting, Berne*, p. 183

26. Bateson, M.C., Bouchier, I.A.D., Trash, D.B., Maudgal, D.P. and Northfield, T.C. (1981). Calcification of radiolucent gallstones during treatment with ursodeoxycholic acid. *Br. Med. J.*, **283**, 645–6

27. Roda, E., Bazzoli, F., Labate, W.M.N. *et al.* (1982). Ursodeoxycholic acid vs chenodeoxycholic acid as cholesterol gallstone dissolving agents: a comparative study. *Hepatology*, **2**, 804–10

28. Fromm, H., Roat, J.N., Gonzales, V., Sarva, R.J. and Farivar, S. (1983). Comparative efficacy and side effects of ursodeoxycholic acid and chenodeoxycholic acid in dissolving gallstones. *Gastoenterology*, **85**, 1257–64

29. Sauerbruch, T., Delius, M., Paumgartner, G *et al.* (1986). Fragmentation of gallstone by extracorporeal shock waves. *N. Engl. J. Med.*, **314**, 818–22

30. Igimi, H. and Carey, M.C. (1980). pH-solubility relation of chenodeoxycholic and ursodeoxycholic acids: physical-chemical basis for dissimilar dissolution and membrane phenomena. *J. Lipid Res.*, **21**, 72–89

31. Schoenfield, L.J. and Lachin, J.M. (1981). The Steering Committee and the National Cooperative Gallstone Study Group. Chenodiol (chenodeoxycholic acid) for dissolution of gallstones: The National Cooperative Gallstone Study. *Ann. Intern. Med.*, **95**, 257–82

32. Toulet, J., Rousselet, J., Viteau, J.M. *et al.* (1983). Dissolutions incomplete des calculs. Calcification, cholecystectomies après traitment de la lithiase vesiculaire par l'acide chenodesoxycholique. *Gastroenterol. Clin. Biol.*, **7**, 969–74

33. Hofmann, A.F. and Cummings, S.A. (1985). Biliary calcium secretion and its relationship to biliary calcium concentration and biliary calcium activity. In: Barbara, L., Dowling, P.H., Hofmann, A.F. and Roda, E. (eds.), *Recent Advances in Bile Acid Research*, pp. 87–108. (New York: Raven Press)

34. Bachrach, W.H. and Hofmann, A.F. (1982). Ursodeoxycholic acid in the treatment of cholesterol cholelithiasis. *Dig. Dis. Sci*, **27**, 833–55

14

Non-Surgical Treatment of Gallstones: Methyl Tert-Butyl Ether

J.L. Thistle
Division of Gastroenterology
Mayo Clinic
Rochester, MN 55905, USA

INTRODUCTION

Cholelithiasis is a major cause of morbidity in the western world and in the United States about 500,000 cholecystectomies are performed annually. Although cholecystectomy provides a safe and effective treatment a non-surgical treatment has been sought for several reasons. The medical expenses and loss of time from the work force have an important impact on the national economy. Many patients fear general anaesthesia and major abdominal surgery, and may find postoperative disability for several weeks an inconvenient and expensive detraction from their vocation.

Most gallstones are composed mostly of cholesterol, a lipid which can be easily dissolved by many organic solvents. The rapid dissolution of cholesterol gallstones in the gallbladder would therefore seem potentially feasible, if a biologically tolerable solvent could be delivered safely and effectively to the gallbladder. Diethyl ether and chloroform were evaluated *in vivo* several decades ago but discarded because they proved to be unpleasant or toxic[1-3]. Mono-octanoin was the first direct contact cholesterol gallstone solvent shown to be practicable[4]. Its major shortcoming is that it solubilises cholesterol very slowly so that the stones must be in contact with the solvent for several days to weeks to dissolve substantially.

We were therefore stimulated to search for a rapidly acting and safe solvent for direct cholesterol gallstone dissolution. An ether which retained the cholesterol solubilising characteristics of diethyl ether but remained liquid at body temperature, methyl tert-butyl ether (MTBE), was identified. MTBE is a laboratory solvent and an octane enhancer for gasoline so that, acute toxicity studies were already available and suggested a very low level

195

of toxicity[5].

METHYL TERT-BUTYL ETHER

Methyl tert-butyl ether is an aliphatic hydrocarbon with a boiling point of 55°C. It is a potentially explosive and flammable agent with a lower limit of explosivity of 1.5 to 2 volumes per cent, but appears to be more stable than diethyl ether partly because it is less likely to form peroxides. Toxicity studies in animals suggest that MTBE and diethyl ether have similar but low toxicity. Intravenous infusion of MTBE in rats can cause intravascular haemolysis. MTBE dissolved 200–300 mg cholesterol gallstones *in vitro* completely within 1 hour[6]. We therefore started studies of its efficacy in animals.

Percutaneous Transhepatic Gallbladder Catheter Placement

A simple, safe, and inexpensive method of introducing the solvent into the gallbladder was the first requirement. By placing a fine catheter through the hepatic parenchyma into the gallbladder via the gallbladder–hepatic attachment, we hoped to be able to safely remove the catheter after one or two days without a major risk of bile leakage. We therefore first tried out in animals a 5 F.G. (1.7 mm diameter) pigtail catheter which we had designed for percutaneous transhepatic gallbladder placement in patients.

Animal Studies

Dogs were prepared by surgically implanting human gallstones and the pigtail catheter into the gallbladder. After healing, MTBE was infused and aspirated for 4–16 hours. Histological examination of the gallbladder mucosa by light microscopy and scanning electron microscopy demonstrated only slight changes. Clinical, laboratory, and histological evaluation revealed no evidence of significant systemic toxicity[7].

Human Studies

Studies in humans have confirmed the efficacy and safety suggested by the *in vitro* and animal studies[8]. Percutaneous transhepatic catheter placement has been accomplished in more than 70 patients without failure. We have found fluoroscopic guidance after oral contrast ingestion most convenient for catheter placement, but we have occasionally used ultrasonography in the absence of adequate opacification of the gallbladder.

The pigtail catheter is placed with at least one full loop of catheter in the gallbladder and the pigtail in the fundus, and as many stones as possible are manipulated into the centre of the pigtail (Figure 1). The volume of radio-

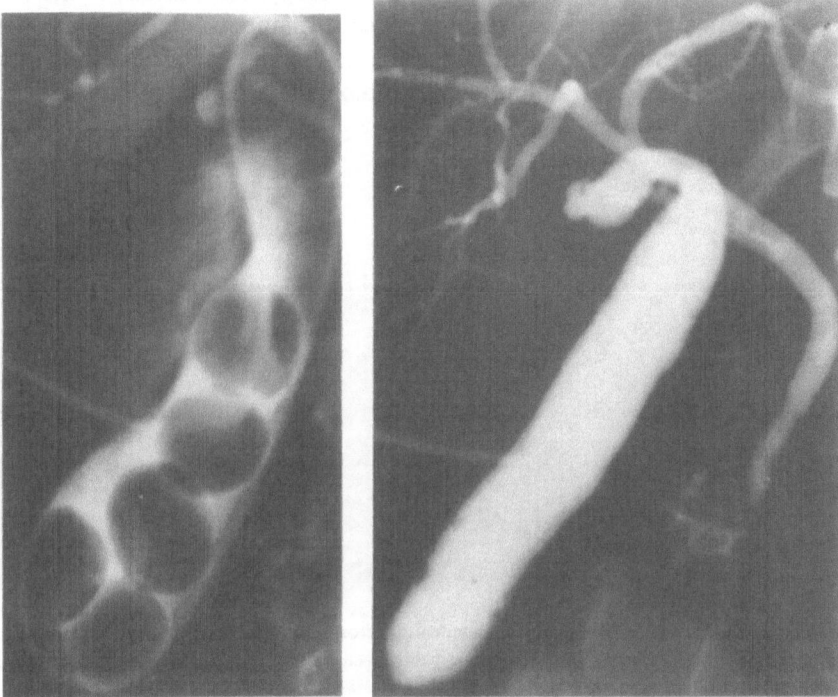

Figure 1 A. Percutaneous transhepatic catheterisation of the gallbladder with full loop of catheter in the gallbladder and pigtail in the fundus. B. Complete dissolution of all five stones and patent normal duct system.

opaque contrast media which envelopes the stones but does not overflow from the gallbladder is determined radiologically and used as the exchange volume for MTBE treatment. Usually 3–5 ml covers the stones well, and the overflow volume is often only 7–15 ml and occasionally less. Excessive overflow of MTBE out of the gallbladder can induce anaesthesia, nausea and vomiting. We have observed duodenitis and intravascular haemolysis in one early patient, in whom overflow persisted throughout the day. These changes caused no symptoms and reversed rapidly, allowing subsequent continuation of therapy[9].

We infuse and aspirate MTBE continuously by hand. An automatic pump designed for this purpose is being developed. All MTBE and bile is removed from the gallbladder at the end of each aspiration, because MTBE floats on bile and bile interferes with the stone-solvent contact. The MTBE is replaced every 10–15 minutes to avoid saturating it with cholesterol. The position of stones within the gallbladder and their size is monitored fluoroscopically every 2–4 hours. Treatment is continued for 1–2 hours after no residual stone material can be seen by fluoroscopy. The patency of the duct system is checked by showing free flow of contrast into the duodenum before removing the catheter. A representative example is illustrated in Figure 1. The five characteristic smooth ovoid radiolucent cholesterol stones were rapidly and completely dissolved.

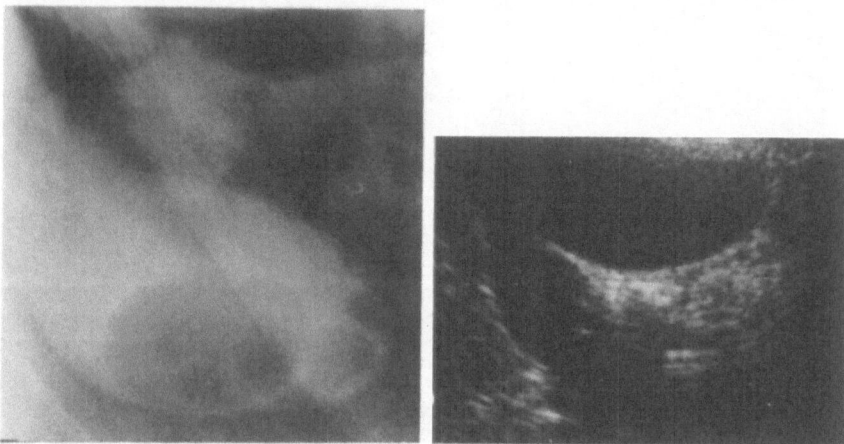

Figure 2   A. Several radiolucent cholesterol gallstones with normal gallbladder opacification at oral cholecystography. B. Ultrasonogram revealing complete stone dissolution without residual non-cholesterol debris.

A little residual debris (1–3 mm diameter) is common but usually detectable only by ultrasound examination. It rarely causes symptoms. Smooth ovoid stones composed mainly of cholesterol can usually be dissolved in one day and often leave no residuum (Figure 2). Multiple large stones filling the gallbladder may need two or three days and often leave a small amount of residual non-cholesterol debris.

Calcified Stones

Stone calcification, even if only apparent on CT scan, often prevents complete dissolution with MTBE. Calcium solvents such as ethylenediamine-tetra-acetic acid are relatively slow, and vigorous prolonged efforts at calcium binding may be prohibited by the dependence of the integrity of mucosal tight junctions on the presence of calcium[10,11]. Fragmentation of calcified cholesterol stones would allow MTBE to reach the lipid-soluble components of the stone and greatly increase the surface area available for dissolution. If fragmentation resulted in particles no larger than 1–2 mm, some of the debris might be aspirated or flushed from the gallbladder. Several fragmentation methods are under investigation[12,13].

We have started to assess the use of shock-wave lithotripsy followed by MTBE fragment dissolution on the same day, initially in animals and most recently in patients with calcified stones[14-16]. The susceptibility of such stones to fragmentation varies widely and the number of shock waves required to fragment a single stone may approach or exceed the total number of shock waves shown to be safe in humans. Although it may become possible to pulverise all stones predictably and completely so that they pass without severe clinical consequences, dissolving the fragments in a few hours before they escape from the gallbladder seems an appealing approach.

SUMMARY

This new method of stone dissolution has rekindled enthusiasm for non-surgical methods of gallstone treatment. Predissolution stone fragmentation may allow its extension to at least partially calcified cholesterol stones. The techniques will importantly extend the practical non-surgical alternatives to cholecystectomy. We must not, in our enthusiasm, however, lose sight of the safety, speed and long-term efficacy of elective cholecystectomy.

REFERENCES

1. Pribam, B.O.C. (1939). Ether treatment of gallstones impacted in the common duct. *Lancet*, i, 1311–3
2. Alfthan, O. and Kohler, R. (1958/1959). Ether treatment of retained postoperative biliary tree stones. *Acta. Chir. Scand.*, 116, 437–49
3. Torresyap, F.C. (1958). Chloroform instillation of common bile duct. *AMA. Arch. Surg.*, 77, 903–7
4. Thistle, J.L., Carlson, G.L., Hofmann, A.F., LaRusso, N.F., MacCarty, R.L., Flynn, G.L., Higuchi, W.L. and Babayan, V.K. (1980). Monooctanoin, a dissolution agent for retained cholesterol bile duct stones: physical properties and clinical application. *Gastroenterology*, 78, 1016–22
5. Little, C.J., Dale, A.D., Wheatley, J.A. and Wickings, J.A. (1979). Methyl tertiary butyl ether: a new chromatographic eluent. *J. Chromatogr*, 169, 381–385
6. Allen, M.J., Borody, T.J. and Thistle, J.L. (1985). In vitro dissolution of cholesterol gallstones. A study of factors influencing rate and a comparison of solvents. *Gastroenterology*, 89, 1097–103
7. Allen, M.J., Borody, T.J., Bugliosi, T.F., May, G.R., LaRusso, N.F. and Thistle, J.L., (1985). Cholelitholysis using methyl tertiary butyl ether. *Gastroenterology*, 88, 122–25
8. Allen, M.J., Borody, T.J., Bugliosi, T.F., May, G.R., LaRusso, N.F. and Thistle, J.L. (1985). Rigid dissolution of gallstones by methyl tert-butyl ether. *N. Engl. J. Med.*, 312, 217–20
9. Thistle, J.L., Nelson, P.E. and May, G.R. (1986). Dissolution of cholesterol gallbladder stones using methyl tert-butyl ether. *Gastroenterology*, 90, 1775
10. Nelson, P.E., Moyer, T.P. and Thistle, J.L. (1987). Gallstone dissolution with methyl tert-butyl ether: radiologic selection criteria. *Gastroenterology*. (In press)
11. Nelson, P.E., Moyer, T.P. and Thistle, J.L. (1987). Dissolution of calcium bilirubinate and calcium carbonate debris remaining after methyl tert-butyl ether dissolution of cholesterol gallstones. *Gastroenterology*. (In press)

12. Sauerbruch, T., Delius, M., Paumgartner, G., Holl, J., Wess, O., Weber, W., Hepp, W. and Brendel, W. (1986). Fragmentation of gallstones by extracorporeal shock waves. *N. Eng. J. Med.*, **314**, 818–22

13. Sackmann, M., Delius, M., Sauerbruch, T., Holl, J., Weber, W., Hagelauer, U., Hepp, W., Brendel, W. and Paumgartner, G. (1987). Extracorporeal shock wave lithotripsy of gallbladder stones: results of 101 treatments. *Gastroenterology*, **92**, 1608

14. Peine, C.J., May, G.R., Nagorney, D.M., Patterson, D.E., Segura, J.W. and Thistle, J.L. (1986). Same day sequential extracorporeal shock wave lithotripsy and methyl tert-butyl ether dissolution of gallstones in dogs: effect on gallbladder mucosa and MTBE absorption. *Hepatology*, **6**, 1206

15. Peine, C.J., Nagorney, D.M., Madson, T.H., Patterson, D.E., Segura, J.W. and Thistle, J.L. (1987). Dissolution of radio-opaque gallstones: safety of alternating methyl tert-butyl ether with EDTA-polysorbate 20 and/or N-acetylcysteine with and without prior extracorporeal shock wave lithotripsy in dogs. *Gastroenterology*, **92**, 1763

16. Peine, C.J., Petersen, B.T., Williams, H.J., Bender, C.E., Patterson, D.E., Segura, J.W., Nagorney, D.M. and Thistle, J.L. (1987). Fragmentation and dissolution of calcified cholesterol gallstones using extracorporeal shock wave lithotripsy and methyl tert-butyl ether in humans *Hepatology*, **7**, 113 (abstract)

15
Non-Surgical Treatment of Gallstones: Lithotripsy

G. Paumgartner, M. Sackmann, J. Holl and T. Sauerbruch
Department of Medicine II
University of Munich
Federal Republic of Germany

INTRODUCTION

Several methods have been developed over the past decades for non-surgical treatment of gallbladder and bile duct stones. One of the major factors limiting the success of these methods has been stone size. The animal experiments of Brendel and Enders[1] have shown that gallstones can be fragmented *in vivo* by shock-waves generated outside the body. We treated the first patients with gallbladder and bile duct stones by extracorporeally generated shock-waves in 1985. Our early experience, published in 1986[2], has now been enlarged by treating more than 250 patients with gallbladder stones and more than 40 patients with bile duct stones.

Principles of Extracorporeal Shock-wave Lithotripsy

Shock-waves are high-pressure waves that obey the laws of acoustics. They can be generated by underwater spark discharge and focussed by an ellipsoidal reflector, to cause focus pressures of about 1000 bar. Such a system achieves a peak pressure within about 30 nanoseconds, and a positive pressure pulse duration of about one microsecond. The shock-waves travel practically unimpeded through water and soft tissue, and do not severely damage these tissues because no major change in acoustical impedance occurs. When an object such as a stone with an acoustical impedance different from water is placed at the shock-wave focus, the shock-wave creates pressure and tensile forces within the stone and cavitation phenomena at the surface of the stone. This leads to fragmentation of the stone.

Shock-wave Lithotripsy of Gallbladder Stones

For treatment of gallbladder stones the patient is placed prone, so that the shock\,196waves enter the abdomen from the ventral aspect. The lithotripter (Dornier MPL 9000) used by our group features a water cushion coupled with the skin by an ultrasonic gel to transmit the shock-waves into the body. The gallbladder and the stones are visualised by ultrasound. Real time ultrasound is also used to guide the positioning of the stones and to monitor the process of fragmentation.

The shock-waves are triggered by the R-waves of a continuously monitored electrocardiogram . On average, 1200 (460–1600) discharges are delivered within about 40 minutes. Early in the development of the procedure, all patients were treated under general anaesthesia. More recently, with the new lithotripter (Dornier MPL 9000) neither general anaesthesia nor epidural anaesthesia are required. Intravenous opiate analgesia with alfentanyl[3] has become the method of choice.

Table 1   Selection of patients with gallbladder stones for extracorporeal shock-wave lithotripsy

Inclusion criteria

1. History of biliary colic
2. Solitary radiolucent stone with a diameter up to 30 mm or up to 3 radiolucent stones with similar total stone volume.
3. Functioning gallbladder as documented by opacification on oral cholecystography
4. Clear detection of stone(s) by ultrasound and positioning in the shock-wave focus must be possible

Exclusion criteria

1. Acute cholecystitis, biliary obstruction or known bile duct stone
2. Gastroduodenal ulcer
3. Acute pancreatitis
4. Cysts or vascular aneurysms in the path of the shock-waves
5. Coagulopathy or current medication with anticoagulants, aspirin or non-steroidal anti-inflammatory drugs
6. Pregnancy (female patients must have lab test to exclude pregnancy)

We have demonstrated *in vitro* that cholesterol stones disintegrate to sand and small fragments that dissolve rapidly in a model bile containing a high percentage of ursodeoxycholic acid[4]. We therefore selected patients with radiolucent (presumed cholesterol) stones for shock-wave treatment plus adjuvant bile acid litholytic therapy to dissolve stone fragments. We used a combination of ursodeoxycholic acid and chenodeoxycholic acid (7–8 mg/kg body weight/day each), started at least one week before shock-wave treatment and continued for up to 3 months after complete disappearance of stone fragments.

Table 1 lists the criteria according to which the patients were selected for shock-wave lithotripsy. The stones were disintegrated by shock-waves in nearly all patients selected according to these criteria. About 50% of patients with solitary stones and 20% of patients with multiple stones were free of fragments 2–4 months after lithotripsy, and about 85% and 40% after 8–12 months bile acid treatment. All patients with solitary stones and about 75% of the patients with multiple stones who have been followed for two years were free of fragments[5].

All patients tolerated shock-wave treatment without serious adverse effects. Laboratory tests (such as aminotransferases, alkaline phosphatase, and bilirubin) showed no evidence of hepatocellular damage or hepatobiliary dysfunction. Cutaneous petechiae occurred in 14% of the patients and transient gross haematuria in 3%. Mild pancreatitis was observed one to six months after shock-wave treatment in about 1% of the patients. It resolved shortly after endoscopic sphincterotomy and extraction of two small stone fragments in one and spontaneously in another patient. Although all patients suffered biliary pain before treatment, only about one third experienced transient colicky pain prior to complete disappearance of stone fragments.

Shock-wave Lithotripsy of Bile Duct Stones

Our technique for fragmentation of bile duct stones was somewhat different from that used to fragment gallbladder stones. We used a Dornier kidney lithotripter. The patient was immersed supine in the water bath and the shock-waves entered the body from the rear[2,6]. This position was chosen to avoid interposition of intestinal gas between the shock-wave source and the stones. Treatment was preceded by endoscopic sphincterotomy and insertion of a nasobiliary catheter, in order to inject contrast medium into the common bile duct to show the common bile duct and the stones. The position and disintegration of the stones was monitored by fluoroscopy using a two-dimensional X-ray system.

Out of 168 patients referred for non-surgical treatment of bile duct stones, 34 patients were selected for extracorporeal shock-wave lithotripsy because their stones could not be removed by endoscopic techniques. Of these patients 25 had extrahepatic stones and nine had intrahepatic stones. The diameters of the stones ranged from 10-55 mm (mean 22 mm). The stones were impacted in most patients, and stone size and/or duct stenosis made endoscopic extraction impossible in the others.

Shock-wave lithotripsy produced stone fragments in 27 of the 34 patients (79%) which could easily be extracted endoscopically (17 patients) or passed spontaneously (10 patients). One patient developed acute cholecystitis after shock-wave lithotripsy and cholecystectomy had to be performed. Another patient suffered rupture of a juxta-papillary diverticulum but this was due to the endoscopic papillotomy performed prior to shock-wave lithotripsy.

Our results demonstrate that gallstones can successfully be treated by extracorporeal shock-wave lithotripsy in selected patients. Our stringent criteria lead to selection of only 28% of patients with gallbladder stones and 20% of patients with common bile duct stones for extracorporeal shock-wave treatment. It appears likely that with more experience, and with recent technical improvements, the indications for this new non-surgical therapeutic modality can be broadened.

SUMMARY

Extracorporeal shock-wave lithotripsy combined with medical dissolution therapy is a safe and effective treatment for selected patients with symptomatic gallbladder stones. Moreover, in about 80% of patients with bile duct stones that could not be removed by endoscopic procedures, extracorporeal shock-wave lithotripsy achieved rapid disappearance of stones and symptoms.

Acknowledgement

This work has been supported by the Koerber Foundation

REFERENCES

1. Brendel, W. and Enders, G. (1983). Shock-waves for gallstones: animal studies. *Lancet*, **1**, 1054
2. Sauerbruch, T., Delius, M., Paumgartner, G., Holl, J., Wess, O., Weber, W., Hepp, W. and Brendel, W. (1986). Fragmentation of gallstones by extracorporeal shock-waves. *N. Engl. J. Med.*, **314**, 818–22
3. Sackmann, M., Weber, W., Delius, M., Holl, J., Hagelauer, U., Sauerbruch, T., Brendel, W. and Paumgartner, G. (1987). Extracorporeal shock-wave lithotripsy of gallstones without general anesthesia: first clinical experience. *Ann. Intern. Med.*, **107**, 347–48
4. Neubrand, M., Sauerbruch, T., Stellaard, F. and Paumgartner, G. (1986). *In vitro* cholesterol gallstone dissolution after fragmentation with shock-waves. *Digestion*, **34**, 51–9
5. Sackmann, M., Delius, M., Sauerbruch, T., Holl, J., Weber, W., Ippisch, E., Hagelauer, U., Wess, O., Hepp, W., Brendel, W. and Paumgartner, G. (1988). Shock-wave lithotripsy of gallbladder stones. The first 175 patients. *N. Engl. J. Med.M*, **318**, 393–7
6. Sauerbruch, T., Holl, J., Sackmann, M., Jocham, D., Delius, M., Brendel, W. and Paumgartner, G. (1987). Treatment of bile duct stones by extracorporeal shock-waves. *Seminars in Ultrasound, CT and MR*, **8**, 155–61

16
Non-surgical Treatment of Gallstones: Overall Strategy

T.C Northfield and R.P. Jazrawi
*Department of Medicine II, St. George's Hospital Medical School,
London SW17 0RE, UK*

INTRODUCTION

The first requirement in tackling this broad subject is a satisfactory definition of strategy. Since the subject concerns the war against gallstone disease, and since this book is an international undertaking, we thought it appropriate to consult the writings of a famous military strategist, Von Clausewitz. He states that 'die Strategie ist der Gebrauch des Gefechts zum Zweck des Krieges'. This is translated as 'strategy is the use of battles for the object of the war'. Thus, strategy consists of relating methods to a clearly defined object. We would define the object of the war against gallstone disease as being 'to ensure that as many gallstone patients as possible are maintained free of gallstones in the long term'. In order to achieve this object, we have at present three non-surgical methods that we can use – a physical approach (fragmentation therapy or extracorporeal shock wave lithotripsy), a chemical approach (the use of chemical solvents, in particular methyl tert-butyl ether) and a physico-chemical approach (bile acid therapy using chenodeoxycholic acid (CDCA) and/or ursodeoxycholic acid UDCA)).

We will attempt here to answer three questions:

(1)   What proportion of gallstone patients is suitable for non-surgical treatment?

(2)   What is the role of bile acid therapy in relation to the new non-surgical therapies?

(3)   What is the best long term strategy for non-surgical therapy?

SUITABILITY FOR NON-SURGICAL TREATMENT

Table 1 predicts what proportion of patients are suitable for surgery and for the three non-surgical approaches to therapy, according to the specific selection criteria for each. The proportions given are based on the excellent Italian epidemiological data on patients with gallbladder stones detected by ultrasonography. We believe that only those patients with symptoms attributable to gallbladder disease should be considered for treatment, because evidence suggests that less than 20% of asymptomatic patients will develop symptoms or complications from their gallstones over the following 20 years[1]. Asymptomatic patients should only be observed.

Table 1 Suitable gallstone patients (%)

Criteria	BA therapy	Fragmentation	MTB	Surgery
Symptoms	33	33	33	33
Radiolucent	70	70	70	100
GB visualisation	70	70	70	100
Diameter <6 mm	10 ⎫	— ⎫	10 ⎫	100
6-15 mm	25 ⎬ 35	25 ⎬ 80	25 ⎬ 90	
5-30 mm	— ⎭	55 ⎭	55 ⎭	
All criteria	6	13	15	33
On therapy in UK	0.03 pa	—	—	1 pa

According to the Italian epidemiological data[2], only one-third of patients with gallstones on ultrasonographic screening have symptoms attributable to gallstones. Of these approximately 70% have radiolucent stones on oral cholecystography, and only these stones can be considered for non-surgical therapy. Symptomatic radio-opaque stones should therefore be considered for surgical treatment. Only 70% of gallstone patients achieve opacification of the gallbladder on oral cholecystography, a further requirement for all the non-surgical therapies. Gallstone diameter is <6 mm in 10% of cases, 6–15 mm in 25%, 15–30 mm in 55% and >30 mm in diameter in 10% of cases. Bile acid therapy is generally considered to be suitable only for small and medium sized stones (<15 mm diameter, 35% of the total), whilst fragmentation therapy is most suitable for stones with a diameter of 6–30 mm (80% of the total) and is not suitable for stones <6 mm in diameter[3]. MTBE is suitable for gallstones up to 30 mm diameter (90% of the total)[4], and of course there is no size limitation for surgery.

If all these criteria are considered together, then the proportion of people with gallstones potentially suitable for bile acid therapy is 6%, and for fragmentation therapy or MTBE 13–15%. All 33% having symptoms are potentially suitable for surgical treatment, but may be considered unfit for surgery due to old age or coexistent medical disease. We believe that the personal preference of the patient must also be taken into consideration.

Data from the Prescription Pricing Authority suggest that in the United Kingdom only 0.03% per annum of people with gallstones are receiving therapy with UDCA or CDCA, assuming that these drugs are being prescribed in the currently recommended doses. On the other hand, hospital discharge and death data for England and Wales[5] suggest that 1% per annum of gallstone patients are treated by cholecystectomy. The discrepancy is very large, and probably arises mainly because in the United Kingdom general practitioners traditionally refer the patient directly to a surgeon rather than to a physician. Surgeons only consider bile acid therapy for patients who are very reluctant to consider surgery, or in whom there are medical contraindications to surgery. The new non-surgical therapies may well change this balance if lithotripsy for renal stones is any guide, since very few of these are still being treated surgically.

OVERALL ROLE OF BILE ACID THERAPY

Gallstone dissolution is more rapid for small than for large gallstones. This is because the surface area/volume ratio is higher for small stones, as illustrated in Figure 1 by the close correspondence between the curve relating observed gallstone dissolution rate to diameter in 40 patients and the theoretical curve relating the surface area/volume ratio to the diameter of a sphere (unpublished observations). It can be seen in Figure 1 that almost all patients (12 out of 14) with gallstones 6 mm or less in diameter achieved more than 50% reduction in gallstone volume over the first 6 months, but only one of the eight patients with a gallstone diameter of 15 mm or more achieved this dissolution rate. Thus, bile acid therapy is most effective for gallstones < 6 mm in diameter. By contrast, fragmentation therapy is not suitable for gallstones < 6 mm diameter, so that in this respect the two methods of treatment are complementary. Indeed, it could be said that lithotripsy is an adjunct to bile acid therapy, and that the object of this form of treatment is to reduce large stones to small fragments that should respond rapidly to bile acid therapy.

Gallstone recurrence is likely to remain a problem with all forms of non-surgical treatment including MTBE. Since prevention of gallstone recurrence cannot be achieved by present methods (Chapter 11), redissolution of recurrent stones is necessary. With regular ultrasound observation, these recurrent stones should be detected when they are still < 6 mm in diameter. This points to a viable long term policy involving intermittent courses of bile acid therapy.

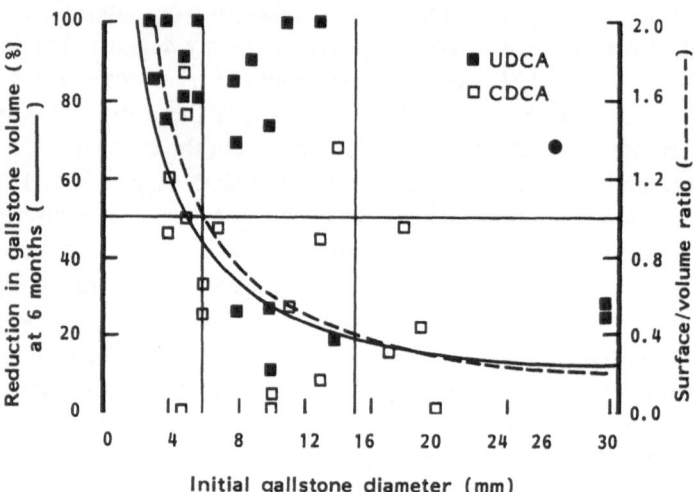

Figure 1 Relationship between initial gallstone diameter and gallstone dissolution rate during UDCA or CDCA (—); comparison with relationship between diameter and surface/volume ratio for a sphere(– – –).

LONG-TERM STRATEGY FOR NON-SURGICAL THERAPY

A mathematical model can be used to predict the proportion of gallstone patients who are free of gallstones at any time during intermittent bile acid therapy. This mathematical model[7] predicts that when a large proportion of a population (in this case gallstone-free patients) is affected by one life event to a small extent (gallstone recurrence), and the remainder of that population (with recurrent gallstones) is affected by an opposing life event to a large extent (gallstone redissolution), a steady state situation will be reached if an adequate follow up period is allowed. If we consider the number of gallstone free patients at time t (F_t), the recurrence rate (R) and the dissolution rate (D), then the number of gallstone–free patients a year later (F_{t+1}) is expressed by the following equation $F_{t+1} = F_t (1–R–D) + D$. When a steady state is reached: $F_{t+1} = F_t = F$

$$F = F (1–R–D) + D$$
$$F = D/(R+D)$$

208

According to this formula, the main factor which affects the proportion of gallstone-free patients when the steady state is reached is the recurrence rate (R). Applying the above equation to a cohort of 100 gallstone patients whose gallstones have dissolved and who are being followed up by annual ultrasonography, with an annual recurrence rate of 20% and an annual redissolution rate of 40%, then the number of gallstone-free patients when a steady state has been reached (F) = 40/(20 + 40) x 100 = 67

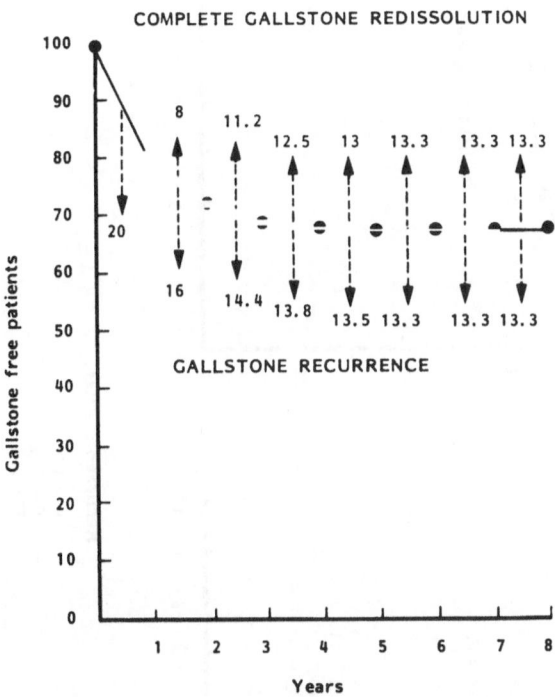

Figure 2 Gallstone-free patients (%), assuming a gallstone recurrence rate of 20% pa and a redissolution rate of 40% pa (reproduced from Northfield and Jazrawi, 1988[12]).

Figure 2 illustrates the course of events during the 5 years necessary to reach a steady state. The downward arrows show the absolute number of patients undergoing gallstone recurrence each year, and the upward arrows the absolute number of patients with gallstone recurrence who are achieving complete gallstone redissolution each year. Once a steady state situation has been reached 67 patients are gallstone free at any given time, as already calculated from the equation above.

In practice, a redissolution rate of 80% may be achievable. This corresponds to our best results for initial dissolution in the first year in a group of patients with radiolucent stones less than 15 mm diameter in an opacify-

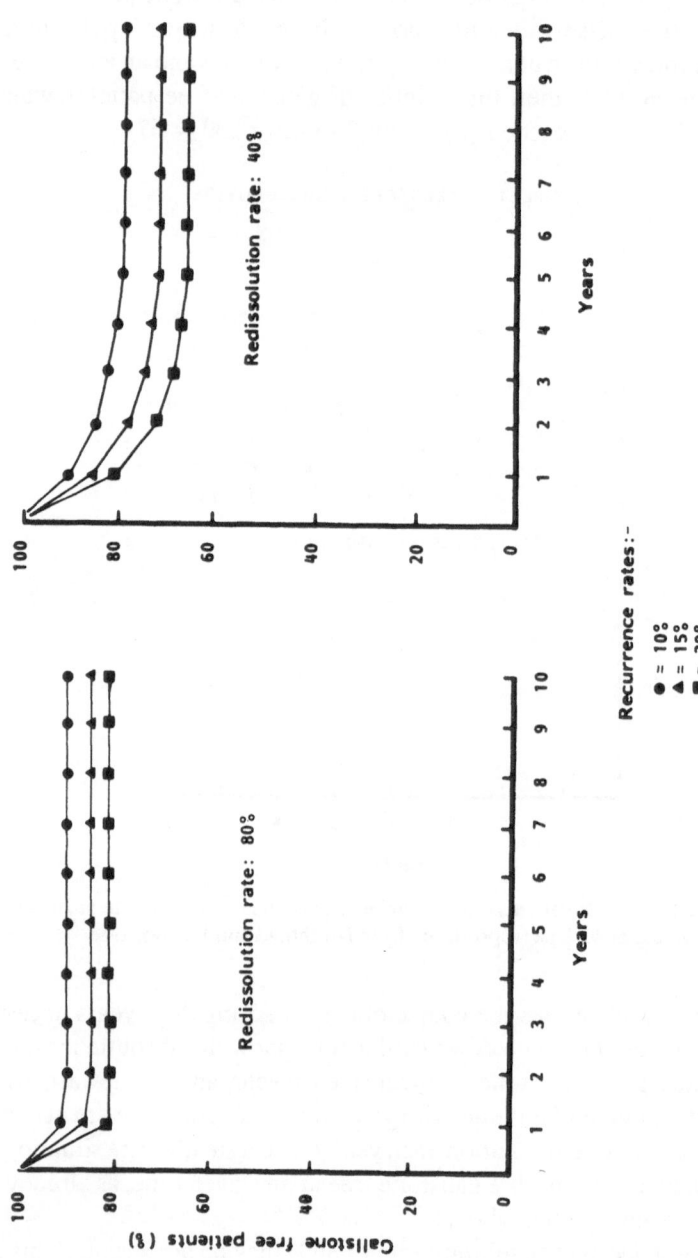

Figure 3 Gallstone-free patients (%) from a range of recurrence rates and redissolution rates (reproduced from Northfield and Jazrawi, 1988[12]).

ing gallbladder, treated with bedtime CDCA and a low cholesterol diet[10]. It is also similar to that predicted for eventual gallstone dissolution by Dowling's group[11] for gallstone patients fitting the ideal selection criteria. For redissolution a higher response rate might be predicted than for initial dissolution, because patients who have not achieved initial gallstone dissolution because of resistance to bile acid therapy or the presence of pigment stones will have been selected out during the initial period of bile acid therapy, and because post-dissolution management should include annual ultrasonography to detect the recurrent stones while they are still very small. At present, very little data is available on gallstone redissolution rate, and these predictions need confirmation in a prospective study.

For a redissolution rate of 80%, the steady state proportion of gallstone-free patients ranges from 80–90%, assuming gallstone recurrence

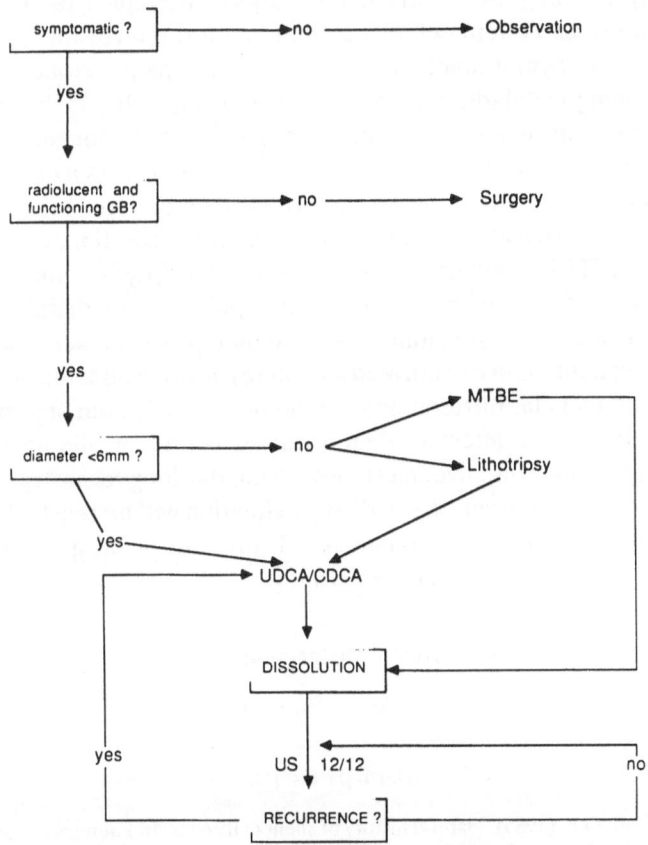

Figure 4 Algorithm for overall strategy for management of gallbladder stones.

rates of 10–20% per annum (Figure 3). For a redissolution rate of 40%, the steady state proportion of gallstone-free patients ranges from approximately 70–80% for the same recurrence rates. The recurrence rates that we have chosen encompass the results of the first year of post-dissolution follow up reported by Ruppin and Dowling[8] and by Lanzini and colleagues[9], as well as those reported in the British/Belgian Gallstone Study Group's post-dissolution trial[6] in Chapter 11. According to these calculations, we will only be treating 10–30% of our gallstone population at any given time. These calculations are independent of drop out rate due to complications and other factors, which will exert their influence via redissolution rate.

SUMMARY

Figure 4 summarises in the form of an algorithm our views on the best overall strategy to integrate different non-surgical therapies for cholesterol gallbladder stones. Patients who are asymptomatic should be managed by observation alone. Symptomatic patients with radioopaque stones or with a non-functioning gallbladder should be treated surgically. If, however, the stones are radiolucent and the gallbladder opacifies, then non-surgical treatment can be considered in relation to other factors such as age, health and patient preference. If the stones are >6 mm in diameter, then the main contenders for non-surgical therapy are lithotripsy or MTBE. If they are <6 mm in diameter MTBE remains a possibility but lithotripsy is contraindicated, whereas bile acid therapy causes relatively rapid gallstone dissolution. Following lithotripsy for larger stones, bile acid therapy will be necessary to dissolve the fragments. Once confirmed complete gallstone dissolution has been achieved, then regular ultrasonography should be carried out at yearly intervals. If recurrence is detected, then a further course of bile acid therapy should be given to redissolve the stones. Using this long term strategy of intermittent bile acid therapy, a steady state situation will be reached in which the majority of patients are maintained gallstone-free at any given time, thus achieving the declared object of our strategy.

Acknowledgements

We are grateful to Miss Marion Amos for secretarial assistance.

REFERENCES

1. Ransohoff, D.F. (1985). Natural history of silent gallstones. In Paumgartner, G., Stiehl, A. and Gerok, W. (eds.) *Enterohepatic Circulation of Bile Acids and Sterol Metabolism*. pp. 277–84 (Lancaster: MTP Press)
2. Attili, A.F. (1986). Natural history and prevention. In Bateson, M. (ed.) *Gallstone Disease and its Management*. pp. 57–70. (Lancaster: MTP Press)

3.   Paumgartner, G. (1988). In Northfield, T.C., Jazrawi, R. and Zentler-Munro, P.L. (eds.) *Bile Acids in Health and Disease*. Ch. 15. (Lancaster: MTP Press)

4.   Thistle, J.L. (1988). In Northfield, T.C., Jazrawi, R. and Zentler-Munro, P.L. (eds.) *Bile Acids in Health and Disease* Ch. 14. (Lancaster: MTP Press)

5.   Hospital in-patient enquiry, 1985. Series HB4 No. 27. DHSS Office of Population Censuses and Surveys. HMSO London, 1987

6.   Pounder, R. (1981). Model of medical treatment for duodenal ulcer. *Lancet*, 1, 29–30

7.   Hood, K. (1988). In Northfield, T.C., Jazrawi, R. and Zentler-Munro, P.L. (eds.) *Bile Acids in Health and Disease*. Ch. 11. (Lancaster: MTP Press)

8.   Kupfer, R.M., Maudgal, D.P. and Northfield, T.C. (1982). Gallstone dissolution rate during chenic acid therapy. Effect of bedtime administration plus low cholesterol diet. *Dig. Dis. Sci.*, 27, 1025–29

9.   Maton, P.N., Iser, J.H., Reuben, A., Saxton, H.M., Murphy, G.M. and Dowling, R.H. (1982). The final outcome of CDCA-treatment in 125 patients with radiolucent gallstones: factors influencing efficacy, withdrawal, symptoms and side effects and post-dissolution recurrence. *Medicine*, 61, 85–96

10. Ruppin, D.C. and Dowling, R.H. (1982). Is recurrence inevitable after gallstone dissolution by bile acid treatment? *Lancet*, 1, 181–5

11. Lanzini, A., Jazrawi, R.P. and Northfield, T.C. (1986). Gallstone recurrence after medical dissolution: an over-estimated threat? *J. Hepatol.*, 3, 241–6

12. Northfield, T.C. and Jasrawi, R.P (1988). Patient selection for bile acid therapy. In Paumgartner, G., Stiehl, A. and Gerok, W. (eds) *Bile Acids and the Liver*. pp. 329–342, (Lancaster: MTP Press)

SECTION E
LIPID DIGESTION
AND BILE ACID
ABSORPTION

17

Fat Digestion and Solubilisation

B. Borgström
Department of Physiological Chemistry
University of Lund
Lund, Sweden

INTRODUCTION

The main outlines of the process of fat digestion and absorption have been fairly well established: after absorption from the intestine dietary triglyceride appears in the milky chyle[1] as triglyceride, bile[2] and pancreatic juice[3] normally being necessary for this process. What takes place in between, however, has long been the subject of great controversy and the details are not yet fully established[4].

Until recently, classical pancreatic lipase was considered to be the main enzyme involved in lipid digestion in the gastrointestinal lumen. Lingual/gastric lipase[5], and the carboxyl ester lipase of pancreatic origin[6], are now also thought to have important co-operative roles in lipid digestion. The lipase of human milk, stimulated by bile salt, is in most respects identical with pancreatic carboxyl ester lipase and probably can substitute for a low pancreatic lipase level in early infancy[7].

During the last decades much interest has been devoted to the physico-chemical form of lipid dispersions in aqueous systems involving bile[8,9] and this knowledge has been applied to systems resembling intestinal content during digestion[10-12]. The work of Dietschy *et al.* and others has indicated that the uptake of lipids from the intestinal lumen takes place from a monomeric solution[13] enhanced by the presence of a mixed micellar phase, but little is known of the role of vesicular or liquid crystalline dispersions in this process[4].

LIPID DIGESTION

Four different enzymes are secreted into the digestive tract which hydrolyse lipid-soluble substrates. Three of these act on dispersed long-chain triglyceride fat and therefore by definition are lipases. The fourth is a phospholipase (A2) secreted in pancreatic juice together with colipase, an activator for classical pancreatic lipase in the presence of bile salt.

Acid Lipases

Intragastric lipolysis of short- and long-chain triglycerides has long been known to occur[14-16] although the source of the lipolytic activity was not known. Otterby *et al.*[17] demonstrated that the enzyme promoting intragastric lipolysis in the ruminant was of preduodenal origin, and Cohen *et al.*[18] showed that gastric aspirate from man contained lipolytic activity that could not be ascribed to pancreatic lipase. This latter enzyme was named gastric lipase and partly characterised. An enzyme with similar properties was later shown in the rat to be present in Von Ebner's glands in the back of the tongue[19,20]. This enzyme was named lingual lipase (or, later, pharyngeal and pregastric lipase). Lingual and gastric lipase have been found to have similar properties and show a high degree of homology in their protein structure. Some species such as the rat, the mouse and the ruminants produce only lingual lipase, some such as the rabbit and the guinea pig produce only gastric lipase, whilst the primates seem to produce both[5]. Due to their great functional and structural similarity, and the fact that they both have acid pH-optima, it has been suggested that these enzymes be called acid lipases[4].

Acid lipases have been purified from man[21] and calf[13] and cloned from the rat[22]. They have molecular weights of around 52 kDa, broad pH optima in the range of 2–6; their physiological substrates are triacylglycerols of various chain-lengths with a maximum for tributyrin, and they hydrolyse primary and secondary esterbonds at identical rates. The specific activity of human gastric lipase is 1160 U/mg and 620 U/mg with tributyrin and triolein as substrate respectively[24]. Human gastric juice contains 40–80 U/ml[24]. Human gastric lipase will also hydrolyse the triglycerides of milk fat globules; it is rapidly inactivated at the surface of a tributyrin emulsion and is protected by the presence of amphiphiles such as bile salts, and phosphatidylcholine, and proteins such as albumin[25].

Pancreatic Lipase and Colipase

Classical pancreatic lipase has been studied for more than a century but due to its easy inactivation during purification it was not obtained in pure form until 1969[26]. The addition of a proteolytic inhibitors now allows the purification of 100 mg batches of lipase – sufficient to allow the amino acid sequencing of porcine pancreatic lipase in 1981[27].

In 1969[28] rat pancreatic juice was shown conclusively to contain a cofactor for lipase; this was partly purified from porcine pancreas and named colipase[29]. It is difficult to separate colipase from lipase[30] and it can therefore be assumed that all studies of lipase before 1969 (and some thereafter) have been performed in the presence of uncontrolled levels of colipase. This is relevant particularly to experiments performed in the presence of bile salts. *In vitro*, lipase is fully active in the absence of colipase which protects it against interfacial inactivation[31]. Lipase attaches to the substrate interface by a combination of ionic and hydrophobic bondings, and in this way forms an enzyme-substrate complex. Bile salts in concentrations around and above their critical micellar concentration (CMC) prevent the binding of lipase to the substrate interface and thereby inhibit lipase by a purely physical means[32–34]. Colipase reverses this inhibition by allowing lipase, or rather its active centre, to reach its substrate in the presence of bile salts[35,36]. Several different mechanisms have been proposed for this function[37,38]. In particular, the products of lipolysis – fatty acid and monoglyceride – increase the binding between lipase, colipase and the substrate interface in the presence of bile salts. One hypothesis is that the binding of colipase to lipase effects a conformational change in lipase, opening up a hydrophobic binding site on lipase for its substrate interface[39].

Pancreatic lipase has been purified from many different species including man[40]. Its molecular weight is around 48–52 kDa, its physiological substrates are water insoluble triacylglycerols with an optimum rate for tributyrin. It is specific for esterbonds with primary hydroxyl groups, and its products are therefore 1,2-di- and 2-monoacylglycerols and fatty acids. Pancreatic lipase also catalyses the hydrolysis of some other esters of biological interest such as retinyl-palmitate. Its specific activity is 7000–10,000 U/mg and 3000–4000 U/mg with tributyrin and triolein as substrate respectively[36], depending on the conditions of the assay. Human intestinal content during the digestion of a lipid-rich meal contains around 1000 U/ml or 0.1 mg/ml, corresponding to a 2×10^{-6} mol/l solution[41].

Pancreatic colipase is secreted into pancreatic juice as a zymogen procolipase[42] which is activated by the cleavage of an N-terminal pentapeptide by trypsin. Colipase has a molecular weight of 10 kDa and its amino acid sequence has been determined except for a small sequence in the C-terminal part[43–45]. The concentration of colipase in human intestinal content during digestion is about 0.04 mg/ml, corresponding to a 4×10^{-6} mol/l solution[41]. Under these experimental conditions the molar ratio of colipase : lipase is about 2, but under other conditions lower figures have been reported[46]. It has been suggested that the colipase concentration in intestinal content is a regulating factor for lipase activity especially at low lipase concentrations[47].

Carboxyl Ester Lipase

This enzyme has many different names: the best known are cholesterol esterase and sterol ester hydrolase and it has also been called carboxyl ester hydrolase, non-specific lipase and bile salt stimulated lipase. The name carboxyl ester lipase (CEL), as suggested by Rudd and Brockman[6], is best because it reflects the enzyme's lack of positional and acyl specificity for the carboxyl ester hydrolysed, whilst being an interfacial enzyme. A closely related enzyme present in milk is usually named bile salt stimulated lipase[48]; although previously believed to be present only in milk of primates, it has now been demonstrated in the milk of other species such as dog and cat[49].

Carboxyl ester lipase requires bile salt for its activity. The preferred physical state for its optimal activity is not known; it may require a rather loose packing at the interface such as is achieved by bile salt[6]. It catalyses the hydrolysis of a wide range of esters; its physiological substrates are acylglycerols, cholesterol esters and esters of vitamin A and D. It has been reported to hydrolyse lysophospholipids in the absence of bile salt[50]. Its hydrolysis of long-chain triacylglycerols (in the presence of bile salt) may not be physiologically important as the presence of phospholipids in the system prevents this action (unpublished by the author). It has been suggested[46] that the product phase of pancreatic lipase in the presence of bile salt acts as the substrate for carboxyl ester lipase, to produce the proper physico-chemical environment for hydrolysis of dietary cholesterol- and fat soluble vitamin esters[6].

The physiological function of the bile salt stimulated lipase in milk has been suggested to be the rapid release of short chain fatty acids from the triacylglycerols in milk fat globules, but these are not directly available to the enzyme. Cholesterol- and vitamin esters may be the main physiological substrates for bile salt stimulated lipase, as for pancreatic carboxyl ester lipase, in co-operation with acid and pancreatic lipase (see below)[51].

Carboxyl ester lipase has been ascribed a role in the absorption of cholesterol. According to this concept, the enzyme is present on both sides of the enterocyte membrane and allows the movement of cholesterol ester over the membrane by a flip-flop mechanism[52]. This concept is not, however, supported by other experimental results[53].

Carboxyl ester lipase has been purified from several species including man[54], and bile salt stimulated lipase from human milk[55]. Their molecular weights are around 60–125 kDa. The enzymes aggregate in the presence of bile salt, their behaviour being different in different species[56]. The specific activity of carboxyl ester lipase is only 1/20 that of pancreatic lipase with tributyrin as substrate; its activity in human intestinal content during digestion is approximately 1/40 that of lipase with tributyrin as substrate (unpublished by the author).

220

Phospholipase A$_2$.

Although this is one of the most extensively studied enzymes of pancreatic juice[57], its role in the intraluminal digestion of fat – beyond the cleaving of phosphatidylcholines to the corresponding lyso compounds – is not clear. Its activity against long-chain phosphoglycerides is dependent on the phosphoglyceride: bile salt ratio, but the conditions have not been well controlled in published studies[4]. The available information indicates that phosphoglycerides in mixed bile salt micellar solution, or in bilayer dispersions, are not good substrates for the enzyme; vesicular dispersions may be better[58].

Co-operation and Substitution in Lipid Digestion

The presence of several lipolytic enzymes in the digestive tract suggest that they have separate roles but may also be able to substitute for each other. Acid lipases affect a partial hydrolysis of triacylglycerols that seems to halt at the diglyceride stage to produce 15–20% free fatty acid. It has been suggested that the presence of free fatty acid in the fat leaving the stomach determines the strength of binding of lipase to procolipase, and reduces the lag time in the start of lipolysis by pancreatic lipase[59–61]. It may be an alternative way of activating the colipase–lipase system in the absence of procolipase activation by trypsin. It has further been suggested that acid lipase could act as substitute for pancreatic lipase in the newborn or premature baby[62], and in pancreatic insufficiency[63]. Pretreatment of milk fat globules *in vitro* with acid lipase makes them more available to bile salt stimulated lipase[64]. Whether acid lipases can, like pancreatic lipase, prepare emulsified solutions of triacylglycerols with cholesterol esters and retinol esters in bile salt dispersions for hydrolysis by carboxyl ester lipase is not known.

Phospholipids inhibit the hydrolysis of triacylglycerol emulsions by pancreatic lipase; this inhibition can be overcome by the addition of colipase, free fatty acids[60] or by phospholipase A$_2$[59]. Phospholipase A$_2$ may act mainly by generating free fatty acids with no specific physiological meaning.

LIPID SOLUBILISATION

Products of Lipolysis

Lipolysis results in the formation of more polar products from the largely non-polar dietary fat, the main end products being fatty acids and 2-monoacylglycerols. The ionisation of the fatty acids depends on the pH of the intestinal content; in the upper small intestine where digestion takes place this varies from moment to moment but is usually slightly acid – around 5.5–

6.5^{65}. In theory two moles of fatty acid should be formed for each mole of 2-monoacylglycerol, assuming that little fat is absorbed as di-acylglycerol and little mono-acylglycerol is hydrolysed – as is normal. Other lipids are present in the diet in small quantities: those present as esters are hydrolysed to the alcohol and the free fatty acid. The reactions catalysed by pancreatic lipase and carboxyl ester lipase have equilibria in which appreciable quantities of ester are present even in aqueous suspensions. This maintains equilibrium states *in vitro* and also under the conditions of intestinal contents during digestion[6,66].

Lipids in Intestinal Contents during Digestion: Chemical Constituents

The first analysis of the lipids in upper intestinal contents of man after the ingestion of a fatty meal[67] showed the presence of a mixture of fatty acids and different glyceride species. The composition of the lipids extracted from 10 samples from the upper jejunum during the first and second postprandial half-hours had a mean total lipid concentration of 7.4 mg/ml with a large range (2.6–16.9). On a molar basis the free fatty acids dominated and the fatty acid:monoglyceride ratio was 4.8:1, higher than the 2:1 ratio expected if the triacylglycerol were hydrolysed to fatty acid and monoglyceride. This could be explained by a preferential absorption of monoglyceride, but not by partial hydrolysis to diglyceride. Other investigations have shown similar or higher fatty acid:monoglyceride ratios, and another explanation is that monoglyceride is hydrolysed after sampling – before and during treatment to inactivate lipase. Lipase inactivation has usually been performed by heating the samples to 75 °C for 10 min. More recently[65] it has been accomplished by acidification to pH 3 but no analysis of the separate glyceride species has been published from these experiments.

Physico-chemical Characteristics

In 1962 Hofmann and Borgström[67,68] separated human postprandial intestinal contents by centrifugation into an emulsified oil phase, containing mostly unchanged triglyceride and diglyceride, and a clear aqueous phase. The latter was rich in fatty acid and monoglyceride and contained bile salts over their critical micellar concentration. The results were consistent with the hypothesis that in the intestine lipids are partitioned between an oil phase and an aqueous mixed lipid micellar phase from which absorption of dietary fat takes place. This 'micellar hypothesis' was generally accepted but results were later obtained indicating that it was an over-simplification and that other phases could also be present. The work by Patton and Carey in 1979[69] can be considered to be a break-through in this field. They watched unstirred lipolysis on a glass slide under the microscope and observed the formation of successive lipolytic product phases: a crystalline phase, followed by a liquid crystalline phase which finally dissolved into an isotropic micellar product phase. The liquid crystalline phase was suggested to be a cubic phase. This work was an impetus to further *in vitro* studies of relevant phase systems. Martin Carey has discussed lipid solubilisation in bile earlier in this volume; and the solubilisation of lipids in intestinal contents represents a special case of the general physico-chemical rules discussed by Carey in chapter 5.

Three different approaches have been chosen to characterise intestinal contents during digestion.

1. *In vitro* study of the phase behaviour of monoolein/oleic acid/water systems has identified three different phases: a cubic phase, a reversed hexagonal phase and an L2-phase or microemulsion. Characterisation of the dispersion properties of these phases in dilute bile salt solutions has shown the cubic phase to be easily dispersed to a micellar solution. Construction of a phase diagram for the monoglyceride/ triglyceride/water system showed increased solubilisation of triglyceride oil or oleic acid in the cubic liquid crystalline phase formed by monoglyceride and water, resulting in the formation of a reversed hexagonal liquid–crystalline phase followed by an L2-phase[10]. A phase diagram of the ternary system monoolein/oleic acid-oleate/sodium taurocholate in 99% water was also constructed but the physical structures of the dispersed phase were not characterised[12] (see Figure 1).

2. The phase equilibria of lipid mixtures patterned after the aqueous luminal lipids have been studied by Stafford *et al.*[70,71] employing different physical methods. They concluded that in duodenal content large bile salt-mixed micelles saturated with lipolytic products coexist with liposomes of the same lipids. These results were published in abstract form in 1981 but have not yet been properly reported.

3. *In vivo* study of the lipids present in human intestinal contents has shown a liquid crystal phase and giant liposomes in jejunal chyme, identified by physical means after ultracentrifugation[72]. These phases were contained in an upper and a lower intermediary phase which together contained around 20% of the fatty acid mass[73]. Holt *et al.*[74], also using ultracentrifugation, isolated a viscous gel-like phase from human intestinal content during rapid lipolysis. This phase, which probably corresponded to the upper intermediary phase of Fine *et al.*[73], was birefringent and therefore contained liquid crystals.

The evidence available therefore indicates that the equilibrium physi-

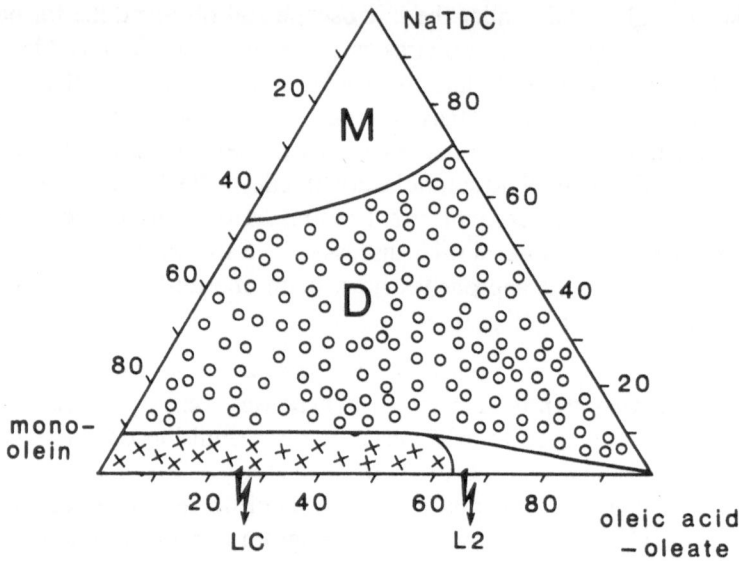

Figure 1 Phase diagram of the ternary system of monoolein/oleic acid–oleate/sodium taurodeoxycholate (NaTDC) in 10 mmol/l Tris–maleate buffer, pH 6.5, in 150 mmol/l NaCl, 0.02% NaN3 at 25 °C. The total amount of the three components is held constant at 1% (weight). Phases formed in excess of aqueous phase are a liquid crystalline phase (LC) (a viscous isotropic phase) and an L2 phase (inverted micelles or microemulsion). With increasing amounts of NaTDC the lipid phases are dispersed (D) in the aqueous phase above the critical micellar concentration. In the area where NaTDC dominates a clear isotropic mixed micellar (M) solution exists. From reference 12.

cal state of intestinal lipids consists of coexisting saturated micellar and liquid crystalline lipid phases dispersed in an aqueous phase containing monomeric bile salts – as predicted by Carey in 1983[75]. It is, however, clear that postprandial upper intestinal content is in a very dynamic state: lipid-containing chyme empties in fractions from the stomach, mixes with pancreatic juice containing bicarbonate and the lipolytic enzymes and almost instantaneously with bile.

The enzyme concentration in this broth is extremely high (lipase sufficient to hydrolyse 1000 μmoles ester bonds per ml per min) but its bile salt concentration rather low (4–7 mmol/l[65]). Taking the figures of Zentler-Munro et al.[65] of a mean lipid content in upper intestinal content of 36 μmol/l as fatty acid (corresponding to 12 μmol/ml triglyceride with two ester bonds available per mole), the lipids in intestinal content could be completely hydrolysed in 1.4 sec (24 x 60/1000). The reaction catalysed by lipase is thus an equilibrium reaction with approximately equimolar amounts of mono, di- and triglycerides present under the intraluminal conditions, ready to generate within seconds any product that is absorbed. The composition of the lipid mixture present at any time depends on the rates of delivery, lipolysis and absorption. No good information is available on the rate of absorption, but with the extremely high rate of hydrolysis it can be expected that absorption is the limiting factor. With the relatively low bile salt concentration, the lipids would therefore be present mainly in the form of vesicles and different liquid crystalline lipid phases. Indications that lipids are absorbed from the intestine in non-micellar form can be found in the older literature[76] and are now appearing again[77].

SUMMARY

An account is given of recent developments in the field of luminal digestion of dietary fat. It is indicated that the lipases involved gastric, pancreatic and carboxyl ester lipase (work in a concerted way to) optimise digestion, the product of one being substrate for the following. The physicochemical state of the lipolytic products of dietary fat in the content of the upper small intestine in discussed with reference to recent developments in this field.

REFERENCES

1. Munk, I. (1900). Zur Frage des Fettresorption. *Z. Physiol.*, **14**, 153–6
2. Bernard, C. (1849). Recherches sur les usages du sac pancreatique dans la digestion. *Acad. Sci.*, **28**, 249–85
3. Dastre, A. (1890). Recherches sur la bile. *Arch. Physiol.*, 5 sereie, **2**, 315–30
4. Borgström, B. and Patton, J.S. (1988). Luminal events in gastrointestinal lipid digestion. *Handbook of Physiology*, In Press)
5. Hamosh, M. (1986). Lingual lipase. *Gastroenterology*, **90**, 1290–7
6. Lindström, M.B., Sternby, B. and Borgström, B. (1988). Concerted action of human carboxyl ester lipase and pancreatic lipase during lipid digestion *in vitro*: importance of the physicochemical state of the substrate. *Biochim. Biophys Acta*, **959**, 178–184
7. Hernell, O., Bläckberg, L., Fredrikzon, B. and Olivecrona, T. (1981). Bile salt stimulated lipase in human milk and lipid digestion during the neonatal period. In Lebenthal, E. (ed.) *Textbook of Gastroenterology and Nutrition of Infancy*, pp. 465–471, (New York: Raven Press)
8. Carey, M.C. (1982). The enterohepatic circulation. In Arias, I., Popper, H., Schachter, D. and Schafritz, D.A. (eds.) *The Liver: Biology and Pathobiology)*, pp. 429–465, (New York: Raven Press)
9. Mazer, N.A., Carey, M.C., Kwasnic, R.F. and Benedek, G.B. (1979). Quasielastic light scattering studies of aqueous biliary lipid systems. Size, shape and thermodynamics of bile salt micelles. *Biochemistry*, **18**, 3064–75
10. Lindström, M., Ljusberg-Wahren, H., Larsson, K. and Borgström, B. (1981). Aqueous lipid phases of relevance to intestinal fat digestion and absorption. *Lipids*, **16**, 749–54
11. Carey, M.C., Small, D.M. and Bliss, C.M. (1983). Lipid digestion and absorption. *Annu. Rev. Physiol.*, **45**, 651–77
12. Borgström, B. (1985). The micellar hypothesis of fat absorption: must it be revisited? *Scand. J. Gastroenterol.*, **20**, 389–94
13. Thomson, A.B.R. and Dietschy, J.M. (1981). In Johnson, C.R. (ed.) *Physiology of the Gastrointestinal Tract.*, pp. 1147–220, (New York: Raven Press)
14. Volhard, F. (1901). Uber das fettspaltende Ferment des Magens. *Z. Klin. Med.*, **42**, 414–

29

15. Borgström, B., Dalqvist, A., Lundh, G. and Sjövall, J. (1957). Studies of intestinal digestion and absorption in the human. *J. Clin. Invest.*, **36**, 1521–36
16. Hamosh, M. (1981). Oral lipases and lipid digestion during the neonatal period. In Lebenthal, E. (ed.) *Textbook of Gastroenterology and Nutrition in Infancy* pp. 445–63 (New York: Raven Press)
17. Otterby, D.E., Ramsey, H.A. and Wise, G.H. (1964). Lipolysis of milk fat by pregastric esterase in the abdomen of the calf. *J. Dairy Sci.*, **47**, 993–7
18. Cohen, M., Morgan, R.G.H. and Hofmann, A.F. (1971). Lipolytic activity of human gastric and duodenal juice against medium and long chain triglycerides. *Gastroenterology*, **60**, 1–15
19. Hamosh, M. (1984). Lingual lipase. In Borgström, B. and Brockman, H.L. (eds.) *Lipases*, pp. 49–82. (Amsterdam: Elsevier)
20. Hamosh, M. (1978). Rat lingual lipase: factors affecting enzyme activity and secretion. *Am. J. Physiol.*, **235**, E416–E421
21. Hamosh, M. and Burns, W.A. (1977). Lipolytic activity of human lingual glands (Ebner). *Lab. Invest.*, **37**, 603–8
22. Docherty, A.J.P., Bodmer, M.W., Angal, S., Verger, R., Riviere, C., Lowe, P.A., Lyons, A., Emtage, J.S. and Harris, T.J.R. (1985). Molecular cloning and nucleotide sequence of rat lingual lipase cDNA. *Nucl. Acids Res.*, **13**, 1891–903
23. Bernbäck, S., Hernell, O. and Bläckberg, L. (1985). Purification and molecular characterisation of bovine pregastric lipase. *Eur. J. Biochem.*, **148**, 233–8
24. Gagouri, Y. Pieroni, G., Riviere, C., Sauniere, J.-F., Lowe, P.A., Sarda, L. and Verger, R. (1986). Kinetic assay of human gastric lipase on short- and long-chain triacylglycerol emulsions. *Gastroenterology*, **91**, 919–25
25. Gargouri, Y., Pieroni, G. Lowe, P.A., Sarda, L. and Verger, R. (1986). Human gastric lipase. The effect of amphiphiles. *Eur. J. Biochem.*, **156**, 305–10
26. Verger, R., De Haas, G.H., Sarda, L. and Desnuelle, P. (1969). Purification from porcine pancreas of two molecular species with lipase activity. *Biochim. Biophys. Acta*, **188**, 272–82
27. De Caro, J., Boudouard, M., Bonicel, J., Goudoni, A., Desnuelle, P. and Rovery, M. (1981). Porcine pancreatic lipase. Completion of the primary structure. *Biochim. Biophys. Acta*, **671**, 129–38
28. Morgan, R.G.H, Barrowman, J. and Borgström, B. (1969). The effect of sodium taurodeoxycholate and pH on the gel filtration behaviour of rat pancreatic protein and lipases. *Biochim Biophys. Acta*, **175**, 65–75
29. Maylie, M.F., Charles, M., Gache, C. and Desnuelle, P. (1971). Isolation and partial purification of a pancreatic colipase. *Biochim. Biophys. Acta*, **229**, 286–9
30. Patton, J.S., Albertsson, P.-Ä., Erlanson, C. and Borgström, B. (1973). Binding of porcine pancreatic lipase and colipase in the absence of substrate studied by two-phase partition and affinity chromatography. *J. Biol. Chem.*, **253**, 4195–202
31. Borgström, B. (1982). The temperature-dependent interfacial inactivation of porcine pancreatic lipase. Effect of colipase and bile salts. *Biochim. Biophys. Acta*, **712**, 490–7
32. Borgström, B. (1975). On the interactions between pancreatic lipase and colipase and the substrate and the importance of bile salts. *J. Lipid Res.*, **16**, 411–17
33. Vandermeers, A., Vandermeers, M.C., Rathe, J. and Christophe, J. (1975). Effect of colipase on adsorption and activity of rat pancreatic lipase on emulsified tributyrine in the presence of bile salts. *FEBS Lett.*, **49**, 334–7
34. Momsen, W.E. and Brockman, H.L. (1976). Effect of colipase and taurodeoxycholate on the catalytic and physical properties of liapse B at an oil-water interface. *J. Biol. Chem.*, **251**, 378–83
35. Borgström, B. and Erlanson, C. (1971). Pancreatic juice colipase: Physiological importance. *Biochim. Biophys. Acta*, **242**, 509–13
36. Borgström, B. and Erlanson-Albertsson, C. (1984). Pancreatic colipase. In Borgström,

B. and Brockman, H.L. (eds.) *Lipases*, pp. 151–83, (Amsterdam: Elsevier)

37.   Patton, J.S. (1981). Gastrointestinal digestion. In Johnson, L.R. (ed.) *Physiology of the Gastrointestinal Tract*, pp. 1123–46. (New York: Raven Press)

38.   Verger, R. (1984). Pancreatic lipase. In Borgström, B. and Brockman, H.L. (eds.) *Lipases*, pp. 83–150, (Amsterdam: Elsevier)

39.   Erlanson-Albertsson, C. and Åkerlund, H.-E (1982). Conformational change in pancreatic lipase induced by colipase. *FEBS Lett.*, **155**, 38–42

40.   Vandermeers, A., Vandermeers-Piret, M.C., Rathe, J. and Christophe, J. (1974). On human pancreatic triacylglycerol lipase: isolation and some properties. *Biochim. Biophys. Acta*, **370**, 257–68

41.   Borgström, B. and Hildebrand, H. (1975). Lipase and colipase activities of human small intestinal contents after a liquid test meal. *Scand. J. Gastroenterol.*, **10**, 585–91

42.   Borgström, B., Wieloch, T. and Erlanson-Albertsson, C. (1979). Evidence for a pancreatic pro-colipase and its activation by trypsin. *FEBS Lett.*, **108**, 407–10

43.   Charles, M., Erlanson, C., Bianchetta, J., Joffre, J., Guidoni, A. and Rovery, M. (1974). The primary structure of porcine colipase II. I. The amino acid sequence. *Biochim. Biophys. Acta*, **359**, 186–97

44.   Erlanson, C., Charles, M., Astier, M. and Desnuelle, P. (1974). The primary structure of porcine colipase II. II The disulphide bridges. *Biochim. Biophys. Acta*, **359**, 198–203

45.   Larsson, A. and Erlanson-Albertsson, C. (1981). The identity of two forms of activated colipase from porcine pancreas. *Biochim. Biophys. Acta*, **664**, 538–48

46.   Gaskin, K.J., Durie, P.R., Hill, R.E., Lee, C.M. and Forstner, G.G. (1982). Colipase and maximally activated pancreatic lipase in normal subjects and patients with steatorrhea. *J. Clin. Invest.*, **69**, 427–34

47.   Gaskin, K.J,, Durie, P.R., Lee, L., Hill, R. and Forstner, G.G. (1984). Colipase and lipase secretion in childhood-onset pancreatic insufficiency. Delineation of patients with steatorrhea secondary to relative colipase deficiency. *Gastroenterology*, **86**, 1–7

48.   Olivecrona, T. and Bengtsson, G. 1984). In Borgström, B. and Brockman, H.L. (eds.) *Lipases*, pp. 205–62, (Amsterdam: Elsevier)

49.   Freed, L.M., York, C.M., Hamosh, M., Sturman, J.A. and Hamosh, P. (1986). Bile salt-stimulated lipase in non-primate milk: Longitudinal variation and lipase characteristics in cat and dog milk. *Biochim. Biophys. Acta*, **878**, 209–15

50.   Lombardo, D., Fauvel, J. and Guy, O. (1980). Studies on the substrate specificity of a carboxyl ester hydrolase from human pancreatic juice. *Biochim. Biophys. Acta*, **611**, 136–46

51.   Hernell, O., Bläckberg, L. and Bernbäck, S. (1987). Milk lipase and in vivo lipolysis. In Lönnerdahl, B. and Atkinson, S. (eds.) *Protein and N-protein Nitrogen in Human Milk*, (CRC Press) (In press)

52.   Bhat, S.G. and Brockman, H.L. (1982). The role of cholesterol ester hydrolysis and synthesis in cholesterol transport across the rat intestinal mucosa membrane; a new concept. *Biochem. Biophys. Res. Commun.*, **109**, 486–92

53.   Watt, S.M. and Simmonds, W.J. (1981). The effect of pancreatic diversion on lymphatic absorption and esterification of cholesterol in the rat. *J. Lipid Res.*, **22**, 157–65

54.   Lombardo, D., Campese, D., Multigner, L., Lafont, H. and De Caro, A. (1983). On the probable involvement on arginine residues in the bile salt-binding site of human pancreatic carboxyl ester hydrolase. *Eur. J. Biochem.*, **133**, 327–33

55.   Bläckberg, L. and Hernell, O. (1981). The bile salt-stimulated lipase in human milk: purification and characterisation. *Eur. J. Biochem.*, **116**, 221–25

56.   Erlanson-Albertsson, C. (1986). Pancreatic carboxyl ester hydrolyse and non-enzymatic constituents of pancreatic juice. In Desnuelle, P., Sjöström, H. and Norén, O. (eds.) *Molecular and Cellular Basis of Digestion*, pp. 297–308, (Amsterdam: Elsevier)

57.   Volwerk, J.J. and De Haas, G. (1982). Pancreatic phospholipase A2: a model for membrane-bound enzymes. In Jost, P.C. and Griffits, O.H. (eds.) *Lipid Protein Interactions*, Vol. 1, pp. 69–149, (New York: Wiley-Interscience)

58. Goormaghtigh, E., van Campenhoud, M. and Ruyss-chaert, J.-M. (1981). Lipid phase. Separation mediates binding of porcine pancreatic phospholipase A_2 to its substrate. *Biochem. Biophys. Res. Commun.*, **101**, 1410–18

59. Borgström, B. (1980). Importance of phospholipids, pancreatic phospholipase A_2 and fatty acid for the digestion of dietary fat. In vitro experiments with the porcine enzymes. *Gastroenterology*, **78**, 954-62

60. Gargouri, Y., Pieroni, G., Riviére, C., Lowe, P.A., Sauniére, J.-F., Sarda, L. and Verger, R. (1986). Importance of human gastric lipase for intestinal lipolysis in an in vitro study. *Biochim. Biophys. Acta*, **879**, 419–23

61. Larsson, A. and Erlanson-Albertsson, C. (1986). Effect of phosphatidylcholine and free fatty acid on the activity of pancreatic lipase-colipase. *Biochim. Biophys. Acta*, **876**, 543–50

62. Hamosh, M., Scanlon, J.W., Ganot, D., Likel, M., Scanlon, K.B. and Hamosh, P. (1981). Fat digestion in the newborn. Characterisation of lipase in gastric aspirates of premature and term infants. *J. Clin. Invest.*, **67**, 838–46

63. Abrams, C.K., Hamosh, M., Hubbard, V.S., Dutta, S.K. and Hamosh, P. (1982). Fat digestion in cystic fibrosis - compensatory role of lingual lipase *Clin. Res.*, **30**, 279A

64. Lombardo, D. and Guy, O. (1980). Studies on the substrate specificity of a carboxyl ester hydrolase from human pancreatic juice. II. Action on cholesterol esters and lipid-soluble vitamin esters. *Biochim. Biophys. Acta*, **611**, 147–55

65. Zentler-Munro, P.L., Fine, D.R., Fitzpatrick, W.J.F. and Northfield, T.C. (1984). Effect of intrajejunal acidity on lipid digestion and aqueous solubilisation of bile acids and lipids in health using a new simple method of lipase inactivation *Gut*, **25**, 491–9

66. Borgström, B. (1964). Influence of bile salt, pH and time on the action of pancreatic lipase; physiological implications *J. Lipid Res.*, **5**, 522–33

67. Hofmann, A.F. and Borgström B. (1964). The intestinal phase of fat digestion in man: The lipid content of the micellar and oil phases of intestinal content obtained during fat digestion and absorption. *J. Clin. Invest.*, **43**, 247–57

68. Hofmann, A.F. and Borgström, B. (1962). Physico-chemical state of lipids in intestinal content during their digestion and absorption. *Fed. Proc.*, **21**, 43–50

69. Patton, J.S. and Carey, M.C. (1979). Watching fat digestion. The formation of visible product phases by pancreatic lipase is described. *Science*, **204**, 145–48

70. Stafford, R.J. and Carey, M.C. (1981). Physical-chemical nature of the aqueous lipids in intestinal content after a fatty meal. Revision of the Hofmann–Borgström Hypothesis. *Clin. Res.*, **28**, 511A

71. Stafford, R.J., Donovan, G.B., Benedek, G.B. and Carey, M.C. (1980). Physical-chemical characteristics of aqueous duodenal content after a fatty meal. *Gastroenterology*, **80**, 1291, Abstr.

72. Fine, D., Brown, C., Fine, M. and Northfield, T.C. (1983). Two new phases in ultracentrifuged chyme. *Clin. Sci.*, **65**, 41P

73. Fine, D., Brown, C. and Northfield, T.C. (1985). Two new phases in ultracentrifuged chyme. *Gastroenterology*, **90**, 202, Abstr.

74. Holt, P.R., Fairchild, B.M. and J. Weiss, J. (1986). A liquid crystalline phase in human intestinal contents during fat digestion. *Lipids*, **21**, 444–6

75. Carey, M.C. (1983). In Barbara, L., Dowling, R.H., Hofmann, A.F. and Roda, E. (eds.) *Bile Acids in Gastroenterology*, pp. 19–56. (Boston: MTP Press)

76. Borgström, B., Barrowman, J.A. and Lindström, M. (1985). Roles of bile acids in intestinal lipid digestion and absorption. In Danielsson, H. and Sjövall, J. (eds.) *Sterols and Bile Acids*, pp. 405–425. (Amsterdam: Elsevier)

77. Reynier, M.O., Crotte, C., Montret, J.C., Sauve, P. and Gerolami, A. (1987). Intestinal cholesterol and oleic acid uptake from solutions supersaturated with lipids *Lipids*, **22**, 28–32

18
Bile Acid Absorption

A. Stiehl
Department of Medicine
University of Heidelberg
Heidelberg
Federal Republic of Germany

INTRODUCTION

Bile acids are formed in the liver from cholesterol. After their excretion in bile a major proportion is reabsorbed from the intestine and recirculates via the portal vein to the liver. Absorption in the intestine is a prerequisite sitesitesitefor the enterohepatic circulation of bile acids.

The bile acid pool of 3–5 g recirculates approximately 8 times daily. Approximately 10–30% of the bile acid pool is lost each day in the faeces, and the same amount (600–800 mg/day), is synthesised in the liver from cholesterol. Less than 2–5% of the bile acid pool is lost with every enterohepatic cycling. This very effective absorption of bile acids from the intestine is necessary for the conservation of the bile acid pool.

The absorption of bile acids occurs mainly in the small intestine[1-5] but there is evidence that the colon also plays a role in the absorption of bile acids[6-10]. In the liver the two primary bile acids cholic acid ($3\alpha,7\alpha,12\alpha$-trihydroxy-5β-cholanoic acid) and chenodeoxycholic acid ($3\alpha,7\alpha$-dihydroxy-5β-cholanoic acid) are conjugated at their carboxyl groups with the amino acids glycine and taurine.

INTESTINAL EVENTS

Duodenal bile acids are almost 100% conjugated. Conjugated bile acids may be absorbed or they may be deconjugated by bacteria and subsequently absorbed. Bacteria are present in incubates of ileal fluid which can rapidly split the conjugate bonds, but analysis of fresh ileal fluid taken directly from an ileostomy has shown that little deamidation occurs[11]. Deconjugation is apparently in progress when the bile acids pass the ileo-caecal valve, and during passage through the colon virtually all the bile acids are deconjugated. After their return to the liver, bile acids are reconjugated with glycine and taurine and then re-excreted into bile.

The anaerobic bacteria of the colon can also dehydroxylate bile acids. 7α-dehydroxylation of cholic acid forms deoxycholic acid ($3\alpha,12\alpha$-dihydroxy-5β-cholanoic acid) which is in part absorbed from the colon[12]. 7α-dehydroxylation of chenodeoxycholic acid forms lithocholic acid (3α-monohydroxy-5β-cholanoic acid) which is poorly soluble in water and therefore hardly absorbed from the colon[13–15]. Under physiological conditions 30–90% of lithocholic acid is sulphated at the 3α-hydroxyl group[16], mainly in the intestinal wall, the liver and the kidneys.

Bile acids can be absorbed from the intestine only when they are in aqueous solution. A bile acid will precipitate out of solution when intraluminal pH is lower than its particular 'precipitation pH'[17,18]. Glycine conjugates precipitate when intraluminal pH is only slightly lower than normal, whereas taurine conjugates do not. Such a situation can occur in the upper small intestine in patients with gastric hypersecretion, or in the colon due to bacterial degradation of intestinal contents.

Absorption in the Jejunum

Bile acids are absorbed in the jejunum by ionic and non-ionic diffusion[3,4]; at physiological pH absorption is mostly by passive ionic diffusion. The rate depends on intraluminal concentration. The diffusion rates of individual bile acids decrease with the addition of hydroxyl, glycine or taurine groups to the sterol nucleus[4]. The passive absorption of dihydroxy bile acids is more efficient than that of trihydroxy bile acids[4,5]; unconjugated bile acids are absorbed more efficiently than glycine conjugates, and the latter more than taurine conjugates[4,5]. In the upper small intestine, therefore, chenodeoxycholic acid and deoxycholic acid conjugates can be absorbed but cholic acid conjugates are only poorly absorbed.

Absorption in the Ileum

Bile acids are absorbed in the ileum by passive diffusion and by active transport[1–5]. Unconjugated bile acids are predominantly absorbed by passive ionic and, to some extent, non-ionic diffusion. Taurine and glycine conjugates are, in contrast, much better absorbed by active transport[4,5]. The rate of active transport in the ileum of individual bile acids also depends on the number of hydroxyl groups: V_{max} values for trihydroxy bile acids are higher than those for dihydroxy bile acids[4,5] while those for monohydroxy bile acids are very low[4]; values for taurine conjugates are higher than those for glycine conjugates[4]. It seems likely that in the small intestine it is the conjugated bile acids that are mainly absorbed. The absorption of trihydroxy bile acid conjugates depends on an intact ileum, since they are only poorly absorbed from the upper small intestine while dihydroxy conjugates can be absorbed there by passive diffusion.

Absorption from the Colon

If the small intestine is intact, approximately 700 mg of bile acids pass the ileo-caecal valve and reach the colon where they are rapidly deconjugated and dehydroxylated by bacteria. This amount increases in patients with small intestinal disease or resection and also after oral administration of bile acids for cholelitholysis. The capacity (per unit length) of the colon to absorb unconjugated bile acids by diffusion is as high[4,8] as that of the ileum, and about twice that of the jejunum[4,8,9]. Bile acids not absorbed in the ileum can therefore be absorbed from the colon: about 200 mg of deoxycholic acid[12] and 20–60 mg of lithocholic acid[13,14] are absorbed from the colon per day. If, however, the concentrations of the dihydroxy bile acids chenodeoxycholic acid and deoxycholic acid increase above a certain level the absorption fails to increase in parallel, and actually decreases[8]. This induces colonic water secretion and then bile acid diarrhoea will follow.

Absorption of Sulphated Bile Acids

Bile acids can be sulphated at their hydroxyl groups[16], usually at the 3α position. Sulphation decreases with the number of hydroxyl groups on the sterol nucleus[19-21]. Under physiological conditions in bile lithocholic acid is 30–90% sulphated but only small amounts of dihydroxy and trihydroxy bile acids are sulphated. In cholestasis the amount of sulphated dihydroxy and trihydroxy bile acid increases[19,20]. The absorption of sulphated bile acid in the intestine is less efficient than that of the unsulphated molecules[22,23], and rates of absorption in the proximal small intestine are lower than in the distal small intestine. Absorption occurs mainly by diffusion[22,23], and only taurochenodeoxy-3-sulphate has been shown to be actively absorbed from the ileum[22,23]. Very little sulphated bile acid is absorbed in the colon[23], but it may be desulphated by bacteria and then absorbed. Bile acid sulphates have a shorter biological half-life than non-sulphated molecules[14,16,24], indicating that desulphation and subsequent absorption in the colon do not compensate for the decreased absorption in the small intestine.

Absorption of Keto Bile Acids

7-ketolithocholic acid is a tertiary bile acid which is formed from ursodeoxycholic acid[25,26]. This bile acid has a single hydroxyl group in the 3α position and a keto group in the 7α position. In rats 7-ketolithocholic acid is absorbed at the same rate from jejunum, ileum and colon as the corresponding dihydroxy bile acids ursodeoxycholic acid and chenodeoxycholic acid[27].

INTESTINAL ABSORPTION OF EXOGENOUS CHENODEOXYCHOLIC AND URSODEOXYCHOLIC ACIDS

Chenodeoxycholic acid is dissolved rapidly at physiological intraluminal pH, and is virtually completely absorbed when administered to patients with gallstones[28,29]. Plasma time-concentration curves indicate that absorption is complete within 2–4 hours of oral administration[29], but may be delayed slightly by the simultaneous ingestion of a test meal[29].

Ursodeoxycholic acid is, in contrast, only poorly soluble in water below pH 8.0[18], and is only partly in solution in the upper small intestine after oral administration[30]. Plasma profiles indicate that ursodeoxycholic acid absorption is not complete up to 10 hours after oral administration[31]. In ileostomy patients, over 50% of an oral 500 mg dose of ursodeoxycholic acid is excreted within 24 hours[32], of which over two-thirds is excreted unconjugated and apparently without prior absorption[32].

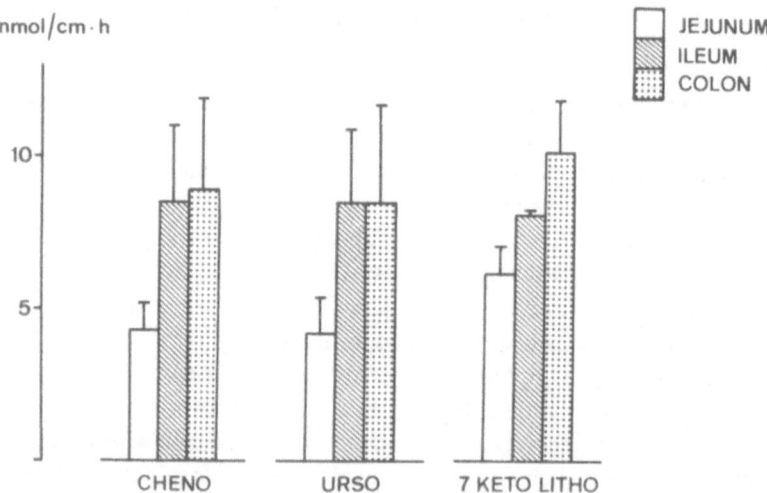

Figure 1 Absorption of bile acids in jejunum, ileum and colon of rat. Data were obtained in perfusion experiments at a perfusion concentration of 25 μmol/l (From *Z. Gastroenterologie* (1985) 23, 681–3). Abbreviations: CHENO = chenodeoxycholic acid; URSO = ursodeoxycholic acid; 7 KETO LITHO = 7-ketolithocholic acid.

In the rat, ursodeoxycholic acid is absorbed from the colon at the same rate as from the ileum[9]. In man, 90% of a 250 mg dose of ursodeoxycholic acid administered into the ascending colon is absorbed within 2 hours[31]. Colonic absorption may be of major importance, since ursodeoxycholic acid is poorly absorbed in the small intestine.

INHIBITION OF BILE ACID ABSORPTION

Many factors can decrease bile acid absorption[33].

Competitive inhibition of the absorption of individual bile acids by other bile acids has been demonstrated in the ileum and confirms the existence of an active transport site. Decreased small intestinal transit time decreases absorption of bile acids in the small intestine which, after passing into the colon, aggravate diarrhoea.

Incorporation of lipids into the micelle decreases the absorption of bile acids. This effect increases the intraluminal concentration of bile acids and thus facilitates micellar solubilisation and subsequent absorption of the lipid. The faecal excretion of bile acids increases in patients on high fat diets[34], but it is not clear whether this results from decreased intestinal bile acid absorption, increased biliary secretion or both. It has been suggested that there may be a causal relationship between high fat diets, high faecal bile acid excretion rates and the development of colon carcinoma.

Binding of bile acid in the intestine decreases absorption, which in turn increases catabolism of cholesterol to bile acids and thus decreases of plasma cholesterol. This is of clinical importance. Fibre has been shown to bind bile acids *in vitro* but initial reports that it greatly increased faecal bile acid excretion have not been confirmed. Ion exchange resins bind approximately ten times as much bile acid per gram as cellulose *in vitro*[35]. Cholestyramine decreases biliary and plasma concentrations of bile acid and increases faecal bile acid excretion[35]. It binds more dihydroxy than trihydroxy bile acid which leads to a particular decrease in the dihydroxy bile acid pool[36]. The decrease in plasma bile acids during cholestyramine treatment is used therapeutically in the treatment of patients with itching due to cholestasis.

SUMMARY

One of the most important steps in the enterohepatic circulation of bile acids is their efficient absorption from the intestine. Absorption occurs by passive diffusion in jejunum, ileum and colon and by active transport in the ileum. Most bile acid is absorbed in the jejunum and ileum; about 20% escapes absorption in the small intestine of which half is absorbed in the colon. Only approximately 10% of the bile acid pool is excreted each day in the faeces.

REFERENCES

1. Lack, L. and Weiner, I.M. (1963). Intestinal absorption of bile salts and some biological implications. *Federation Proc.*, **22**, 1334–8
2. Holt, P.R. (1963). Intestinal absorption of bile salts in the rat. *Am. J. Physiol.*, **207**, 1–7
3. Dietschy, J.M., Salomon, H.S. and Siperstein, M.D. (1966). Bile acid metabolism. I. Studies on the mechanisms of intestinal transport. *J. Clin. Invest.*, **45**, 832–46
4. Schiff, E.R., Small, N.C. and Dietschy, J.M. (1972). Characterisation of the kinetics of the passive and active transport mechanisms for bile acid absorption in the small intestine and colon of the rat. *J. Clin. Invest.*, **51**, 1351–62
5. Krag, E. and Phillips, S.F. (1974). Active and passive bile acid absorption in man. Perfusion studies of the ileum and jejunum. *J. Clin. Invest.* **53**, 1686–94
6. Samuel, P., Saypol, G.M., Meilman, E., Mosbach, E. and Chafizadeh, M. (1968). Absorption of bile acids from the large bowel in man. *J. Clin. Invest.*, **47**, 2070–8
7. Morris, J.S. and Heaton, K.W. (1974). The fate of labelled bile acids introduced into the colon. *Scand. J. Gastroent.* **9**, 33–9
8. Mekhjian, H.S., Phillips, S.F. and Hofmann, A.F. (1979). Colonic absorption of unconjugated bile acids. Perfusion studies in man. *Dig. Dis. Sci.*, **24**, 545–50
9. Walker, S., Stiehl, A., Raedsch, R., Kloters, P. and Kommerell, B. (1985). Absorption of urso- and chenodeoxycholic acid and their taurine and glycine conjugates in rat jejunum, ileum and colon. *Digestion* **32**, 47–52
10. Holmquist, L., Anderson, H. and Rudic, N. (1986). Bile acid malabsorption in children and adolescents with chronic colitis. *Scand. J. Gastroent.* **21**, 87–92
11. Huibregtse, F., Hoek, F., Sanders, G.T.B. and Tytgat, G.N.J. (1977). Bile acid metabolism in ileostomy patients. *Eur. J. Clin. Invest.*, **7**, 137–40
12. Hepner, G.W., Hofmann, A.F. and Thomas, P.J. (1972). Metabolism of steroid and amino acid moieties of conjugated bile acids in man. I. Cholylglycine (glycocholic acid). *J. Clin. Invest.*, **51**, 1889–97
13. Hepner, G.H., Hofmann, A.F. and Thomas, P.J. (1972). Metabolism of steroid and amino acid moieties of conjugated bile acids in man. II. Glycine-conjugated dihydroxy bile acids. *J. Clin. Invest.*, **51**, 1898–905
14. Cowen, A.E., Korman, M.G., Hofmann, A.F., Cass, O.W., and Coffin, S.B. (1975). Metabolism of lithocholate in healthy man. II. Enterohepatic circulation. *Gastroenterology*, **69**, 67–76
15. Allan, R.N., Thistle, J.L. and Hofmann, A.F. (1976). Lithocholate metabolism during chenotherapy for gallstone dissolution. 2. Absorption and sulphation. *Gut*, **17**, 413–19
16. Palmer, R.H. (1971). Bile acid sulphates. II. Formation metabolism, and excretion of lithocholate sulphates in rat. *J. Lipid. Res.*, **12**, 680–7
17. Carey, M.C. (1982). The enterohepatic circulation. In Arias, I.M., Popper, H., Schachter, D., Shafritz, D.A. (eds). The Liver. *Biology and Pathobiology*, 429–66, (New York: Raven Press)
18. Igimi, H. and Carey, C. (1980). PH-solubility relations of chenodeoxycholic and ursodeoxycholic acids: physical-chemical basis for dissimilar solution and membrane phenomena. *J. Lipid. Res.*, **21** 72–90
19. Stiehl, A. (1972). Bile salt sulphates in intra- and extrahepatic cholestasis. In Back, P. and Gerok, W. (eds). *Bile Acids in Human Diseases*, pp. 73–77, (Stuttgart–New York: FK Schattauer)
20. Stiehl, A. (1974). Bile salt sulphates in cholestasis. *Eur. J. Clin. Invest.*, **4**, 59–63
21. Stiehl, A., Earnest, D. and Admirand, W.H. (1975). Sulphation and renal excretion of bile salts in patients with cirrhosis of the liver. *Gastroenterology*, **68**, 534–44
22. DeWitt, E. and Lack, L. (1980). Effects of sulphation patterns on intestinal transport of bile acids sulphates. *Am. J. Physiol.*, **138**, G34–G39
23. Walker, S., Stiehl, A., Raedsch, R., Kloters, P. and Kommerell, B. (1986). Colonic absorption of sulphated and nonsulphated bile acids in rat. *Digestion*, **33**, 1–6

234

24. Stiehl, A., Ast, E., Czygan, P., Frohling, W., Raedsch, R. and Kommerell, B. (1978). Pool size synthesis, and turnover of sulphated and nonsulphated cholic acid and chenodeoxycholic acid in patients with cirrhosis of the liver. *Gastroenterology*, 75, 1016–20

25. Fedorowski, T., Salen, G., Colallilo, A., Tint, G.S. and Mosbach, E.H., (1977). Metabolism of ursodeoxycholate in man. *Gastroenterology*, 73, 1131–7

26. Fromm, H., Carlson, G.L., Hofmann, A.F., Farrivar, S. and Amin, P. (1980). Metabolism in man of 7-ketolithocholic acid: precursor of cheno- and ursodeoxycholic acids. *Am. J. Physiol.*, 239, G161–G166

27. Walker, S., Stiehl, A., Raedsch, R., Kloters, P. and Kommerell, B. (1985). Absorption of 7-ketolithocholic acid in rat jejunum, ileum and colon. *Z. Gastroenterologie*, 23, 681–3

28. Mok, H.Y. and Grundy, S.M. (1980). Cholesterol and bile acid absorption during bile acid therapy in obese subjects undergoing weight reduction. *Gastroenterology*, 78, 62–7

29. van Berge-Hengouwen, G.P. and Hofmann, A.F. (1977). Pharmacology of chenodeoxycholic acid. II. Absorption and metabolism. *Gastroenterology*, 73, 300–9

30. Parquet, M., Metman, E.H., Raizman, A., Ramband, J.C., Berthaux, N. and Infante, R. (1985). Bioavailability, gastrointestinal transit, solubilization and faecal excretion of ursodeoxycholic acid in man. *Eur. J. Clin. Invest.*, 15, 171–8

31. Stiehl, A., Raedsch, R., Walker, S., Rudolph, G. and Kloters, P. (1988). Colonic absorption of ursodeoxycholic acid in man. In Paumgartner, G., Stiehl, A. and Gerok, W. (eds). Bile Acids and the Liver. (Lancaster: MTP Press)

32. Stiehl, A., Raedsch, R. and Rudolph, G. (1988). Ileal excretion of bile acids: comparison to bile composition and effect of ursodeoxycholic acid treatment. *Gastroenterology*, 94, 1201–6

33. Stiehl, A., Walker, S. and Raedsch, R. (1983). Inhibition of cholesterol and bile acid absorption. In Creutzfeldt, W. and Folsch, U.R. (eds). Delaying Absorption as a Therapeutic Principle in Metabolic Diseases. (Stuttgart–New York: G. Thieme)

34. Brussaard, J.H., Katan, M.B. and Hautvast, G.A.J. (1983). Faecal excretion of bile acids and neutral steroids on diets differing in type and amount of dietary fat in young healthy persons. *Eur. J. Clin. Invest.*, 13, 115–22

35. Stanley, M.M., Paul, D., Gacke, D. and Murphy, J. (1973). Effect of cholestyramine, metamucil and cellulose on faecal bile salt excretion in man. *Gastroenterology*, 65, 889–94

36. van der Linden, W. and Nakayama, F. (1969). Change of bile composition in man after administration of cholestyramine (a gallstone dissolving agent in hamsters). *Acta Chir. Scand.*, 135, 433–8

SECTION F
LIPID MALDIGESTION AND BILE ACID MALABSORPTION

19

Fat Digestion and Solubilisation in Disease

P.L. Zentler-Munro*, D.R. Fine** and T.C. Northfield
*Department of Medicine, St. George's Hospital Medical School
London SW17 0RE, UK*

INTRODUCTION

Most foods contain large quantities of various fats, some of which are essential to life. Fat is not miscible with water. The assimilation of fat into a mainly watery organism therefore requires processes far more complex than those required for protein and carbohydrate assimilation. These processes are conveniently grouped under three headings: digestion, solubilisation and absorption. Digestion is an essentially chemical process comprising the hydrolysis of dietary fats – mainly long–chain triglycerides – into more polar lipolytic products – fatty acids and monoglycerides (the solutes). Solubilisation is an essentially physical process comprising the incorporation of these amphiphilic molecules into water-soluble particles formed by biliary amphipathic lipids (the solvent), so rendering previously insoluble lipids dispersible into aqueous solution. Absorption comprises the delivery of these water-soluble particles down a concentration gradient through the mucosal unstirred water layer to the intestinal mucosal cell membrane; it is not considered further here.

Professor Borgström has, in a previous chapter, discussed the many distinct but interdependent functions of each organ involved in the normal digestion and solubilisation of fat. He has shown how the combined effects of some of the processes described *in vitro* by Professor Carey can be identified in health. Observations in health tell us little, however, of the importance of each process taken on its own. The observation of diseases effecting each of these organs would, it might be hoped, reveal their precise contribu-

* Present address: Raigmore Hospital, Inverness
** Present address: Southampton General Hospital

tions and might also show how the body adapts itself to disruption of such a co-ordinated process. Many of the common disorders of fat assimilation involve several organs either directly or secondarily. This means that common features can be seen at work in most such diseases.

These common features devolve from certain characteristics of the five mediators of fat digestion and solubilisation; lingual lipase, pancreatic lipase, colipase, phospholipase, and biliary bile acid. The important characteristics of these compounds, in this context, are as follows. Lingual lipase is active down to about pH 3[1] but is inhibited by biliary amphipathic molecules such as bile acid but not phospholipid[2]. Pancreatic lipase is irreversibly inactivated below pH 5[3], and its inhibition by bile acid and lecithin can be overcome only by pancreatic colipase[4] and phospholipase[5] respectively. Phospholipase is also inactivated below pH 5[6]. Bile acids precipitate out of solution at a pH below their pKa[7], which for glycine-conjugated and free bile acids is around pH 5–6, and cannot then function as solubilisers. All bile acids can also be removed from aqueous solution by being bound to undigested protein[8], a process which is itself pH-dependent[9].

In this chapter, we shall discuss diseases affecting the five principal organs directly or indirectly involved in the digestion and solubilisation of fat: the tongue, the stomach, the pancreas, the biliary system and the small intestine. We shall show how a study of their pathophysiology has illuminated normal physiology, adaptive physiology and therapeutics.

THE TONGUE

The tongue secretes lingual lipase, an acid resistant enzyme capable of hydrolysing long-chain triglyceride to fatty acids and diglyceride[1]. Its role is probably to generate small amounts of fatty acid which promote emulsification in the stomach[10], and a co-ordinated action of pancreatic lipase and colipase in the duodenum[2,5]. Insufficiency of lingual lipase has not been described in man, but its contribution has been demonstrated by showing impairment of fat absorption in babies fed by nasogastric intubation rather than by suckling[11], and in rats subjected to oesophageal diversion[12]. It would be interesting to study fat absorption in patients subjected to glossectomy. The adaptive and therapeutic role of this enzyme in pancreatic disease will be discussed shortly.

THE STOMACH

The stomach also secretes an acid-resistant lipase whose actions have not been separated from those of lingual lipase. More importantly, its churning action is responsible for emulsifying dietary triglyceride with lecithin and protein, whilst its reservoir function is responsible for releasing this emulsion at an appropriately controlled rate into the duodenum[13]. Despite the commonness of total gastrectomy, the precise contribution to these functions has not been characterised.

The main contribution of the stomach to fat digestion is a negative one; it secretes large quantities of acid. This acid has to be neutralised in the duodenum by pancreatic bicarbonate in order to restore the neutral environment required for the remaining intraluminal processes involved in fat assimilation. This neutralisation is not completely effective even in health; in our study in healthy subjects[14], 20% of a meal entered the jejunum at a pH below 5, at which both lipase inactivation and bile acid precipitation were detected and shown to limit fat solubilisation.

The failure of this process of neutralisation is best seen in Zollinger-Ellison syndrome. In this disorder, massive gastric hypersection overwhelms the neutralising capacity of the pancreas and intrajejunal pH falls markedly.

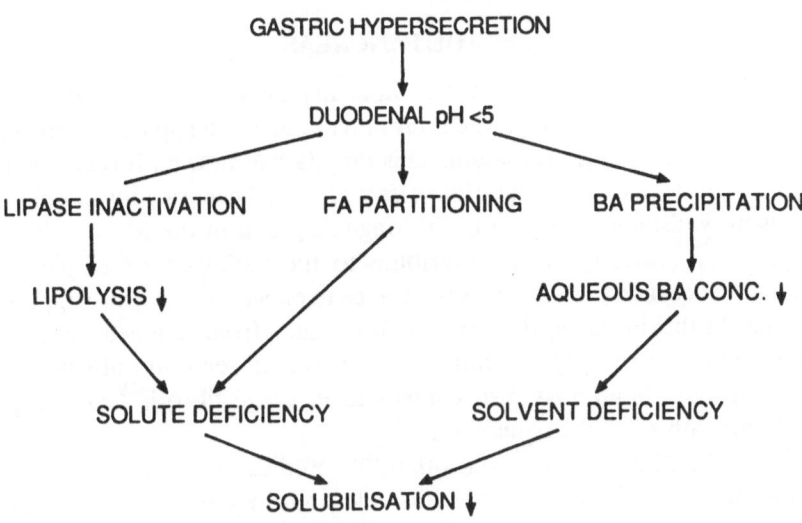

Figure 1   Intraluminal processes in Zollinger–Ellison syndrome

Go et al.[15], in a detailed study of intraluminal events in a patient with steatorrhoea due to Zollinger-Ellison syndrome, set the pace for future studies of this kind. By pooling and analysing separately postprandial chyme aspirated at pHs below 2.5 and above 5.5, they showed that endogenous pancreatic lipase – already diluted by the high volume of gastric secretion – was inactivated in the acidic samples. This inactivation directly impaired lipolysis and the formation of solute for solubilisation; it could not be reversed by neutralising the acidic samples *in vitro*. Bile acids were also present in sub-normal concentration, but in the acidic samples 50% of the available bile acid was precipitated out of solution. This process further reduced aqueous-phase concentrations of solvent but was, however, reversible *in vitro*. As a result of both processes, only 3% of the fatty acids were solubilised in the aqueous phase of the acidic samples of chyme, compared with 40% in the neutral samples – a proportion similar to that in healthy controls.

This study demonstrated, for the first time, the importance of in-traluminal pH in determining the efficiency of the chemical and physical processes of fat assimilation. Another factor the study did not examine was the direct effect of pH on the solubility of fatty acids in micellar solution. Fatty acids, like bile acids, are protonated at a pH below their pKa – around 6 – and pass out of micellar solution into an oil phase[16]. The process is like-ly to have contributed to impairment of lipid solubilisation in the acidic samples.

THE PANCREAS

Classical teaching has it that steatorrhoea in pancreatic exocrine insufficien-cy is due simply to the impaired secretion of pancreatic lipase and the resul-tant failure of solute formation. This dogma had not, until recently, been adequately tested. The deleterious effect of jejunal hyperacidity in Zollinger-Ellison syndrome suggested to Di Magno's group in the Mayo Clinic that jejunal hyperacidity might contribute to the pathogenesis of pancreatic steatorrhoea, and perhaps to its resistance to pancreatic enzyme supplemen-tation. In this instance, the hyperacidity results from reduced secretion of pancreatic bicarbonate[17,18] rather than increased secretion of gastric acid, although the latter may also contribute in cystic fibrosis[19] and in some patients with alcoholic pancreatitis[20].

The Mayo Clinic[21] and other[22,23] studies in alcoholic pancreatitis have shown that intrajejunal pH falls below 5 for a substantial proportion of the postprandial period, whilst our study in cystic fibrosis[24] has shown that the major proportion of a meal enters the jejunum below this pH. Inactiva-tion of endogenous lipase is irrelevant in the absence of this enzyme, but studies in both diseases[24,25] have demonstrated precipitation of a substantial proportion of the available bile acid, and a parallel impairment of lipid solubilisation. Our study[24] showed, using a mathematical model, that fatty acid protonation below pH 6 also limited lipid solubilisation, and that factor increased in importance when the formation of fatty acids was greatly promoted by administration of pancreatin[26]. It also showed that a rise in intrajejunal pH above 6 (by administration of cimetidine before the meal)

242

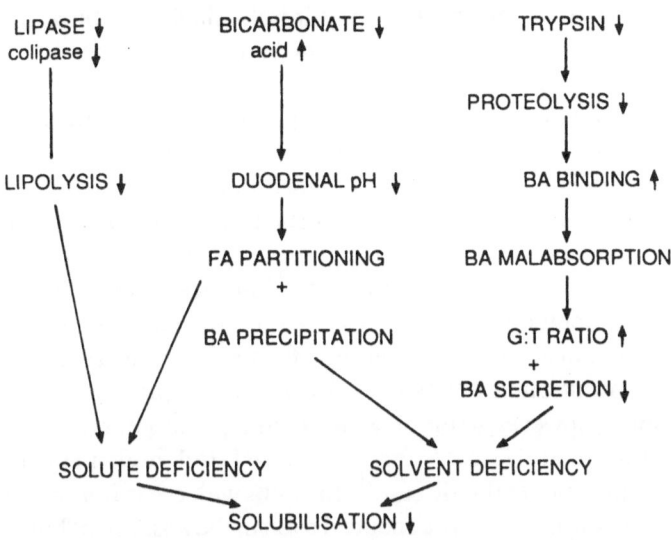

Figure 2   Intraluminal processes in pancreatic insufficiency

reduced bile acid precipitation and improved lipid solubilisation in the absence of administered lipase. These studies in both diseases showed a much greater improvement in fat solubilisation when these intrajejunal pH-dependent factors, as well as intragastric enzyme inactivation, were prevented by treating patients with cimetidine as an adjunct to pancreatic enzyme supplementation. Alteration in the formulation and coating of pancreatic enzyme supplements cannot restore fat absorption to normal when it is limited by such intrajejunal pH-dependent processes. These studies have shown, therefore, how pathophysiology has helped therapeutics.

Pancreatic colipase secretion is also reduced in pancreatic exocrine insufficiency. A careful study in cystic fibrosis[27] has shown that in patients with borderline lipase deficiency, the secretion of colipase determines the presence or absence of steatorrhoea. It is therefore important now to determine whether commercial pancreatic enzyme supplements contain sufficient colipase to saturate the available lipase. Individuals with deficient secretion of colipase alone have been reported[28]. These individuals have steatorrhoea, but the disturbances in their intraluminal processes have not yet been characterised.

The pathophysiology of pancreatic steatorrhoea may also involve deficient secretion of pancreatic proteases. We were surprised to find, in our study of cystic fibrosis[24], that bile acid precipitation was apparent in samples aspirated above pH 6, well above the pKa for all conjugated bile acids. Treatment with cimetidine, although raising intraluminal pH above 6, did not abolish this precipitation. We attributed this reduction in aqueous-phase bile acid concentration to the binding of bile acids to undigested protein, and subsequently showed quantitatively similar binding to the identical protein *in vitro* [9]. The abolition of both precipitation and binding by treatment with pancreatin in addition to cimetidine supports this model.

Protein-binding of bile acids affects both glycine and taurine conjugates alike, and increases as pH falls. It may explain[29] the marked increase in faecal bile acid excretion in cystic fibrosis[30] and in alcoholic pancreatitis[31]. This well-documented interruption of the enterohepatic circulation is not usually sufficient in cystic fibrosis children to impair bile acid secretion or intraluminal concentration unless liver disease is also present[32]. It probably does contribute, however, to the elevation of lithogenic index in cystic fibrosis patients with steatorrhoea[33] and the associated high prevalence of cholesterol gallstones in this disease[29]. In adults with cystic fibrosis, however, bile acid secretion appears to be reduced even in the absence of both steatorrhoea and liver disease[34], a finding attributed to impaired gallbladder motility. Intraluminal concentration, however, remains normal[24,34] but the interruption in the enterohepatic circulation leads to an increase in the proportion of glycine-congugated bile acids[24,35] which, with their much higher pKa, are more prone to pH-dependent precipitation. The administration of taurine reverses this trend and can reduce steatorrhoea by about 20%[36].

Cystic fibrosis has more recently revealed further problems with lipid solubilisation. In our study[24] we demonstrated that despite the marked reduction in lipolysis, concentrations of lipids in the aqueous phase were only slightly and not significantly reduced in comparison with healthy controls. The deficit in the Mayo Clinic study[25] is also surprisingly small. Our subsequent study[37], using ultracentrifugation to separate postprandial chyme into different physical phases, has demonstrated that this unexpected lipid can be accounted for by an increased concentration of endogenous biliary phospholipid in the aqueous phase. This results in a micellar phase which is unsaturated by the criteria of Mazer *et al.*[38]. Such unsaturated micellar phases decrease rather than promote fat absorption[39]. The situation probably arises from the absence of pancreatic phospholipase, which in health hydrolyses lecithin to yield lysolecithin. The latter is a more hydrophilic molecule which has a lower affinity for micellar solubilisation. This study also demonstrated two additional aqueous phases in health: a phase intermediate in density between the isotropic micellar phase and the oil phase, which contains liquid crystals, and a phase intermediate between the micellar phase and precipitate, which contains vesicles. The existence of these phases could be predicted from the *in vitro* work of Professor Carey and others[40], and inferred from mathematical analysis of existing data[41]. In patients with steatorrhoea due to cystic fibrosis the liquid crystalline phase is absent. In health this phase consists mainly of fatty acid and monoglyceride and its absence reflects reduced lipolysis. The vesicular phase is present, however, and contains the same concentration of fatty acid as in health, suggesting that it preferentially sequesters such fatty acid as is available. Whether absorption can occur from this phase is unknown, but on theoretical grounds[39] it is likely to be less efficient in promoting fat absorption than the micellar phase.

The study of cystic fibrosis has thus provided interesting insights into the pathophysiology of fat and bile acid malabsorption and their interactions. It has also revealed methods by which the body can compensate for pancreatic insufficiency.

Most patients with pancreatic achylia are able to absorb some fat. In our study[24] we found low levels of lipolysis despite the complete absence of pancreatic lipase. Subsequent studies have shown that this degree of lipolysis can be attributed to lingual lipase which, with its acid resistance, can act both in the stomach and in the hyperacidic duodenum. This enzyme is now known to act in this way in cystic fibrosis well beyond the period of its conventional role in infancy[42]. Our own studies[43] have suggested that its secretion may be increased in adults with cystic fibrosis, perhaps in compensation to provide greater intragastric lipolysis than was seen in health. No such increase has been identified in alcoholic pancreatic insufficiency[44]. Lingual lipase generates predominantly diglyceride rather than monoglyceride and fatty acid, and is unlikely therefore to drive fat digestion to completion. The enzyme has recently been biosynthesised but is likely to prove expensive to exploit commercially. Certain fungi produce similar enzymes which have been subjected to preliminary clinical trials, as an adjunct to conventional pancreatic supplements, with mixed results[45].

THE HEPATOBILIARY SYSTEM

Given the central role assigned to bile acid in acting as a solvent for fat solubilisation, steatorrhoea is seldom as prominent as might be expected in diseases of the organ where bile acid is synthesised. Steatorrhoea can complicate many forms of hepatic cirrhosis, but usually occurs only in the later stages of the disease when cholestasis develops, or when cirrhosis is associated with pancreatic exocrine insufficiency.

There had been little work on the effect of liver disease on fat solubilisation until Badley's classic study[46]. Patients with non-alcoholic cirrhosis were selected, in order that pancreatic insufficiency might not complicate the picture. In these patients, lipolysis was normal but the concentration

245

of bile acid in postprandial chyme was greatly reduced in patients with steatorrhoea, with a corresponding reduction in the micellar solubilisation of lipid. Cirrhotic patients without steatorrhoea were normal in both respects. Bile salt concentrations in the steatorrhoea patients were mostly below 4 mmol/l, a concentration that the same group had shown in an earlier

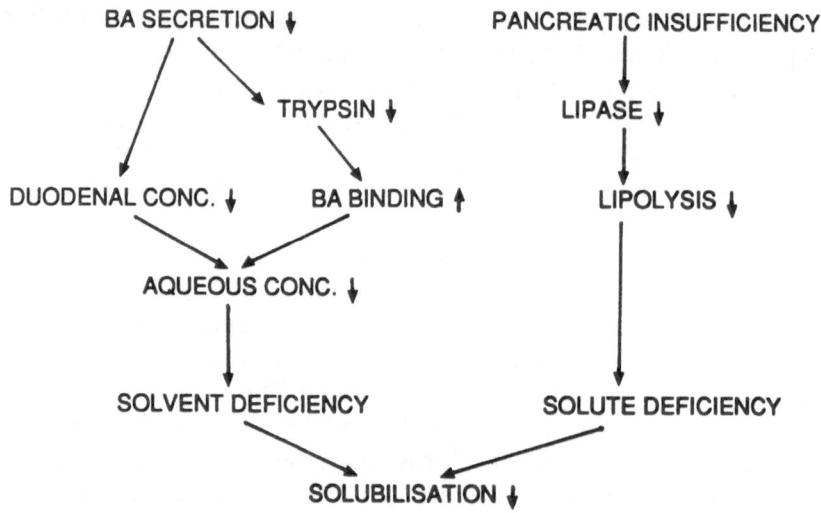

Figure 3   Intraluninal processes in hepatic cirrhosis

in vitro experiment[47] to be the minimum required to solubilise a normal dietary load of fat. This critical physiological concentration is somewhat higher than the critical micellar concentration of the bile acids involved in simple model solutions.

A more recent study of intraluminal events in patients with primary biliary cirrhosis from Barcelona[48] has confirmed this finding, and also illustrated the interaction between pancreatic exocrine insufficiency and cirrhosis. Earlier work had suggested that some patients with primary biliary cirrhosis also have pancreatic exocrine insufficiency. The Barcelona group analysed chyme from primary biliary cirrhosis patients with normal fat absorption, with steatorrhoea but normal pancreatic function as defined by trypsin output, and from a single patient with steatorrhoea and severe pancreatic insufficiency. Most patients with steatorrhoea had cholestasis 'as defined by hyperbilirubinaemia' and a significantly lower intraluminal concentration of bile acid than in the patients without steatorrhoea and in the healthy controls. There was, however, an even greater reduction in aqueous phase bile acid concentration in the patients with steatorrhoea, a value of 3 mmol/l precisely separating them from the patients without steatorrhoea. This reduction could not be attributed to pH-dependent precipitation, since the jejunum was hyperacidic only in the patient with pancreatic insufficiency. The authors demonstrated a direct correlation between intraluminal bile acid concentration and tryptic activity, and it may be that they were observing the effect of bile acid deficiency impairing trypsinogen activation and thus of impaired proteolysis on the binding of bile acid to undigested protein. All patients (except the one with pancreatic insufficiency) had normal lipolysis, but those with steatorrhoea had reduced fat solubilisation by comparison with non-steatorrhoeic patients and in healthy controls. The authors demonstrated an exponential relationship between aqueous phase bile acid concentration and faecal fat (reminiscent of Di Magno's enzyme : faecal fat curves), such that a concentration of 3 mmol/l clearly separated steatorrhoeic from non-steatorrhoeic patients – a value close to Badley's critical physiological concentration.

The intrahepatic cholestasis which characterises primary biliary cirrhosis occurs relatively early in the usually prolonged course of this disease, and is followed by the development of increasingly severe steatorrhoea. The situation forms an interesting contrast with extrahepatic cholestasis, as in pancreatic or bile duct carcinoma, where despite severe cholestasis – unaccompanied by cirrhosis – steatorrhoea is seldom severe. The pathophysiology of extrahepatic cholestasis has not been explored, but an early study of patients with external biliary fistulae[49] showed that small but significant quantities of fat can be absorbed in the complete absence of bile acid, and despite an associated marked reduction in fat solubilisation. Bile acids are now considered to speed the passage of lipid across the unstirred water layer by concentrating it in mixed micelles within the aqueous phase of intestinal contents. The more recent *in vitro* work already cited suggests that there are other methods of concentrating fat in the aqueous phase, and presumably these methods compensate for bile acid deficiency in cholestasis.

THE SMALL INTESTINE

Bile acid deficiency can also occur when disease or resection of the lower ileum impairs the reabsorption of bile acid from the intestine, reduces their return to the liver and thus interrupts the enterohepatic circulation. The liver is able to compensate for the loss of bile acid in the faeces by increasing synthesis to a certain extent, beyond which bile acid pool size and secretion rate fall[50]. In the classic Mayo Clinic study of ileectomy steatorrhoea[51], patients who had lost more than 100 cm of ileum had significant lower intraluminal bile acid concentrations than those with smaller ileal resections, and significantly worse steatorrhoea. Bile acid precipitation was apparent in these patients, and further reduced the amount of bile acid available for solubilisation. The authors were able to show a correlation between aqueous phase bile acid and lipid concentrations which, interestingly, extended linearly over the whole range of bile acid concentrations to the critical micellar concentration. In a study of patients with lesser degrees of resection[52], we confirmed the presence of pH-dependent precipitation of glycine-conjugated bile acids, but found no evidence of a fall in jejunal pH below the levels found in health. Treatment with cimetidine, nevertheless, reduced bile acid precipitation and improved lipid solubilisation.

As with other diseases, steatorrhoea in ileal resection is seldom total. This again suggests the presence of a compensatory mechanism. A study of patients with sufficient ileal disease or resection to cause a gross interruption of enterohepatic circulation but minimal or no steatorrhoea[53] was unable to identify any compensatory mechanism in terms of a change in micellar composition, or the presence of non-micellar forms of lipid solubilisation. This study, alone among those cited in this chapter, used ultrafiltration rather than ultracentrifugation to separate the different molecular forms of lipid present in postprandial chyme.

In conclusion, it is apparent that biochemistry, physical chemistry and experimental medicine are all coming together to contribute to the understanding of the common physiological processes that interact in different ways to produce steatorrhoea or to minimise it, in diseases effecting each of the organs involved in fat digestion and absorption.

SUMMARY

Recent advances in physiology have shown that the preparation of dietary fat for absorption is more complex than the classical model of pancreatic lipolysis and micellar solubilisation. Digestion also involves lingual lipase and pancreatic colipase, whilst solubilisation also involves the formation of vesicles and liquid crystals. Pancreatic bicarbonate provides the neutral environment required for digestion and solubilisation.

The pathogenesis of steatorrhoea in its various forms is, correspondingly, more complex than is classically taught. Three diseases illustrate how these processes interact.

In Zollinger-Ellison syndrome, the greatly increased secretion of gastric acid results in severe duodenal hyperacidity. Pancreatic lipase and trypsin are inactivated, so impairing lipolysis and proteolysis. Bile acids are precipitated, greatly diminishing aqueous phase concentrations, and fatty acids partition out of micellar solution.

In pancreatic steatorrhoea, the secretion of colipase determines whether steatorrhoea occurs when pancreatic lipase secretion is borderline.

248

Pancreatic bicarbonate deficiency leads to duodenal hyperacidity, which in turn leads to bile acid precipitation and fatty acid protonation – thus disrupting the whole process of solubilisation. Bile acids are bound to undigested protein and so excreted in faeces. This interruption of the enterohepatic circulation is compensated by an increase in bile acid synthesis so that bile acid secretion is maintained, but the proportion of glycine conjugates increases, thus predisposing to precipitation. What lipid is hydrolysed may be sequestered in vesicles and unsaturated micelles.

In cirrhosis, bile acid secretion is reduced so that intraluminal concentrations may become inadequate. Bile acid deficiency also impairs trypsinogen activation: the resulting undigested protein binds bile acid thus further decreasing their concentration in the aqueous phase of chyme. In primary biliary cirrhosis, true pancreatic insufficiency may also occur.

Despite these severe disturbances, fat absorption is seldom zero in these diseases – suggesting the presence of compensatory mechanisms. In pancreatic insufficiency, the persistence of lingual lipase allows some lipolysis, whilst in cirrhosis, liquid crystals and liposomes might act as an alternative means of lipid solubilisation when bile acid levels are inadequate.

REFERENCES

1. Hamosh, M., Klaeveman, H.L., Wolf, R.O., Scow, R.O. (1975). Pharyngeal lipase and digestion of dietary triglyceride in man. *J. Clin. Invest.*, **55**, 908–13
2. Carey, M.C. (1983). Role of lecithin in the absorption of dietary fat. In: Avogaro, P. *et al.*(eds.), *Phospholipids and Atherosclerosis*, Plenum Press, New York, pp. 33–62
3. Legg, E.F., Spencer, A.M. (1975). Studies on the stability of pancreatic enzymes in duodenal fluid to storage temperature and pH. *Clin. Chim. Acta 1*, **65**, 175–79
4. Hofmann, A.F. (1978). Lipase, colipase, amphipathic dietary proteins, and bile acdis: new interactions at an old interface (editorial). *Gastroenterology*, **75**, 530–32
5. Borgström, B. (1980). Importance of phospholipids, pancreatic phospholipase A2, and fatty acids for the digestion of dietary fat: *in vitro* experiments with the porcine enzymes. *Gastroenterology*, **78**, 954–62
6. Ihse, I. and Arnesjö, B. (1973). The phospholipase A2 activity of human small intestinal contents. *Acta Chem. Scand.*, **27**, 2749–56
7   Hofmann, A.F. (1983). The role of bile salts in fat absorption: the solvent properties of dilute, micellar solutions of conjugated bile salts. *Biochem. J.*, **89**, 57–68
8. Eastwood, M.A. and Hamilton, D. (1968). Studies on the absorption of bile salts to non-absorbed components of diet. *Biochem. Biophys. Acta*, **152**, 165–73
9. Lanzini, A., Fitzpatrick, W.J.F., Pigozzi, M.G. and Northfield, T.C. (1987). Bile acid binding to dietary casein: a study *in vitro* and *in vivo*. *Clin. Sci.*, **73**, 343–50
10. Hamosh, M., Scow, R.O. (1973). Lingual lipase and its role in the digestion of dietary fat. *J. Clin. Invest.*, **52**, 88–95
11. Hamosh, M., Scanlon, J.W., Ganot, D., Likel, M., Scanlon, K.B. and Hamosh, P. (1981). Fat digestion in the newborn – characterisation of lipase in gastric aspirates of premature and term infants. *J. Clin. Invest.*, **67**, 838–46
12. Roy, C.C., Roulet, M., Lefebvre, D., Chartrand, L., Lepage, G. and Fournier, L.A. (1979). The role of gastric lipolysis on fat absorption and bile acid metabolism in the rat. *Lipids,* **14**, 811–15

13. Miller, L.J., Malagelada, J.R. and Go, V.L. (1978). Postprandial duodenal function in man. *Gut,* 19, 699–736
14. Zentler-Munro, P.L., Fine, D.R., Fitzpatrick, W.J.F. and Northfield, T.C. (1984). Effect of intrajejunal acidity on lipid digestion and aqueous solubilisation of bile acids and lipids in health, using a new simple method of lipase inactivation. *Gut,* 25, 491–99
15. Go, V.L., Poley, J.R., Hofmann, A.F., Summerskill, W.H. (1970). Disturbance in fat digestion induced by acidic jejunal pH due to gastric hypersecretion in man. *Gastroenterology,* 58, 638–46
16. Borgström, B. (1967). Partition of lipids between emulsified oil and micellar phases of glyceride–bile salt dispersions. *J. Lipid Res.,* 8, 598–608
17. Regan, P.T., Malagelada, J.R., Dimagno, E.P., Go, V.L. (1979). Postprandial gastric function in pancreatic insufficiency. *Gut,* 20, 249–54
18. Dutta, S.K., Russell, R.M. and Iber, F.L. (1979). Impaired acid neutralisation in the duodenum in pancreatic insufficiency. *Dig. Dis. Sci.,* 24, 775–80
19. Cox, K.L., Isenberg, J.N. and Ament, M.E. (1982). Gastric acid hypersecretion in cystic fibrosis. *J. Pediatr. Gastroenterol. Nutr.,* 1, 559–65
20. Saunders, J.H., Cargill, J.M. and Wormsley, K.G. (1978). Gastric secretion of acid in patients with pancreatic disease. *Digestion,* 17, 365–69
21. Regan, P.T., Malagelada, J.R., DiMagno, E.P., Glanzman, S.L. and Go, V.L. (1977). Comparative effects of antacids, cimetidine and enteric coating on the therapeutic response to oral enzymes in severe pancreatic insufficiency. *N. Engl. J. Med.,* 297, 854–58
22. Dutta, S.K., Russell, R.M. and Iber, F.L. (1979). Influence of exocrine pancreatic insufficiency on the intraluminal pH of the proximal small intestine. *Dig Dis Sci* 24, 529–34
23. Bommelaer, G., Benque, A., Moreau, J., Bouisson, M. and Ribet, A. (1984). pH-metrie duodenale durant 24 heures dans les pancreatites chroniqes. *Gastroenterol. Clin. Biol.,* 8, 403–6
24. Zentler-Munro, P.L., Fitzpatrick, W.J.F., Batten, J.C. and Northfield, T.C. (1984). Effect of intrajejunal acidity on aqueous-phase bile acid and lipid concentrations in pancreatic steatorrhoea due to cystic fibrosis. *Gut,* 25, 500–7
25. Regan, P.T., Malagelada, J.R., DiMagno, E.P. and Go, V.L. (1979). Reduced intraluminal bile acid concentrations and fat maldigestion in pancreatic insufficiency: correction by treatment. *Gastroenterology,* 77, 285–89
26. Zentler-Munro, P.L., Fine, D.R., Batten, J.C. and Northfield, T.C. (1985). Effect of cimetidine on enzyme inactivation, bile acid precipitation and lipid solubilisation in pancreatic steatorrhoea due to cystic fibrosis. *Gut,* 26, 892–901
27. Gaskin, K.J., Durie, P.R., Lee, L., Hill, R., Forstner, G.G. (1984). Colipase and lipase secretion in childhood-onset pancreatic insufficiency. *Gastroenterology,* 86, 1–7
28. Hildebrand, H., Brogström, B., Bekassy, A., Erlanson-Albertsson, C. and Helin, I. (1982). Isolated colipase deficiency in two brothers. *Gut,* 23, 243–46
29. Zentler-Munro, P.L. (1987). Cystic fibrosis – a gastroenterological cornucopia. *Gut,* 28, 1531–47
30. Watkins, J.B., Tercyak, A.M., Szczepanik, P. and Klein, P.D. (1977). Bile salt kinetics in cystic fibrosis: influence of pancreatic enzyme replacement. *Gastroenterology,* 73, 1023-28
31. Dutta, S.K., Anand, K. and Gadacz, T.R. (1986). Bile salt malabsorption in pancreatic insufficiency secondary to alcoholic pancreatitis. *Gastroenterology,* 91, 1243–49
32. Robb, T.A., Davidson, G.P. and Kirubakaran, C. (1985). Conjugated bile acids in serum and secretions in response to cholecystokinin–secretion stimulation in children with cystic fibrosis. *Gut,* 26, 1246–56
33. Roy, C.C., Weber, A.M., Morin, C.L., Combes, J.C., Nusslé, D., Mégevand, A. and Lasalle, R. (1977). Abnormal biliary lipid composition in cystic fibrosis. Effect of pancreatic enzymes. *N. Engl. J. Med.,* 297, 1301–5
34. Weizman, Z., Durie, P.R., Kopelman, H.R., Vesely, S.M. and Forstner, G.G. (1986).

Bile acid secretion in cystic fibrosis: evidence for a defect unrelated to fat malabsorption. *Gut*, 27, 1043–48

35. Harries, J.T., Muller, D.P., McCollum, J.P., Lipson, A., Roma, E. and Norman, A.P. (1979). Intestinal bile salts in cystic fibrosis: studies in the patient and experimental animal. *Arch. Dis. Child.*, 54, 19–24

36. Darling, P.B., Lepage, G., Leroy, C., Masson, P. and Roy, C.C. (1985). Effect of taurine supplements on fat absorption in cystic fibrosis. *Pediatr. Res.*, 19, 578–82

37. Fine, D.R., Brown, C., Zentler-Munro, P.L., Bala, K., Batten, J.C. and Northfield, T.C. (1985). Composition and distribution of lipids in chyme from patients with pancreatic steatorrhoea. *Gut*, 26, 652 (abstract)

38. Mazer, N.A., Benedek, G.B. and Carey, M.C. (1980). Quasi-elastic light-scattering studies of aqueous biliary lipid systems. Mixed micelle formation in bile salt–lecithin solutions. *Biochemistry*, 19, 601–15

39. Westergaard, H. and Dietschy, J.M. (1976). The mechanism whereby bile acid micelles increase the rate of fatty acid and cholesterol uptake into the intestinal mucosa cell. *J. Clin. Invest.*, 58, 97–108

40. Lindström, M., Ljusberg Wahren, H., Larsson, K. and Borgström, B. (1981). Aqueous lipid phases of relevance to intestinal fat digestion and absorption. *Lipids*, 16, 749–54

41. Borgström, B. (1985). The micellar hypothesis of fat absorption: must it be revisited? *Scand. J. Gastroenterol.*, 20, 389–94

42. Abrams, C.K., Hamosh, M., Hubbard, V.S., Dutta, S.K. and Hamosh, P. (1984). Lingual lipase in cystic fibrosis. Quantitation of enzyme activity in the upper small intestine of patients with exocrine pancreatic insufficiency. *J. Clin. Invest.*, 73, 374–82

43. Balasubramanian, K., Brown, C., Fine, D., Batten, J.C. and Northfield, T.C. (1985). Compensatory increase in lingual lipase activity and intragastric lipolysis in pancreatic steatorrhoea caused by cystic fibrosis. *Gut*, 26, 576 (abstract)

44. Abrams, C.K., Hamosh, M., Dutta, S.K., Hubbard, V.S. and Hamosh, P. (1987). Role of nonpancreatic lipolytic activity in exocrine pancreatic insufficiency. *Gastroenterology*, 92, 125–29

45. Zentler-Munro, P.L. and Northfield, T.C. (1987). Pancreatic enzyme replacement – applied physiology and pharmacology. *Aliment. Pharmacol. Ther.*, 1, 575–92

46. Badley, B.W., Murphy, G.M., Bouchier, I.A. and Sherlock, S. (1970). Diminished micellar phase lipid in patients with chronic nonalcoholic live disease and steatorrhoea. *Gastroentrology*, 58, 781–89

47. Badley, B.W., Murphy, G.M. and Bouchier, I.A. (1969). Intraluminal bile salt deficiency in the pathogenesis of steatorrhoea. *Lancet*, 2, 400–2

48. Ros, E., García-Pugés, A., Reixach, M., Cusó, E. and Rodés, J. (1984). Fat digestion and exocrine pancreatic insufficiency in primary biliary cirrhosis. *Gastroenterology*, 87, 180–7

49. Porter, H.P., Saunders, D.R., Tytgat, G., Brunser, O. and Rubin, C.E. (1971). Fat absorption in bile fistula man. A morphological and biochemical study. *Gastroenterology*, 60, 1008–19

50. Dowling, R.H., Mack, E. and Small, D.M. (1970). Effects of conrolled interruption of enterohepatic circulation of bile salts by biliary diversion and by ileal resection on bile salt secretion, synthesis and pool-size in Rhesus monkey. *J. Clin. Invest.*, 49, 232–42

51. Poley, J.R. and Hofmann, A.F. (1976). Role of fat maldigestion in pathogenesis of steatorrhoea in ileal resection. *Gastroenterology*, 71, 38–44

52. Fitzpatrick, W.J.F., Zentler-Munro, P.L. and Northfield, T.C. (1986). Ileal resection: effect of cimetidine and taurine on intrajejunal bile acid precipitation and lipid solubilisation. *Gut*, 27, 66–72

53. Manbach, C.M., Newton, D., Stevens, R.D. (1980). Fat digestion in patients with bile acid malabsorption but minimal steatorrhoea. *Dig. Dis. Sci.*, 25, 353–62

20

Bile Acid Malabsorption, Diarrhoea and Steatorrhoea

H.V. Ammon
Division of Gastroenterology
Henry Ford Hospital
2799 W. Grand Blvd.
Detroit, MI 48202, USA

INTRODUCTION

Interruption of the enterohepatic circulation by ileal resection or ileal disease causes bile acid malabsorption and diarrhoea. Large ileal resection (> 100 cm) causes, in addition to bile acid malabsorption, significant steatorrhoea[1-4]. As a rule, the diarrhoea caused by short ileal resections responds to treatment with a bile acid binding resin, such as cholestyramine, while that caused by large ileal resections does not[1,2,5]. Faecal weight can sometimes be reduced by replacement of dietary fat with medium chain triglycerides[2]. These observations, together with experiments demonstrating that dihydroxy bile acids and fatty acids adversely affect intestinal electrolyte and water transport, have led to the concepts of 'bile acid' and 'fatty acid' diarrhoea[6].

Although these concepts are now well established, their mechanisms are only incompletely understood. The role of increased faecal bile acid loss in diarrhoeal syndromes unassociated with any demonstrated defect in the ileal transport of bile acids is still controversial[7,8]. This chapter discusses how bile acids and fatty acids induce diarrhoea, and how bile acid malabsorption can lead to diarrhoea and steatorrhoea. For a review of the diagnosis of bile acid diarrhoea the reader is referred to specific reports[9,10], and review articles[9-13].

BIOCHEMISTRY AND PHYSIOLOGY

Bacterial Modification of Bile Acids

Bile acids are normally actively reabsorbed in the ileum and only a small amount enters the colon in healthy individuals. This loss is compensated for by synthesis of new bile acids in the liver (0.2–0.6g/day). The hepatic synthesis rate can increase about ten times in response to interruption of the enterohepatic circulation[14].

Bile acids entering the colon undergo metabolic transformation. Taurine and glycine are removed to yield free bile acids which have a higher pK_a, and so are less water soluble and can be absorbed by non-ionic diffusion. In a second step the 7α-hydroxyl group is removed from the sterol nucleus, to form deoxycholate from cholate and lithocholate from chenodeoxycholate[14].

Effects of Bile Acids and Fatty Acids on Intestinal Transport:

Structure–Activity Relationships

The dihydroxy bile acids, chenodeoxycholate and deoxycholate and their glycine and taurine conjugates inhibit absorption and induce secretion of water and electrolytes in the jejunum, ileum and colon of experimental animals and man[15–19]. Bacterial metabolism of cholic acid thus results in the formation of a cathartic bile acid, deoxycholic acid. Effective secretory concentrations in man are 1–2 mmol/l in the ileum and 3 mmol/l in the colon[16,17]. The effects of lithocholic acid on intestinal transport have not been tested because of its poor aqueous solubility.

Structure–activity studies indicate that two hydroxyl groups in the alpha position are required to confer a secretory effect on a bile acid. Chenodeoxycholate ($3\alpha,7\alpha$-hydroxycholanoic acid) and deoxycholic acid ($3\alpha,12\alpha$-hydroxycholanoic acid) thus induce secretion, but ursodeoxycholate ($3\alpha,7\beta$-hydroxycholanoic acid) has no effect[15–19]. These experimental observations are in agreement with the clinical observation that patients receiving ursodeoxycholate for the dissolution of gallstones do not experience the diarrhoea sometimes suffered by patients receiving chenodeoxycholate. Conjugated bile acids are less active than unconjugated bile acids and conjugates of cholate have no effect[20,21]. These *in vivo* structure–activity relationships are reflected in the ability of bile acids to bind to brush border membranes[22] and to destroy liposomes[23]. These data suggest that an interaction with the lipid portion of the enterocyte membrane is the first event in the induction of intestinal secretion.

Unsaturated long-chain fatty acids also undergo bacterial modification with the formation of hydroxy fatty acids (10-hydroxy stearic acid from oleic acid). The structural similarity of 10-hydroxy stearic acid with a known cathartic fatty acid, ricinoleic acid (12-hydroxy- Δ9,10-octadecenoic acid), the active component of castor oil, led to the hypothesis that hydroxy fatty acids might be responsible for the diarrhoea associated with steatorrhoea[24]. At low concentrations (1–2 mmol/l) both hydroxy fatty acids have a greater effect on water transport than oleic acid[25], but all fatty acids with a chain length of ten carbon atoms or longer can adversely affect intestinal water transport, whether or not they have a hydroxyl group[26]. Because of its poor aqueous solubility 10-hydroxy stearic acid probably does not contribute much to the diarrhoea associated with steatorrhoea.

Structure–activity studies of fatty acids are difficult to interpret because of the limited solubility of fatty acids. When experiments are performed in the presence of bile acids, the results reflect not only the ability of the fatty acids to interact with the enterocyte membrane, but presumably also the monomer concentration of the bile acid in mixed micellar solutions. Fatty acids can have paradoxical effects *in vivo*. When added to taurocholate, oleate induces secretion[21], but the addition of 2 mmol/l oleate to a solution containing 2 mmol/l deoxycholate reduces the secretory effect of the bile acid[27]. Bile acids and fatty acids also stimulate mucus secretion and it is not clear how their interaction with mucus modifies the structure–activity relations.

Detergent Effects

Bile acids and fatty acids have detergent properties and all detergents or amphipaths tested so far affect intestinal transport. Of physiological or clinical interest are dioctyl sodium sulfosuccinate, (a widely used laxative)[28], lysophosphatidyl choline[29] and monoolein[30]. It seems reasonable to consider the effects of biles acid and fatty acids on intestinal transport as detergent effects. Detergents interact with cell membranes in many ways: from simple partition into the lipid portion of the bilayer at low concentrations, to complete membrane dissolution. The intermediate steps involve micellar solubilisation of membrane lipids, and binding to certain membrane proteins[31].

A complete analysis of the mechanisms by which bile acids and fatty acids affect intestinal transport is further complicated by the fact that the intestine is a highly integrated organ made up of many different cell types. Areas of absorption and secretion are anatomically separated in crypts and villi[32]. The intestine also has cells not directly involved in electrolyte and water transport such as goblet cells, enterochromaffin cells, and cells mediating immune and inflammatory responses. Electrolyte and water transport is modulated by intramural and extrinsic neural pathways, prostaglandins and possibly by serotonin and Vascoactive Intestinal Polypeptide[32]. It is therefore not surprising that bile acids and fatty acids have many complex effects on the intestine. In analysing experimental results, it is important not to ascribe the events leading to electrolyte and water secretion to a single mechanism. A detailed study of the cellular mechanisms may require the use of model epithelia grown in tissue culture (e.g. T$_{84}$ cells)[33].

Mechanisms of Action

Several hypotheses have attempted to explain the effects of bile acids and fatty acids on intestinal electrolyte and water transport. These include direct mucosal injury[18,34], enhancement of mucosal permeability[34,35], stimulation of production of cyclic-AMP[36-38], stimulation of prostaglandin synthesis[39], stimulation of calcium influx[40], and stimulation of local neural enteric reflexes[41].

Enhancement of Mucosal Permeability

The fluid secretion induced by dihydroxy bile acids and fatty acids in the intestine is generally associated with an increase in mucosal permeability – as shown by the enhanced absorption of oxalate[42] and low molecular ethylene glycols in the colon[43] and of mannitol and horseradish peroxidase in the small intestine[44,45], by the enhanced plasma to lumen clearance of urea, creatinine and inulin, and by the presence of ricinoleate or dihydroxy bile acids in the colon[34,43]. It has been postulated that the increased permeability, in combination with normal hydrostatic pressure, explains the electrolyte and fluid secretion induced by bile acids[35]. This hypothesis, however, does not explain the active electrolyte secretion observed in Ussing chamber experiments[38,46]. Nor does it explain why pretreatment of rats with propranolol inhibits fluid secretion induced by deoxycholate and ricinoleate, even though mucosal permeability remains increased[47]. Amphotericin B, which enhances mucosal permeability, actually enhances electrolyte and water absorption[47]. The threshold for an effect of bile acids on short circuit current (I_{sc} in Ussing chambers is lower on the serosal than on the mucosal side. An effect during mucosal application is only observed in association with an increase in permeability[48,49]. These findings suggest that enhancement of mucosal permeability provides the access for these compounds to the basolateral membrane, where they exert their secretory stimulus.

Mucosal Injury

Mucosal injury has been observed during perfusion of bile acids and fatty acids[18,3]4, but fluid secretion can occur in the absence of detectable injury[19,45]. The effects on intestinal transport are moreover readily reversible in the face of persisting mucosal injury[50]. Other agents capable of causing severe mucosal injury such as salicylates do not induce fluid secretion in the intestine[51]. These observations suggest that mucosal injury is not the direct cause for the electrolyte and water secretion.

Inhibition of Na^+-K^+-ATPase

Any inhibition of absorption by the mucosal villi would increase the net effect of electrolyte and water secretion by the crypt. Several studies indicate that bile acids inhibit Na^+-K^+-ATPase and it has been suggested that inhibition of this enzyme might impair absorption[52,53]. Since this enzyme is located at the basolateral membrane, enhancement of mucosal permeability is again a prerequisite for this effect. Inhibition of Na^+-K^+-ATPase does not explain the active chloride secretion observed *in vitro*, because ouabain actually abolishes the I_{sc} response to taurodeoxycholate in T_{84} cells[49].

Effects on Transport of Organic Solutes

The effects of bile acids on absorption of water and electrolytes are associated with changes in the absorption of organic solutes. Although irrelevant to the mechanism by which bile acids and fatty acids induce intestinal secretion, these effects are relevant to associated clinical complications such as hyperoxaluria, and to a complete description of the effects of bile acids and fatty acids on intestinal transport.

Bile acids and fatty acids decrease the absorption of glucose[15,21], xylose[21], amino acids[21,54], folic acid[21], and oxalate[55] in jejunal perfusion experiments. Ricinoleate and deoxycholate enhance the absorption of low molecular weight polyethylene glycol and oxalate in the colon[56]; the latter explains the development of hyperoxaluria in patients with malabsorption syndromes. The effects of fatty acids and bile acids on the absorption of actively transported compounds such as glucose and amino acids have been attributed to inhibition of active transport[54]. Their effects on the transport of organic solutes could, however, reflect the net results of two independent effects – enhancement of mucosal permeability and induction of fluid secretion. Using either cholera toxin or a hypertonic perfusate to stimulate secretion and amphotericin B to enhance mucosal permeability, we were able to reproduce qualitatively the effects of bile acids and fatty acids on organic solute transport[44]. Whilst amphotericin B alone enhances the absorption of glucose and low molecular weight polyethylene glycols, the superimposed stimulation of secretion by cholera toxin or the hypertoxic perfusate reduced net absorption of solute in the rat jejunum. In the colon, conversely, the same combination still induced net fluid secretion, but enhanced the absorption of solutes. This model reproduces the effects of bile acids and fatty acids on intestinal organic solute transport but does not explain their effect on electrolyte or fluid transport.

Stimulation of cAMP Production

Several investigators have observed an increase in mucosal cAMP content after exposing the intestine to bile acids or fatty acids[36-38], but not after exposing isolated enterocytes despite a response to PGE_1[56]. Similarly, we have not observed any rise in cAMP or cGMP content in confluent monolayers of T_{84} cells during exposure to 0.5 mmol/l taurodeoxycholate on the serosal side[49] which caused a short circuit rise due to active chloride secretion. In this model, both VIP and PGE_1 stimulated chloride secretion and short circuit current, in association with a rise in cAMP; heat-stable *E. coli* enterotoxin (ST) stimulated chloride secretion in association with a rise in cGMP. The effects of taurodeoxycholate and PGE_1 or heat-stable *E. coli* enterotoxin were additive, suggesting that they might be mediated by different mechanisms. Carbachol, which stimulates active chloride secretion in association with an increase in intracellular calcium activity, did not increase the short circuit response to TDC[49].

Stimulation of Prostaglandin Synthesis

Perfusion of ricinoleic acid or deoxycholate enhances intestinal prostaglandin output. It has therefore been proposed that the release of prostaglandins might mediate the effects of bile acids and fatty acids on electrolyte and water secretion[39]. In such perfusion experiments, the concentration of prostaglandins in the effluent from the rat colon was, however, lower by a factor of 10^4 than that needed to induce colonic secretion[51]. Pretreatment with indomethacin, moreover, reduced prostaglandin E output in response to deoxycholate by 87% but had no significant effect on fluid secretion. Thus, it is unlikely that prostaglandins play a role in mediating bile acid and fatty acid induced secretion.

Stimulation of Calcium Uptake

Bile acids and fatty acids enhance calcium uptake by brush-border membrane vesicles. It has therefore been suggested that calcium entry into the cell might mediate bile acid and fatty acid induced secretion[40]. Since bile acids are more effective during application to the serosal side calcium influx across the brush-border membrane is not likely to be a secretory stimulus. Taurodeoxycholate stimulates calcium absorption *in vivo* without a concomitant increase in fluid secretion[58]. On the other hand, removal of calcium from the serosal bathing medium abolished the I_{sc} response to serosal application of taurodeoxycholate, and measurement of intracellular calcium (using fura-2 fluorescence) suggested that taurodeoxycholate increased the intracellular

258

free calcium signal in T84 cells[49]. Analysis of the effect of various secretory stimuli on protein phosphorylation patterns in confluent monolayers of T84 cells suggests that the response to taurodeoxycholate represents the pattern seen in response to carbachol[59]. These findings, however, are only indirect evidence for a role of calcium in the events leading to bile acid stimulated chloride secretion.

Neural Mediators

Studies by Karlström *et al.* suggest that a significant portion of bile acid and fatty acid induced intestinal secretion is mediated by a local autonomous reflex arch[41]. In the denervated rat intestine fluid secretion induced by perfusion of deoxycholate or ricinoleate can be greatly reduced by serosal application of tetrodotoxin, or by intravenous hexamethonium, but not atropine. The authors suggest that bile acids and fatty acids stimulate an intramural neuroenteric reflex arch with a non-cholinergic postsynaptic neurotransmitter responsible for fluid secretion. Several neurotransmitters, such as VIP, stimulate cAMP production. This theory would explain the rise in cAMP observed in intact tissues but not in isolated cells or in tissue culture. Neural controls must differ between species because Kvietys *et al.* found that atropine inhibited oleate induced fluid secretion in the canine jejunum[60]. No *in vitro* study has yet been performed to confirm these *in vivo* observations.

Effects on Motility

The role of altered motility in the pathogenesis of bile acid and fatty acid diarrhoea is only poorly understood. Although altered transit time will not induce active secretion it could reduce water absorption. Bile acids and fatty acids can affect colonic motility *in vitro* [61] and *in vivo* [62], but whether they have a significant effect on colonic transit is not clear. There has been no direct comparison *in vivo* of the threshold concentrations for the effects on transport and motility.

CLINICAL STUDIES

Bile Acid Diarrhoea

The original concept of bile acid induced diarrhoea was based on clinical observations in patients who had lost the active ileal transport site by surgical resection. A rough correlation exists between the length of ileal resection and faecal bile acid loss. Faecal bile acid excretion rate is limited by hepatic synthesis[14]. The observation that faecal bile acid loss decreased in a few patients with large ileal resection[2] has not been supported by the results of other studies[3,4,63]. When patients with ileal resection and diarrhoea were treated with cholestyramine, only the diarrhoea of patients with ileal resection of < 100 cm improved. Patients with ileal resection > 100 cm had steatorrhoea (faecal fat > 20 g/24 hours), and their diarrhoea improved when dietary intake of long-chain triglyceride was reduced[2].

Bile acid diarrhoea due to loss or disease of the active transport site has been classified as Type I bile acid malabsorption[10] to distinguish it from conditions where bile acid malabsorption occurs in the presence of an intact ileum. Type II describes patients with chronic idiopathic diarrhoea, and excess faecal bile acid loss who respond to treatment with cholestyramine. The syndrome has been described in children and in adults[64,65] but is very rare. Detailed studies in two boys demonstrated a defect in the uptake of bile acids by the ileal mucosa[66]. A recent report described three adults with 'idiopathic bile acid malabsorption' who had normal vitamin B_{12} absorption and normal small bowel X-rays but microscopic abnormalities in the ileal mucosa comprising absent villi and crypt hyperplasia[67]. This study demonstrates how patients can be incorrectly classified unless fully investigated.

Type III bile acid malabsorption describes patients with diarrhoea attributed to bile acid malabsorption following cholecystectomy or vagotomy[68-70]. The mechanisms of bile acid malabsorption in this group are not clear. One hypothesis is that these patients had a marginal absorptive capacity for bile acids prior to surgery, which did not permit compensation for changes in intestinal transit or bile acid load after surgery.

Bile acids and fatty acids have to be in aqueous solution to affect electrolyte and water transport. Bile acids are deconjugated by colonic bacteria and free bile acids are less soluble at the prevailing faecal pH. In addition, significant amounts of bile acids are bound to fibre in the stool[71]. In patients with bile acid malabsorption the concentrations of dihydroxy bile acids in the aqueous phase of stool are frequently below those necessary to induce secretion in intestinal perfusion studies. The role of bile acid malabsorption in the pathogenesis of diarrhoea in these two groups of patients remains controversial[7,8].

Two other points have to be considered in interpreting these observations. Unconjugated bile acids are readily absorbed in the colon by passive non-ionic diffusion[72], whilst bile acid output into the colon is discontinuous and related to meals. Colonic bile acid concentrations may therefore reach higher levels at peak times, which might transiently affect colonic transport and possibly motility. These fluctuations would not be detected in stools pooled over 24 hours or longer. Thus, bile acid concentrations in faecal water below those 'effective' under experimental conditions may still contribute to the pathogenesis of the diarrhoea.

Fatty Acid Diarrhoea

The concept of fatty acid diarrhoea was originally based on studies of patients with steatorrhoea due to ileal resection, but applies to all forms of steatorrhoea. The relationship between faecal fat content and faecal weight is poor, because only fatty acids in aqueous solution can interfere with colonic water transport, whilst other factors may influence intraluminal events, such as the degree of lipolysis, the presence of bile acids, concurrent malabsorption of carbohydrates, changes in faecal pH, and formation of calcium soaps. In a preliminary report, the concentration of fatty acids in faecal water was surprisingly high but did not correlate with the presence or absence of diarrhoea[73].

The severity of steatorrhoea increases roughly with the length of intestinal resection. Most patients with ileal resections of > 100 cm excrete > 20 g of fat per 24 h[2-4,63]. The steatorrhoea of patients with large ileal resection can be attributed to several factors.

Bile acid output in these patients decreases throughout the day, and is accompanied by falling jejunal bile acid concentration as bile acid losses exceed hepatic synthesis rate[74]. During overnight fasting hepatic synthesis restores the bile acid pool to some extent, so that intrajejunal bile acid concentration during the first meal may be above the critical micellar concentration. This explains the clinical observation that bile acid diarrhoea often decreases in the course of a day, and that many patients with short ileal resection and diarrhoea require cholestyramine only with the morning meal.

When unconjugated bile acids absorbed from the colon return to the liver, they are conjugated with glycine and taurine. In the process of deconjugation taurine (an essential amino acid) is lost. This increases the ratio of glycine to taurine conjugated bile acids from 3:1 to 8:1. Glycine conjugated bile acids have a high pK_a and are therefore poorly soluble at the prevailing pH of the duodenum[75]. As a result the aqueous phase concentration of bile acids in the duodenum in patients with ileal resection is even lower than the already reduced total bile acid concentration[76]. These two factors lead to a decrease in the jejunal bile acid concentration below the critical micellar concentration which impairs fat absorption[74,76,77].

The loss of compensatory absorptive surface due to the large ileal resection also contributes. Normally dietary fat is absorbed in the proximal jejunum. With impaired solubilisation fat absorption is delayed and the distal jejunum and ileum are recruited as additional absorptive surface area. When this compensatory surface area is lost, significant steatorrhoea develops. The importance of the compensatory absorptive surface is confirmed by the finding that patients with a short ileal resection may also have low jejunal bile acid concentrations but only mild steatorrhoea[76].

261

SUMMARY

Interruption of the enterohepatic circulation of bile acids can lead to diarrhoea and steatorrhoea. The diarrhoea is caused by the effects of dihydroxy bile acids and fatty acids on colonic electrolyte and water transport. Steatorrhoea occurs when bile acid loss exceeds the capacity of the liver to synthesise new bile acids, so that output decreases and jejunal bile acid concentration falls below the critical micellar concentration. The loss of compensatory absorptive surface due to ileal resection results in steatorrhoea. The cathartic properties of bile acids and fatty acids can be attributed to their detergent effects on the intestinal mucosa. Many other effects on the intestine have been described, but a clear understanding of the mechanisms by which bile acids and fatty acids affect intestinal electrolyte and water transport has still not emerged. Detergents enhance mucosal permeability and thereby get access to the basolateral membrane of the enterocytes where they stimulate active chloride secretion. Inhibition of absorption may also unmask concurrent normal secretion. A significant proportion of the secretory response may be mediated by neural mechanisms. Whether changes in intestinal motility induced by these agents contribute to the diarrhoea has not been defined. The concept of bile acid diarrhoea has been extended to other syndromes of diarrhoea with increased faecal bile acid loss such as cases of idiopathic diarrhoea, and post-cholecystectomy or post-vagotomy diarrhoea. The significance of increased faecal bile acid loss in the pathogenesis of diarrhoea under these circumstances is controversial.

Acknowledgements

Worked performed in the author's laboratory was supported by NIH Grant AM 17941 and DK 38428, and by the Research Service of the Veterans Administration.

REFERENCES

1. Hofmann, A.F. and Poley, J.R. (1969). Cholestyramine treatment of diarrhoea associated with ileal resection. *N. Engl. J. Med.*, **281**, 397–401
2. Hofmann, A.F. and Poley, J.R. (1972). Role of bile acid malabsorption in pathogenesis of diarrhoea and steatorrhoea in patients with ileal resection. *Gastroenterology*, **62**, 918–34
3. McJunkin, R., Fromm, H., Sarva, R.P. and Amin, P. (1981). Factors in the mechanism of diarrhoea in bile acid malabsorption: Faecal pH - a key determinant. *Gastroenterology*, **80**, 1454–64
4. Aldini, R., Roda, A., Festi, D., Sama, C., Mazzalle, G., Bazzoli, F., Morselli, A.M., Roda, E. and Barbara, L. (1982). Bile acid malabsorption and bile acid diarhoea in intestinal resection. *Dig. Dis. Sci.*, **27**, 495–502
5. Poley, J.R. and Hofmann, A.F. (1976). Role of fat maldigestion in pathogenesis of steatorrhoea in ileal resection. *Gastroenterology*, **71**, 38–44

6. Hofmann, A.F. (1972). Bile acid malabsorption caused by ileal resection. *Arch. Intern. Med.*, **130**, 597–605

7. Fromm, H., Tunuguntla, A.K., Malavolti, M., Sherman, C. and Ceryak, S. (1987). Absence of significant role of bile acids in diarrhoea of a heterogeneous group of postcholecystectomy patients. *Dig. Dis. Sci.*, **32**, 33–44

8. Schiller, L.R., Hogan, R.B., Morawki, S.G., Santa Ana, C.A., Bern, M.J., Norgaard, R.P., Bo-Linn, G.W. and Fordtran, J.S. (1987). Studies of the prevalence and significance of radiolabelled bile acid malabsorption in a group of patients with idiopathic chronic diarrhoea. *Gastroenterology*, **92**, 151–60

9. Balistreri, W.F., Heubi, J.E. and Suchy, F.J. (1983). Bile acid metabolism: Relationship of bile acid malabsorption and diarrhoea. *J. Pediatr. Gastroenterol. Nutr.*, **2**, 105–21

10. Fromm, H. and Malavolti, M. (1986). Bile acid-induced diarrhoea. *Clin. Gastroenterol.*, **15**, 567–82

11. Binder, H.J. (1980). Pathophysiology of bile-acid- and fatty acid-induced diarrhoea. In: Field, M., Fordtran, J.S. and Schultz S.G. (eds.) *Secretory Diarrhoea.*, pp. 159–76, (Baltimore, Maryland: Waverly Press, Inc)

12. Dowling, R.H. (1983). Bile acids in constipation and diarrhoea. In: Barbara, L., Dowling, R.H., Hoffmann and Roda, E. (eds) *Bile Acids in Gastroenterology*, pp. 157–71, (Lancaster: MTP Press)

13. Ammon, H.V. (1985). Effects of fatty acids on intestinal transport. In: Kabara, JJ. (eds.) *The Pharmacological Effect of Lipids II*, pp. 173–81, (Champaign, IL: The American Oil Chemists' Society)

14. Carey, M.C. (1982). The enterohepatic circulation. In: Arias, I., Popper, H., Schachter, D. and Shafritz D.A. (eds) *The Liver: Biology and Pathobiology*, pp. 429–65, (New York: Raven Press)

15. Wingate, D.L., Phillips, S.F., and Hofmann, A.F. (1973). Effect of glycine-conjugated bile acids with and without lecithin on water and glucose absorption in perfused human jejunum. *J. Clin. Invest.*, **52**, 1230–6

16. Krag, E. and Phillips S.F. (1974). Effect of free and conjugated bile acids on net water, electrolyte and glucose movement in the perfused human ileum. *J. Lab. Clin. Med.*, **83**, 947–56

17. Mekhjian, H.S., Phillips, S.F. and Hofmann, A.F. (1971). Colonic secretion of water and electrolytes induced by bile acids: Perfusion studies in man. *J. Clin. Invest.*, **50**, 1569–77

18. Chadwick, V.S., Gaginella, T.S., Carlson, G.L., Debongnie, J.-C., Philips, S.F. and Hofmann, A.F. (1979). Effect of molecular structure on bile acid-induced alterations in absorptive function, permeability, morphology in the perfused rabbit colon. *J. Lab. Clin. Med.*, **94**, 661–74

19. Mekhjian, H.S. and Phillips S.F. (1970). Perfusion of the canine colon with unconjugated bile acids. *Gastroenterology*, **59**, 120–9

20. Harries, J.T. and Sladen, G.E. (1972). The effects of different bile salts on the absorption of fluid, electrolytes, monosaccharides in the small intestine in the rat *in vivo*. *Gut*, **13**, 596–603

21. Ammon, H.V., Thomas, P.J. and Phillips, S.F. (1974). Effects of long-chain fatty acids on solute absorption: Perfusion studies in the human jejunum. *Gut*, **18**, 805–13

22. Wilson, F.A. and Treanor, L.L. (1977). Characterisation of bile acid binding to rat intestinal brush-border membranes. *J. Membr. Biol.*, **33**, 213–30

23. Ammon, H.V. and Charaf, U.K. (1985). Effects of bile acids and fatty acids on the integrity of large unilamellar lipsomes. *Gastroenterology*, **88**, 1646 (abstract)

24. James, A.T., Webb, J.P.W. and Kellock, T.D. (1961). The occurrence of unusual fatty acids in faecal lipids from human beings with normal and abnormal fat absorption. *Biochem. J.*, **78**, 333–9

25. Ammon, H.V. and Phillips, S.F. (1973). Inhibition of colonic water and electrolyte absorption by fatty acids in man. *Gastroenterology*, **65**, 744–9

26. Ammon, H.V. and Phillips, S.F. (1974). Inhibition of ileal water absorption by in-

traluminal fatty acids. *J. Clin. Invest.*, **53**, 205–10

27. Lamabadusuriya, S.P., Guiraldes, E. and Harries, J.T. (1975). Influence of mixtures of taurocholate, fatty acids and monolein on the toxic effects of deoxycholate in rat jejunum *in vivo*. *Gastroenterology*, **69**, 463–9

28. Sund, R.B. and Matheson, I. (1978). Glucose and cation transport in rat jejunum, ileum and colon *in vivo*: Effect of anionic and nonionic surfactants and of deoxycholate. *Acta Pharmacol. Toxicol.*, **42**, 253–8

29. Ammon, H.V., Luedtke, L.A. and Andrade, M.A. (1983). Effects of lysophosphatidyl choline on jejunal water and solute transport in the rat *in vivo*. *Lipids*, **18**, 428–33

30. Ammon, H.V., Kozlov, N., Reilly, K. and Wappler, N. (1987). Effects of monoolein on water and solute transport in the human jejunum and cultured model epithlium. *Gastroenterology*, **92**, 1295 (abstract)

31. Helenius, A. and Simons, K. (1975). Solubilisation of membranes by detergents. *Biochim. Biophys. Acta*, **415**, 29–79

32. Donowitz, M. and Welsh, J. (1987). Regulation of mammalian small intestinal electrolyte secretion. In Johnson, LR (ed.) *Physiology of the Gastrointestinal Tract*, pp. 1351–88, (New York: Raven Press)

33. Dharmsathaphorn K., Mandel, K.G., McRoberts, J.A., Cartwright, C.A. and Masui, H. (1983). Utilization of a human colonic tumour cell line as a model to study electrolyte transport in the intestine. In: Skadhauge, E. and Heintze, K. (eds) *Intestinal Absorption and Secretion*, pp. 325–33, (Lancaster: MTP Press)

34. Cline, W.S., Lorenzsonn, V., Benz, L., Bass, P. and Olsen, W.A. (1976). The effects of sodium ricinoleate on small intestinal function and structure. *J. Clin. Invest.*, **58**, 380–90

35. Nell, G. and Rummel, W. (1984). Action mechanisms of secretagogue drugs. In: Csaky, TZ (ed.) *Handbook of Experimental Pharmacology*, pp. 461–508, (Berlin: Springer-Verlag)

36. Binder, H.J., Filburn, C. and Volpe, B.T. (1975). Bile salt alteration of colonic electrolyte transport: role of cyclic adenosine monophosphate. *Gastroenterology*, **68**, 503–8

37. Conley, D.R., Coyne, M.J., Bonorris, G.G., Chung, A. and Schoenfield, L.J. (1976). Bile acid stimulation of colon adenylate cyclase and secretion in the rabbit. *Am. J. Dig. Dis.*, **21**, 453–8

38. Racusen, L.C. and Binder, H.J. (1979). Ricinoleic acid stimulation of active anion secretion in colonic mucosa of the rat. *J. Clin. Invest.*, **63**, 743–9

39. Beubler, E. and Juan, H. (1979). Effect of ricinoleic acid and other laxatives on net water flux and prostaglandin E release by the rat colon. *J. Pharm. Pharmacol.*, **31**, 681–5

40. Maenz, D.D. and Forsyth, G.W. (1982). Ricinoleate and deoxycholate are calcium ionophores in jejunal brush-border vesicles. *J. Membrane Biol.*, **70**, 125–33

41. Karlstrom, L., Cassuto, J., Jodal, M. and Lundgren, O. (1983). The importance of the enteric nervous system for the bile-salt induced secretion in the small intestine of the rat. *Scand. J. Gastroenterol.*, **18**, 117–23

42. Dobbins, J.W. and Binder, H.J. (1976). Effect of bile salts and fatty acids on the colonic absorption of oxalate. *Gastroenterology*, **70**, 1096–100

43. Gaginella, T.S., Chadwick, V.S., Debongnie, J.C., Lewis, J.C. and Phillips, S.F. (1977). Perfusion of rabbit colon with ricinoleic acid: Dose related mucosal injury, fluid secretion and increased permeability. *Gastroenterology*, **73**, 95–101

44. Ammon, H.V., Walter, L.G. and Loeffler, R.F. (1983). Effects of amphotericin B and cholera toxin on intestinal transport in the rat. *J. Lab. Clin. Med.*, **102**, 509–21

45. Teichberg, S., McGarvey, E., Bayne, M. and Lifshitz, F. (1983). Altered jejunal macromolecular barrier induced by α-dihydroxy deconjugated bile salts. *Am. J. Physiol.*, **245**, G122–32

46. Binder, H.J. and Rawlins, C.L. (1973). Effect of conjugated dihydroxy bile salts on electrolyte transport in rat colon. *J. Clin. Invest.*, **52**, 1460–6

47. Binder, H.J., Dobbins, J.W., Racusen, L.C. and Whiting, D.S. (1978). Effect of propranolol on ricinoleic acid- and deoxycholic acid-induced changes of intestinal

electrolyte movement and mucosal permeability. *Gastroenterology*, 75, 668–73

48. Freel, R.W., Hatch, M., Earnest, D.L. and Goldner, A.M. (1983). Dihydroxy bile salt-induced alterations in NaCl transport across the rabbit colon. *Am. J. Physiol.*, 245, G808–15

49. Ammon, H.V. and Dharmsathaphorn, K. (1986). Mechanism of action of bile salts on colonic Cl– secretion: A study based on a cultured epithelial model. *Clin. Res.*, 34, 436A (abstract)

50. Teem, M.V. and Phillips, S.F. (1972). Perfusion of the hamster jejunum with conjugated and unconjugated bile acids: inhibition of water absorption and effects of morphology. *Gastroenterology*, 62, 261–7

51. Satterfield, S.T, Ammon, H.V., Komoroski, R.A. and Loeffler, R.F. (1985). Effect of salicylic acid on jejunal transport and morphology: Dissociation of mucosal damage and fluid secretion. *Gastroenterology*, 88, 1572 (abstract)

52. Guiraldes, E., Lamabadusuriya, S.P., Oyesiku, J.E., Whitfield, A.E. and Harries, J.T. (1975). A comparative study on the effects of different bile salts on mucosal ATPase and transport in the rat jejunum *in vivo*. *Biochim. Biophys. Acta*, 389, 495–505

53. Hafkenscheid, J.C.M. (1977). Influence of bile acids on the (Na^+-K^+)-activated and Mg^2-activated ATP-ase of rat colon. *Pflüger's Arch.*, 369, 203–6

54. Caspary, W.F. (1974). Inhibition of active hexose and amino acid transport by conjugated bile salts in rat ileum. *Eur. J. Clin. Invest.*, 4, 17–24

55. Saunders, D.R., Sillery, J. and McDonald, G.B. (1975). Regional differences in oxalate absorption by rat intestine: Evidence for excessive absorption by the colon in steatorrhoea. *Gut*, 16, 543–54

56. Gaginella, T.S., Phillips, S.F., Dozois, R.R. and Go, V.L.W. (1978). Stimulation of adenylate cyclase in homogenates of isolated intestinal epithelial cells from hamsters. *Gastroenterology*, 74, 11'5

57. Rampton, D.S., Breuer, N.F., Vaja, S.G.H., Sladen, G.E. and Dowling, R.H. (1981). Role of prostaglandins in bile salt-induced changes in rat colonic structure and function. *Clin. Sci.*, 61, 641–8

58. Ammon, H.V., Cho, D.S., Loeffler, R.L. and Reetz, K.L. (1986). Effects of taurodeoxycholate on *in vivo* water and solute transport in rat jejunum in absence and presence of calcium. *Am J. Phyisol.*, 250, (Gastrointest Liver Physiol 13): G248–51

59. Cohn, J. and Dougherty, N. (1987). Distinct protein phosphorylation effects of calcium and cAMP-mediated secretagogues in T84 cell monolayers. *Gastroenterology*, 92, 1350 (abstract)

60. Kvietys, P.R., Wilborn, W.H. and Granger, D.N. (1981). Effect of atropine on bile-oleic acid-induced alteration in dog jejunal hemodynamics, oxygenation and net transmucosal water movement. *Gastroenterology*, 80, 31–8

61. Christensen, J. (1987). Motility of the colon. In: Johnson, L.R. (ed.) *Physiology of the Gastrointestinal Tract*, pp. 665–93, (New York: Raven Press)

62. Stewart, J.J. and Bass, P. (1976). Effect of ricinoleic and oleic acids on the digestive contractile activity of the canine small and large bowel. *Gastroenterology*, 70, 37–6

63. Woodbury, J.F. and Kern, F. (1971). Faecal excretion of bile acids: A new technique for studying bile acid kinetics in patients with ileal resection. *J. Clin. Invest.*, 50, 2531–40

64. Thaysen, E.G.H. and Pedersen, L. (1976). Idiopathic bile acid catharsis. *Gut*, 17, 965–70

65. Heubi, J.E., Balistreri, W.F., Partin, J.C. and Schubert, W.E.K. (1979). Refractory infantile diarrhoea due to primary bile acid malabsorption. *J. Pediatr.*, 94, 546–61

66. Heubi, J.E., Balistreri, W.F., Fondacaro, J.D., Partin, J.C. and Schubert, W.K. (1982). Primary bile acid malabsorption: Defective in vitro ileal active bile acid transport. *Gastroenterology*, 83, 804–11

67. Popovic, O.S., Kostic, K.M., Milovic, V.B., Milutinovic-Djuriic, S., Miletic, V.D., Sesic, L., Djordjevic, M., Bulajic, M., Bojic, P. Rubinic, M. and Borisavljevic, N. (1987). Primary bile acid malabsorption. Histologic and immunologic study in three patients.

Gastroenterology, **92**, 1851–8

68. Hutcheon, D.F., Bayless, T.M. and Gadacz, T.R. (1979). Postcholecystectomy diarrhoea. *J. Am. Med. Assoc.*, **241**, 823–4

69. Duncombe, V.M., Bolin, T.D. and David, A.E. (1977). Double-blind trial of cholestyramine in postvagotomy diarrhoea. *Gut*, **18**, 531–59

70 Allan, J.G., Gerskowitch, V.P. and Russell, R.I. The role of bile acids in the pathogenesis of postvagotomy diarrhoea. *Br. J. Surg.*, **51**, 516–8

71. Eastwood, M.A. and Hamilton, D. (1968). Studies on the adsorption of bile salt to non absorbed components of diet. *Biochem. Biophys. Acta*, **151**, 165–73

72. Mekhjian, H.S., Phillips, S.F. and Hofmann, A.F. (1979). Colonic absorption of unconjugated bile acids. Perfusion studies in man *Dig. Dis. Sci.*, **24**, 545–50

73. Bliss, C.M., Small, D.M. and Donaldson, R.M. (1973). Water phase fatty acid excretion in diarrhoea. *Gastroenterology*, **64**, 701 (abstract)

74. Van Deest, B.W., Fordtran, J.S., Morawski, S.G. and Wilson, J.D. (1968). Bile salt and micellar fat concentration in proximal small bowel contents in ilectomy patients. *J. Clin. Invest.*, **47** 1314–24

75. Abaurre, R., Grodon, S.G., Mann, J.G. and Kern, F. (1969). Fasting bile salt pool size and composition after ileal resection. *Gastroenterology*, **57**, 679–88

76. Mansbach, C.M., Newton, D. and Stevens, R.D. (1980). Fat digestion in patients with bile acid malabsorption but minimal steatorrhoea. *Dig. Dis. Sci.*, **25**, 353–62

77. Poley, J.R. and Hofmann, A.F. (1976). Role of fat maldigestion in pathogenesis of steatorrhoea of ileal resection. *Gastroenterology*, **71**, 38–44

21

Bile Acids in Irritable Bowel Syndrome

M. Eastwood* and M. Merrick**
*Wolfson Laboratories
Gastrointestinal Unit
**Department of Nuclear Medicine
Western General Hospital
Edinburgh, EH4 2XU, UK

INTRODUCTION

An holistic view of the irritable bowel syndrome postulates the problem developing from three sources:[1] physical factors including deficiency of dietary fibre or undiagnosed or early organic disease such as Crohn's disease; adverse life events which lead to feelings of hopelessness and hence anxiety; and the patient's personality.

These factors form a triangle, the shape of which is dependent on their relative importance in each individual and his or her personality. Indeed the proportions of the triangle may vary in the same subject, along with alterations in the relative contributions of the individual factors, over a period of time.

It is possible to examine whether there is any reason for regarding any of the three main factors in the irritable bowel syndrome – emotional, personality and physical factors – as contributing at least to the diarrhoea through a mechanism mediated by bile acids.

EMOTIONAL FACTORS

Many clinicians have been impressed by the psychological characteristics associated with the irritable bowel syndrome. It is possible that this condition is often a part of and prolonged by psychiatric illness[2]; stress factors or threatening life events appear to be involved in its production and maintenance. Irritable bowel syndrome patients appear to have suffered more bereavements and illnesses in early life. The biological mechanisms of this relationship between emotion and bowel function has yet to be described.

The relationship between stool weight and bile acid content is well established. The wide variation in the amounts of stool passed by healthy individuals could either, directly or by unknown secondary mechanisms, alter faecal bile acid excretion. We know of no data, however, relating faecal bile acid output with emotional state.

Personality strongly influences stool weight and frequency independently of diet[3]. This emotional influence could account for as much variation in stool output as, perhaps, dietary fibre. It has been suggested that persons who are more socially outgoing, more energetic and optimistic, less anxious, less socially and ideationally autistic, and who describe themselves in favourable terms without grossly distorting the truth produce heavier stools. Individuals who describe themselves in favourable terms tend to produce more frequent stools. These observations suggest that, in addition to dietary factors, psychological factors are important in stool production. It is yet to be shown whether stool weight changes coincide with changes in faecal bile acids. In diverticular disease, a condition which has never been suggested to have an emotional content to it, the stool is somewhat concentrated and colonic motility is increased but faecal bile acid excretion does not differ much from normal[4]. Mood changes food intake, however, and this may account for these changes. The ingestion of wheatbran increases stool weight but decreases colonic motility and faecal bile acid concentration, (so that the total bile acid mass remains unchanged)[5,6].

PHYSICAL FACTORS

Faecal Composition

Several studies have found patients with irritable bowel syndrome to have faecal weights and faecal constituents very similar to those of a control group, and hypolactasia plays only a minor role in the aetiology of irritable bowel syndrome, at least in Britain. In the Edinburgh study[7] all patients had normal breath hydrogen tests in response to ingested lactose, and faecal weight was moderately increased in irritable bowel syndrome (116 ± 3 vs. 84 ± 5 g/day in a matched control group). The irritable bowel syndrome patients, however, passed stools more frequently than the control subjects. The concentrations of bile acid, fat, long and short chain fatty acid and neutral sterol in the faeces did not differ significantly between patients and controls. Colonic motility was only modestly increased, both under basal conditions and when stimulated by foods. There was a weak correlation between the concentrations of total bile acids and of deoxycholic and lithocholic acids, and motility index.

An Italian study[8] showed that the diarrhoea of the irritable bowel syndrome is unassociated with any changes in serum electrolytes and acid–

base balance. Faecal weight was only moderately increased (235 vs 147 g/day), and the concentrations of sodium, potassium and chloride in faecal water were almost identical to those in normal subjects. The faecal concentration of all major short-chain fatty acids was slightly but not significantly increased in the patients, but the proportions of individual short-chain fatty acids were almost identical with those in normal controls. The total lactic acid concentration was higher in the patients but there was a large overlap. Patients with the irritable bowel syndrome and diarrhoea often mention that they see food in their stool and this suggests that their intestinal transit is accelerated. We have looked, in a study of nine normal individuals eating a typical British diet aged 26–38, at the relationship between transit time and faecal weight and constituents[6]. Five of the subjects had a short transit time (measured with barium impregnated pellets) of under 30 hours, whilst 4 had a prolonged transit time of more than 40 hours. There was no significant difference in stool weight, total bile acid concentration and daily excretion, and percentage of deoxycholic acid between the fast and slow transit groups.

Colonic Motility

The diarrhoea, pain and character of stool in the irritable bowel syndrome suggest an alteration in intestinal and colonic motility. The ingestion of food stimulates motor activity throughout the gastrointestinal tract, partly by a hormonal mechanism which could involve gastrin (which has a choleretic action) or cholecystokinin (which stimulates gallbladder contraction) through the agency of bile (which stimulates intestinal motor activity[9]). Colonic motility is increased in cholerrheoic enteropathy, a condition in which faecal bile acids are markedly elevated, partly as a result of the stimulation of fluid secretion caused by bile salts on the colonic mucosa[10].

Dihydroxy bile acids strongly inhibit electrolyte and water absorption in the colon. Patients with ileal resection diarrhoea excrete mainly primary bile acids and have a significantly greater motility index than patients with other types of diarrhoea who excrete mainly secondary bile acids. Patients with diarrhoea and increased faecal bile acid excretion also have a significantly higher colonic motility index after-food or prostigmine, suggesting that bile acids may contribute to abnormal motility[9]. It seems possible that abnormally large amounts of bile acids in the human colon, particularly dihydroxy bile acids, cause diarrhoea not only by inhibiting water and electrolyte absorption, but also by stimulating colonic motor activity[9]. In the rabbit, an infusion of the dihydroxy bile salt sodium deoxycholate stimulates colonic motor activity, but infusions of the trihydroxy salt sodium glycocholate or of deionised water do not[9]. These changes in motility are not due only to mucosal damage caused by bile acid, rabbits treated with sodium glycocholate develop mucosal changes but no motor response[11].

Flynn and his colleagues[10] found that when faecal bile acids were repeatedly measured over a year, there was a significantly reduced level of faecal deoxycholic acid in patients with irritable bowel syndrome. They suggested that deoxycholic acid was reabsorbed in the colon to a greater extent in these patients, and hence greater concentrations of the bile acid would come into prolonged contact with colonic smooth muscle. This could result in the characteristic slow wave electrical pattern recognised in irritable bowel syndrome. In another study[13] various bile acids at different concentrations were perfused into the sigmoid colon of both normal subjects and patients with irritable bowel syndrome. Only deoxycholic acid was found to stimulated colonic motility in both the normal subjects and the patients, but at a lower concentration (5 mmol/l) in the patients than in the controls (15 mmol/l).

Bile Acid Malabsorption

Idiopathic bile acid malabsorption is generally considered an extremely rare condition associated with continuous diarrhoea similar to that observed following ileal resection. The number of published cases identified by classical techniques of faecal bile acid measurement is small, the largest reported experience in a single centre – well known for its interest in this condition – being 12 cases accumulated over 14 years[14]. Our experience using SeHCAT to measure bile acid retention[15] suggests that it is much less rare, especially in patients previously diagnosed as the diarrhoeal form of irritable bowel syndrome. Some of these patients, especially those with a 7-day SeHCAT retention of less than 3%, had classical symptoms. Others had intermittent symptoms or even alternating diarrhoea and constipation.

In irritable bowel syndrome 7-day SeHCAT retentions vary from zero to more than 80%[15]. None of 200 consecutive subjects with various conditions in our current series with a retention of 15% or greater had evidence of bile acid malabsorption either initially or on follow up[16]; in those with lower values, SeHCAT retention was strongly correlated with faecal bile acid excretion and the severity of symptoms. Milder degrees of bile acid malabsorption were associated with intermittent diarrhoea alternating with periods of normal or even reduced bowel frequency. Patients who retained less than 3% at one week were almost always helped by cholestyramine, although it was often necessary to adjust the dose from time to time to maintain a comfortable balance between diarrhoea and constipation. In those with more mild symptoms it was often difficult to achieve a maintenance does which could hold the balance between diarrhoea and constipation, and frequent adjustment of dose was necessary.

There is no satisfactory explanation for the fluctuating severity of the symptoms. In patients with post-vagotomy diarrhoea the daily variations in faecal bile acid excretion correlates with fluctuations in the severity of diarrhoea[17]. No comparable studies have been reported in irritable bowel syndrome. Changes in the composition of bile, such as an increase in the percentage of the non-secretory bile acids such as cholic and ursodeoxycholic acids or a decrease in the quantity of the secretory dihydroxy acids might produce such fluctuations in symptoms. Such changes have not been reported within this short time scale, and would only lead to the question of why such variations take place. Bile acid malabsorption should be considered when the diarrhoea of irritable bowel syndrome fails to respond to simple conservative measures, including loperamide, and the patient continues to be troubled by the symptoms. Using these as the principal criteria for performing a SeHCAT test, we have identified 26 cases of bile acid malabsorption in 131 patients with the diarrhoeal form of irritable bowel syndrome over the past four years. One case has been described in whom bile acid malabsorption was apparently present from birth and is therefore presumably congenital[18]. The majority are adults who have an insidious onset, and no identifiable cause. No single precipitating factor has been recognised; one of our cases appears to have been preceded by an episode of gastroenteritis, although the responsible organism was not isolated. If accelerated transit of the contents through the ileum is a contributory factor, it is a minor one. Some of the 20 patients in our series with a 7-day SeHCAT retention just below normal (10–15%) gained some relief from transit slowing agents, those with retention less than 10% did not. The bile acid malabsorption seen in these patients is not simply a consequence of a motility disorder. Despite a dogmatic assertion to the contrary[19], we can find no recorded case of, nor have we observed, any patient with proven bile acid malabsorption who responded to loperamide alone.

No current therapeutic agent is ideal. Cholestyramine is probably too efficient at sequestering bile acids in the less severely affected patients, in whom less powerful adsorbents such as Aludrox are sometime helpful.

SUMMARY

The irritable bowel syndrome is a label for a variety of conditions which manifest themselves in one of two symptomatic ways, either the diarrhoeal form or the spastic colon type. It is possible that the association of bile acids with these conditions is equally complex. While the faecal bile acid excretion of the spastic type of irritable bowel is indistinguishable from normal, there is circumstantial evidence that secondary bile acids stimulate motility in the sensitive colon and hence give rise to this form of the condition. On the other hand the diarrhoeal form of the irritable bowel, like ileal resection diarrhoea, seems to be associated with the primary bile acids, possibly through inhibition or electrolyte and water absorption. Our experience shows that up to 20% of patients with the diarrhoeal form of irritable bowel have clinically significant bile acid malabsorption, recognised only by application of the SeHCAT test.

REFERENCES

1. Eastwood, M.A., Eastwood, J. and Ford, M.J. (1987). The irritable bowel syndrome, a disease or a response? *J. R. Soc. Med.*, **80**, 219–21
2. Young, S.J., Alpers, D.H., Norland, C.C. and Woodruff, R.A. (1976). Psychiatric illness and the irritable bowel syndrome. Practical implications for the practising physicians. *Gastroenterology*, **70**, 162–6
3. Eastwood, M.A., Brydon, W.G., Baird, J.D., Elton, R.A., Smith, J.H. and Pritchard, J.L. (1984). Faecal weight and composition, serum lipids and diet among subjects aged 18–80 years not seeking health care. *Am. J. Clin. Nutr.*, **40**, 628–34
4. Tucker, D.M., Standstead, H.H., Logan, Jr. G.M., Klevay, L.M., Mahalko, J., Johnson, L.K., Inman, L. and Inglett, G.E. (1981). Dietary fiber and personality factors as determinants of stool output. *Gastroenterology*, **81**, 879–83
5. Findlay, J.M., Smith, A.N., Mitchell, W.D. and Anderson, J. (1974). Effects of unprocessed bran on colon function in normal subjects and in diverticular disease. *Lancet*, **1**, 146–9
6. Smith, A.N., Drummond, E. and Eastwood, M.A. (1981). The effect of coarse and fine Canadian Red Spring Wheat and French Soft Wheat bran on colonic motility in patients with diverticular disease. *Am. J. Clin. Nutr.*, **34**, 2460–3
7. Eastwood, M.A., Walton, B.A., Brydon, W.G. and Anderson, J.R. (1984). Faecal weight, constituents, colonic motility and lactose tolerance in the irritable bowel syndrome. *Digestion*, **3**, 7–12
8. Vernia, P., Latella, G. Magliocca, F.M., Mancuso, G. and Caprilli, R. (1987). Seeking clues for a positive diagnosis of the irritable bowel syndrome. *Eur. J. Clin. Invest.*, **17**, 189–93
9. Kirwan, W.O., Smith, A.N., Mitchell, W.D., Falconer, J.D. and Eastwood, M.A. (1975). Bile acids and colonic motility in the rabbit and the human. *Gut*, **16**, 894–902
10. Mekhijian, H.S., Phillips, S.F. and Hofmann, A.F. (1971). Colonic secretion of water and electrolytes induced by bile acids: perfusion studies in man. *J. Clin. Invest.*, **50**, 1569–77
11. Falconer, J.D., Smith, A.N. and Eastwood, M.A. (1980). The effect of bile acids on colonic motility in the rabbit. *Q. J. Exp. Physiol.*, **65**, 135–41
12. Flynn, M., Darby, C., Hammond, P. and Taylor, I. (1981). Faecal bile acids and the irritable bowel syndrome. *Digestion*, **22**, 144–9
13. Taylor, I., Basu, P., Hammond, P., Darby, C. and Flynn, M. (1980). Effect of bile acid perfusion on colonic motor function in patients with irritable colon syndrome. *Gut*, **21**, 843–7
14. Thaysen, E.H. (1986). Idiopathic bile acid diarrhoea reconsidered. *Scand. J. Gastroenterol.*, **20**, 452–6
15. Merrick, M.V., Eastwood, M.A. and Ford, M.J. (1985). Is bile acid malabsorption underdiagnosed? An evaluation of accuracy of diagnosis by measurement of SeHCAT retention. *Br. Med. J.*, **290**, 665–8
16. Nyhlin, H., Merrick, M.V., Eastwood, M.A. and Brydon, W.G. (1983). Evaluation of ileal function using 23-selena-25,-homotaurocholate, a gamma-labelled conjugated bile acic. *Gastroenterology*, **84**, 63–8

17. Anderson, H., Filipsson, S. and Hulten, L. (1978). Determination of the fecal excretion of labelled bile salts after IV administration of ^{14}C cholic acid. *Scand. J. Gastroenterol.*, **13**, 249–255

18. Jonas, A., Driver-Haber, A. and Avigad, S. (1986). Well compensated primary bile acid malabsorption presenting as chronic non-specific diarrhoea. *J. Paediatr. Gastroenterol. Nutr.*, **5**, 143–6

19. Heaton, K.W. (1986). Staying cool with a hot test. *Br. Med. J.*, **292**, 1480.

SECTION G
DIAGNOSIS OF BILE ACID MALABSORPTION – ROLE OF ^{75}SeHCAT

22

[75]SeHCAT: An Overview of Physiological Properties and Clinical Value

R.P. Jazrawi, R. Ferraris and T.C. Northfield
Department of Medicine
St George's Hospital Medical School
London, SW17 ORE, UK

INTRODUCTION

[75]SeHCAT ([75]Selenium-HomoCholic Acid Taurine) is a synthetic analogue of the natural conjugated bile acid taurocholic acid, incorporating a γ emitter ^{75}Se in the side chain. The word homo signifies that the molecular structure of the side chain is a mirror image of the natural bile acid.

The fact that it is a bile acid makes it a potentially useful substance to measure bile acid absorption. The fact that it is γ-labelled gives us the possibility for the first time of visualising the enterohepatic circulation (EHC) of bile acids by external gamma camera scanning.

In this chapter we shall discuss the behaviour of [75]SeHCAT, comparing it with its natural counterpart taurocholic acid in the enterohepatic circulation, and the physiological properties that enable [75]SeHCAT to be used to measure bile acid absorption and to test ileal function. We shall also review clinical [75]SeHCAT tests, the problems with these tests, and the methods of overcoming these problems.

PHYSIOLOGICAL PROPERTIES OF [75]SeHCAT

Dynamics of [75]SeHCAT in the EHC

[75]SeHCAT has been shown to undergo enteroheptic circulation. Following oral administration of [75]SeHCAT to healthy subjects activity starts to appear in the gallbladder within a mean of 60 minutes (Figure 1). After 24 hours, about 50% of the [75]SeHCAT detected in the abdomen is concentrated in the gallbladder in the fasting state[1]. This value is similar to the proportion of the natural bile acid pool stored in the fasting-state gallbladder[2]. In a dual isotope

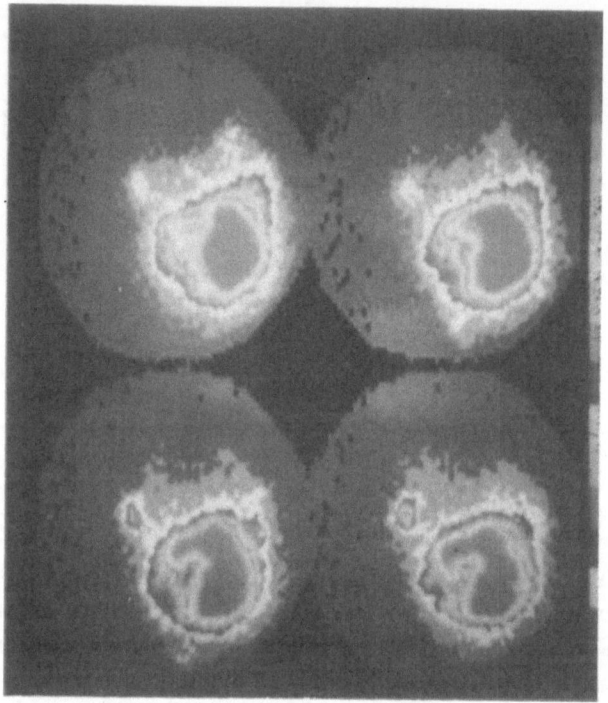

Figure 1 Four frames of abdominal γ-camera scans. Each frame comprises 15 minute continuous data acquisition. The first frame (top left) shows the bulk of [75]SeHCAT activity in the intestine except for an area of faint activity (top left area of frame) which is [75]SeHCAT within the gallbladder. In the following successive 15 minute frames (top right, bottom left, and bottom right) [75]SeHCAT activity within the gallbladder increases as more [75]SeHCAT is being stored there in the fasting state. Taking the gallbladder as the region of interest to generate a time activity relationship the mean time of arrival of the head of colum of [75]SeHCAT to the gallbladder was 60 minutes following its oral administration.

study[1], [75]SeHCAT and ^{99m}Tc-HIDA (a non-absorbable γ-labelled hepato-scintigraphic isotope) were both concentrated within the gallbladder in the fasting state in normal subjects. The gallbladder was then stimulated to contract and the activity of both isotopes over the gallbladder area was followed simultaneously by continuous γ-camera imaging. There was a period of rapid emptying in which the activities of both isotopes over the gallbladder area declined in parallel followed by slow emptying, where the two time–activity curves diverged: [75]SeHCAT activity started to increase, indicating that the synthetic bile acid had completed an enterohepatic cycle and started refilling the gallbladder, whilst ^{99m}Tc–HIDA activity continued to decline (Figure 2).

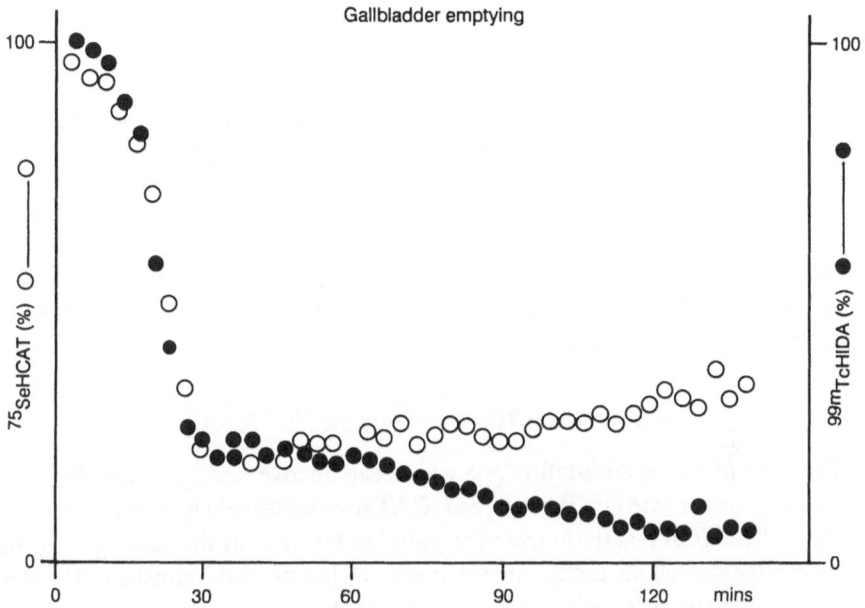

Figure 2 Simultaneous dual isotope scanning over the gallbladder area in a healthy subject starting (top left) with both [75]SeHCAT (an absorbable isotope) and ^{99m}Tc-HIDA (a non-absorbable isotope) concentrated within the gallbladder. Following gallbladder contraction (at time 0) the activities of both isotopes decline in parallel during the rapid emptying phase (time 0-30 min). This is followed by divergence of the two time activity curves so that, whereas the gallbladder activity of ^{99m}Tc-HIDA continues to decline, that of [75]SeHCAT starts to increase. This indicates that some of the SeHCAT that had left the gallbladder at the beginning of this study has now completed an enterohepatic cycle and is starting to refill the gallbladder.

Like natural bile acids, [75]SeHCAT is confined to the EHC[3]. Less than 1% of the administered dose was detected outside the EHC in animal studies at 4, 8 and 24 hours[3].

Hepatic Handling of [75]SeHCAT

Following its oral administration both to rats with bile duct cannulae and to patients with a bile duct T-tube, Merrick et al.[4] demonstrated that more than 90% of the [75]SeHCAT activity was recovered in bile within 24 hours. Galatola et al.[5] demonstrated that [75]SeHCAT recovery in bile parallelled that of its natural counterpart taurocholic acid labelled with [14]C ([14]CAT) when both isotopes were administered simultaneously by mouth. In another study, Galatola et al.[6] demonstrated that following intravenous injection, the plasma disappearance of [75]SeHCAT could be accounted for entirely by its hepatic uptake, whereas for ^{99m}Tc-HIDA only 50% of the plasma disappearance could be accounted for by hepatic uptake. Furthermore, both the plasma disappearance and hepatic uptake for ^{75}SeHCAT were significantly more rapid than those for ^{99m}Tc-HIDA, the hepatic transit time shorter and net excretory rate higher. These results suggest that the liver handles ^{75}SeHCAT more specifically and efficiently than ^{99m}Tc-HIDA.

Faecal Excretion of ^{75}SeHCAT

Following the simultaneous oral administration of ^{75}SeHCAT and ^{14}CAT, Delhez et al.[7] found identical quantities of each excreted in stools collected over successive 24 hour periods for 7 days.

Fractional Turnover Rate for ^{75}SeHCAT

The enterohepatic circulation as a whole can be assessed by measuring fractional turnover rate (FTR) for ^{75}SeHCAT non-invasively by γ-camera imaging of ^{75}SeHCAT activity over the gallbladder area in the fasting state on successive days. This technique assumes – as has been demonstrated[8] – that a constant proportion of the bile acid pool is stored in the fasting gallbladder over successive days. Hence, the slope of the exponential decline of ^{75}SeHCAT gallbladder activity can be used to derive FTR. In five healthy subjects, the overall FTR for ^{75}SeHCAT was found to be similar to that of taurocholate measured by the classical Linstedt technique[9]. The fractional deconjugation rate for ^{75}SeHCAT was, however, very small (2%/day, compared with 12%/day for taurocholate). This suggested that SeHCAT could not be deconjugated by intestinal bacteria. Its absorption should therefore be confined only to the active ileal transport site, since only deconjugated bile acids can be absorbed elsewhere by passive non-ionic diffusion. If ^{75}SeHCAT absorption by the terminal ileum is also efficient, it should therefore provide a more specific test of terminal ileal function than natural bile acids. The observation that the overall FTR of ^{75}SeHCAT was similar to that of taurocholate despite the difference in colonic deconjugation is probably due to the fact that the deconjugated taurocholate will be reconjugated with glycine in the liver and will therefore be no longer part of the taurocholate pool.

Efficiency of Intestinal Absorption for ^{75}SeHCAT

Several studies have provided indirect evidence that the terminal ileum absorbs ^{75}SeHCAT efficiently, by measuring its recovery in bile following oral administration[3,4,11]. We have performed a direct assessment in six healthy subjects of first pass ileal clearance for ^{75}SeHCAT[5] (ileal absorption efficiency/cycle), by installing ^{75}SeHCAT (with bile as cold carrier) via a naso-jejunal tube distal to an inflated jejunal balloon (to prevent a second cycle). The activity of ^{75}SeHCAT proximal to the balloon was then monitored using a γ-camera until a plateau was reached indicating completion of one cycle. The unabsorbed ^{75}SeHCAT was then collected by intestinal lavage distal to the inflated balloon and corrected for incomplete recovery using an unabsorbable recovery marker ^{51}CrCl$_3$ administered simultaneously with ^{75}SeHCAT. Over 95% of the administered dose was absorbed in all six subjects, confirming the very efficient ileal absorption of ^{75}SeHCAT in health[5].

OVERVIEW OF CLINICAL ^{75}SeHCAT TESTS

Retention Tests

Clinical tests of ileal function using ^{75}SeHCAT retention fall into three categories:

(1)   Whole body retention of ^{75}SeHCAT[12–16]

In brief, this technique involves measuring the activity of ^{75}SeHCAT by a whole body counter immediately after oral ingestion, and again after a period of time – usually 7 days, although a 4 day retention period has been used. The retained activity of ^{75}SeHCAT (expressed as a percent of the administered dose) is calculated and the value below a lower limit of normal established in healthy people is used to identify patients with malabsorption.

(2)   Abdominal retention of ^{75}SeHCAT – using a γ-camera scan of the whole abdomen[14,17–20]. This technique involves the valid assumption that ^{75}SeHCAT is not distributed outside the abdomen. ^{75}SeHCAT activity is measured at the time of administration and after 3–7 days, and the retained activity calculated.

(3)   Faecal Excretion of ^{75}SeHCAT[7]

This technique does not require a whole body counter or a γ-camera, but simply a γ-counter. It depends on collecting all stools for 4–7 days following the oral administration of ^{75}SeHCAT, from which the retained ^{75}SeHCAT (100– % excreted) can be calculated.

Absorption Tests[21–23]

1.   Ileal absorption efficiency for ^{75}SeHCAT (abdominal method)[21]

2.   Ileal absorption efficiency for ^{75}SeHCAT (faecal method)[21]

3. $t_{1/2}$ for [75]SeHCAT[22,23]

These three methods will be discussed in detail later in the chapter.

PROBLEMS WITH [75]SeHCAT RETENTION TESTS
Colonic Retention of [75]SeHCAT

With each enterohepatic cycle, the small proportion of [75]SeHCAT that is not actively absorbed by the terminal ileum passes into the colon. Unlike natural bile acids, bacterial metabolism of [75]SeHCAT in the colon is minimal, so that it will remain conjugated in the colon and cannot be reabsorbed by passive non-ionic diffusion. None of the [75]SeHCAT retention tests discriminate between absorbed [75]SeHCAT and colonic [75]SeHCAT, and all assume that the total [75]SeHCAT activity in the whole body or the abdomen or not in the faeces, is within the enterohepatic circulation. Their results may therefore overestimate absorption of [75]SeHCAT to a variable extent depending on the degree of colonic retention in the individual, and on the proportion of [75]SeHCAT passing into the colon. Bias should therefore be greater in patients with bile acid malabsorption.

Ferraris *et al.*[21,24] measured the colonic retention of [75]SeHCAT by the simultaneous administration of the ^{51}Cr-labelled non-absorbable marker [51]CrCl3.

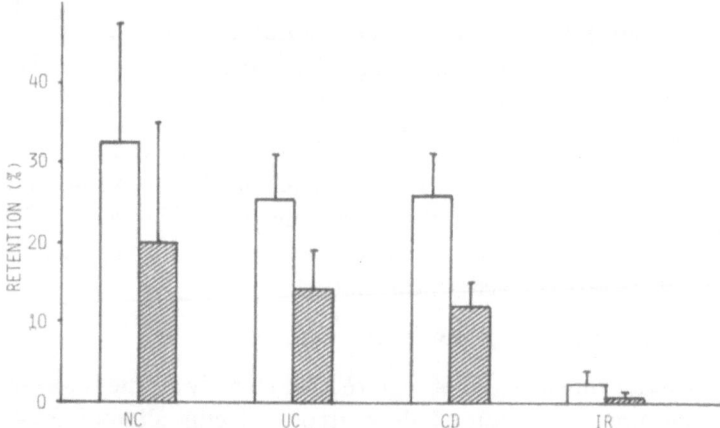

Figure 3   Colonic retention (mean ± SEM) of the γ-labelled non absorbable marker [51]CrCl3, expressed as % of the administered dose of [51]CrCl3 that was detected by abdominal γ-camera scanning at 5 (open columns) and 7 (hatched columns) days in four groups of subjects. NC: normal controls, $n = 8$; UC: ulcerative colitis, $n = 16$; Crohn's disease, $n = 16$ and IR: ileal resection, $n = 8$). There was a systematic difference between the groups in that the IR patients had significantly (p 0.05) less colonic retention than the other three groups. There were also large differences between individuals in each group as indicated by the large standard error lines. This implies that it is necessary to correct for colonic retention in every individual case.

They found that it varied, between individuals, from 0% to 68% per day, and between groups of subjects, being lowest in the group with the most severe diarrhoea.

Colonic retention of $^{51}CrCl_3$ [the proportion of the administered dose of $^{51}CrCl_3$ detected in the abdomen after 5 days of oral ingestion of the marker, Figure 3] at 5 and 7 days was measured in the same groups of subjects above. Similar individual variations were found in the four groups as indicated by the large standard error bars, as well as systematic difference between the groups. The findings emphasise the importance of correcting for colonic retention in individual subjects.

Incomplete Stool Collection

This problem occurs with the faecal excretion technique, and is worse in patients with severe watery diarrhoea who open their bowels very frequently. Stool collection for 4 or 7 days then becomes a serious problem for all concerned, especially if the test is to be carried out on an out-patient basis.

Availability of Equipment

The most sensitive apparatus to measure $^{75}SeHCAT$ activity is the whole body counter. It allows the use of a dose of 1 μCi $^{75}SeHCAT$ (one tenth of that needed with a γ-camera). Whole body counters are very expensive and are therefore available in very few centres. The use of a γ-camera or γ-counter probe[19] is sufficiently sensitive if a larger (but still relatively low) dose of $^{75}SeHCAT$ is used (10 μCi).

Quantitation

$^{75}SeHCAT$ retention tests (whole-body, or abdominal) are semiquantitative. They describe a cut off point which separates reliably normal absorption from malabsorption. They also describe an equivocal range around that cut off point within which the results are said to be not definitely positive or negative. $^{75}SeHCAT$ tests should be of most value in patients with mild bile acid malabsorption, e.g. to detect patients with Crohn's disease involving a short segment of the terminal ileum. Yet, it is in these particular patients that results of the available $^{75}SeHCAT$ retention tests will fall in the equivocal range.

METHODS OF OVERCOMING PROBLEMS

Correction for Colonic Retention

This can be achieved by the simultaneous administration of a non-absorbable marker such as ^{51}CrCl$_3$. In the absence of colonic retention ^{51}CrCl$_3$ activity should be absent from the abdomen 24 hours after administration. Its abdominal activity thus indicates the degree of colonic retention and can be used to correct the abdominal ^{75}SeHCAT activity. In the same way ^{75}SeHCAT studies that depend on stool collection can be corrected for colonic retention and for incomplete stool collection using ^{51}CrCl$_3$.

The validity of using this technique for correction is based on the finding that colonic retention of ^{75}SeHCAT is identical to that of ^{51}CrCl$_3$. Correction for colonic retention improves the sensitivity of ^{75}SeHCAT tests considerably. In our faecal studies by γ-counter and abdominal studies by γ-camera the sensitivity rises from about 35% to >90%. We have found a good correlation between these two independent methods[21] (Figure 4) providing internal validation for the correction procedure.

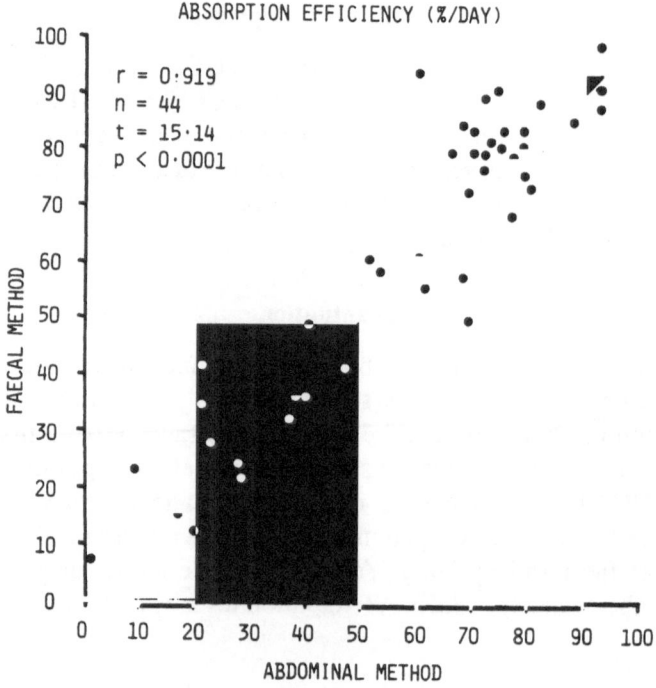

Figure 4 Correlation between the faecal method and abdominal method for measuring daily absorption efficiency for ^{75}SeHCAT both corrected for colonic retention of ^{75}SeHCAT using ^{51}CrCl$_3$ (reproduced from reference 21 with permission).

^{75}SeHCAT Activity over the Gallbladder Area

This subject will be discussed in detail by Dr Ferraris in Chapter 24. The procedure depends on the valid assumptions that the activity of ^{75}SeHCAT over the fasting gallbladder area represents the activity of ^{75}SeHCAT within the enterohepatic circulation and is therefore independent of colonic retention, and that a constant proportion of the bile acid pool is stored in the gallbladder on successive days in normal subjects. The method does not therefore require the use of a non-absorbable correction marker. It does, however, require good anatomical separation of ^{75}SeHCAT activity in the gallbladder area from that within the adjacent colon. Ferraris et al.[21] assessed this aspect in patients receiving both ^{75}SeHCAT and ^{51}CrCl3 by scanning for ^{51}CrCl3 activity within the gallbladder area: since all activity of the non-absorbable marker should be in the colon, any activity detected within the gallbladder area would represent overlapping colonic activity. They reported no contamination of gallbladder ^{Se}HCAT with ^{51}CrCl3 activity. The procedure requires 4–5 gallbladder area scans carried out in the fasting state on successive days, from which a $t_{1/2}$ for ^{75}SeHCAT in the enterohepatic circulation can be derived as an index of bile acid absorption. The finding that the $t_{1/2}$ of ^{75}SeHCAT is identical to $t_{1/2}$ of ^{14}CAT in normal subjects validates the technique. Whether the same findings hold for patients with bile acid malabsorption has still to be clarified.

Schroth et al.[23] have also employed the gallbladder ^{75}SeHCAT method but have carried out only one gallbladder scan a set time after oral administration of ^{75}SeHCAT. Although this technique is more accurate than other ^{75}SeHCAT retention techniques because it is independent of colonic retention, it remains a semiquantitative index and is therefore not as sensitive as determining $t_{1/2}$ (above) by successive gallbladder γ-camera scans. Unfortunately, neither method can be used in patients who have had a cholecystectomy.

Ileal Absorption Efficiency

This measurement can be carried out by one of two methods; the faecal method using a γ-counter and the abdominal method using a γ-camera. Both methods involve simultaneous administration of ^{75}SeHCAT and ^{51}CrCl3 by mouth together with a test meal on the first day of the study and sequential scanning and/or stool collection for 4–5 successive days. ^{51}CrCl3 is used to correct for colonic retention of ^{75}SeHCAT. This technique provides an index of the daily percent absorption of ^{75}SeHCAT, instead of retention, and is therefore more quantitative.

In the faecal method whole stool specimens are counted each day for

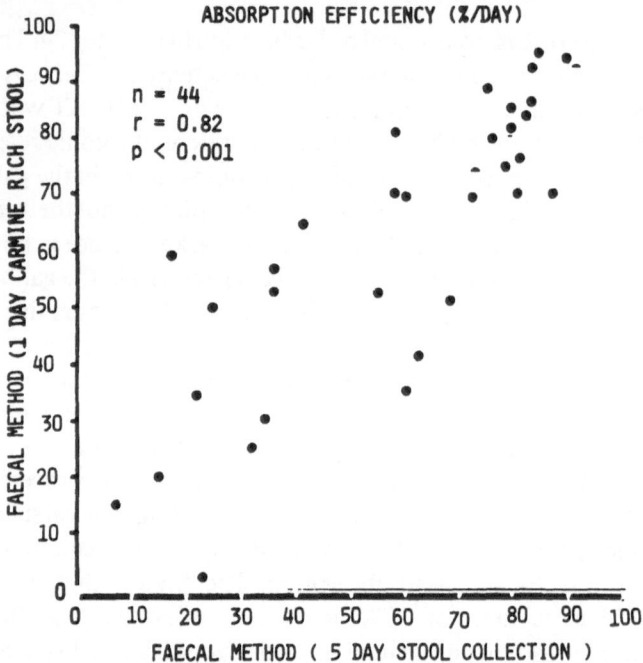

Figure 5 Daily absorption efficiency for ^{75}SeHCAT (faecal method): correlation between values obtained from a single carmine rich day's stool collection and those obtained from a complete stool collection (reproduced from reference 21 with permission).

^{75}SeHCAT and ^{51}CrCl$_3$ using separate windows of a γ-counter. The accumulated amount of the isotope that had been excreted is subtracted from the amount administered, the natural logarithm of the amount remaining is plotted against time to obtain the slope K. The percent absorption is derived using the following formula:

$$\% \text{ ABS} = \left[1 - \frac{\ln K\ ^{75}\text{Se}}{\ln K\ ^{51}\text{Cr}} \right] \times 100\%$$

where K in each case is the slope of the decline of activity of the respective isotope with time.

The test can be simplified by giving carmine-red with ^{75}SeHCAT and ^{51}CrCl$_3$ to identify visibly the stool most likely to contain a large proportion of the correction marker ^{51}CrCl$_3$. This allows counting of only one stool. We found a good correlation between the results of ^{75}SeHCAT daily absorption efficiency [using the 5–day stool collection method] with the results of the 1-day carmine rich stool absorption index in 44 subjects[21]. It appeared that collection could be limited to 48 hours, as stool containing the carmine red had almost always been passed within that period.

In the abdominal method, ^{75}SeHCAT and ^{51}CrCl$_3$ are counted separately on 4–5 successive days by a γ-camera. Counts are corrected for crosstalk and decay and the absorption efficiency is calculated according to the following formula:

$$\% \text{ ABS} = \left[1 - \frac{\ln K^{51}\text{Cr} - \ln K^{75}\text{Se}}{\ln K^{51}\text{Cr}} \right] \times 100\%$$

We have compared the sensitivity and specificity of ^{75}SeHCAT daily absorption efficiency (both faecal and abdominal methods) with the measurement of ^{14}C-faecal radioactivity following ^{14}C-glycocholate, which is still considered the best conventional test of ileal function, in a total of 62 patients (13 healthy controls, 21 with ileal Crohn's disease, 17 with ulcerative colitis and 11 with ileal resection). There was no difference in the sensitivity between ^{75}SeHCAT tests (91% for the faecal method and 96% for abdominal method) and ^{14}C-faecal radioactivity (95%). Nor was there a difference in specificity for both faecal (95%) and abdominal (97%) ^{75}SeHCAT test and ^{14}C-faecal radioactivity (94%). The ^{75}SeHCAT tests however have the advantage of providing a quantitative estimate of ileal absorption, and of requiring apparatus that is simpler and more widely available than faecal ^{14}C radioactivity measurement which requires a combustion chamber.

SUMMARY

^{75}SeHCAT allows for the first time non-invasive assessment of the enterohepatic circulation of bile acids in health and in disease. It behaves like a natural bile acid with regard to enterohepatic cycling, hepatic handling, active absorption from the terminal ileum, faecal excretion and overall turnover in the enterohepatic circulation. It differs from natural bile acids in that it undergoes negligible deconjuation by colonic bacteria. Its absorption is therefore confined to the active transport site in the terminal ileum, by contrast with natural bile acids. It provides an ideal substance for testing terminal ileal function. The early conventional retention tests do not correct for colonic retention of ^{75}SeHCAT and are only semiquantitative. Correction for colonic retention, and the measurement of daily absorption efficiency improves the sensitivity of ^{75}SeHCAT tests to match that of ^{14}C-faecal radioactivity following oral administration of ^{14}C-Glycocholate.

REFERENCES

1. Jazrawi, R.P., Lanzini, A., Britten, A., Meller, S.T. and Northfield, T.C. (1984). Dynamics of gallbladder function and of the enterohepatic circulation studied by a γ-

labelled bile acid. *Clin. Sci.*, **66**, 10P

2.   Van Berge Henegouwen, G.P. and Hofmann, A.F. (1978). Nocturnal gallbladder storage and emptying in gallstone patients and healthy subjects. *Gastroenterology*, **75**, 879–85

3.   Soundy, R.G., Simpson, J.D., McL Ross, H. and Merrick, M.V. (1982). Absorbed dose to man from the Se-75 labelled bile salt SeHCAT. *J. Nucl. Med.* **23**, 157–61

4.   Merrick, M.V., Eastwood, M.A., Anderson, J.R. and McL Ross, J. (1982). Enterohepatic circulation in man of a gamma-emitting bile acid conjugate, 23-selena-25-homocholic acid taurine (SeHCAT). *J. Nucl. Med.* **23**, 126–30

5.   Galatola, G., Jazrawi, R.P., Bridges, C., Joseph, A.E.A. and Northfield, T.C. (1986). First pass ileal clearance of bile acid in man. *Clin. Sci.* **13**, 71P

6.   Galatola, G., Jazrawi, R.P., Bridges, C., Joseph, A.E.A. and Northfield, T.C. (1988). Hepatic handling of the synthetic-labelled bile acid SeHCAT. *Gastroenterology*, **94**, 771–8

7.   Delhez, H., Van den Berg, J.W.O., Van Blankenstein, M. and Meerwaldt, J.H. (1982). New method for the determination of bile acid turnover using ^{75}Se-homocholic acid taurine. *Eur. J. Nucl. Med.* **7**, 269–71

8.   Jazrawi, R.P., Bridges, C., Joseph, A.E.A. and Northfield, T.C. (1986). Effects of artificial depletion of the bile acid pool in man. *Gut*, **27**, 771–7

9.   Lindstedt, S. (1957). The turnover of bile acid in man. *Acta Physiol. Scand.*, **40**, 1–9

10.   Jazrawi, R.P., Ferraris, R., Bridges, C. and Northfield, T.C. (1988). Kinetics for the synthetic bile acid ^{75}SeHCAT in man: Comparison with ^{14}C-taurocholate. *Gastroenterology*, (In press)

11.   Boyd, G.S., Merrick, M.V., Monks, R. and Thomas, I.L. (1981). Se-75 labeled bile acid analogs, new radiopharmaceuticals for investigation. *J. Nucl. Med.*, **22**, 720–5

12.   Nyhlin, H., Merrick, M.V., Eastwood, M.A. and Boydon, W.G. (1983). Evaluation of ileal function using 23-selena-25-homo-taurocholate, a γ-labelled conjugated bile acid. *Gastroenterology*, **84**, 63–8

13.   Merrick, M.V., Eastwood, M.A. and Ford, M.J. (1985). Is bile acid malabsorption underdiagnosed? An evaluation of accuracy of diagnosis by measurement of SeHCAT retention. *Br. Med. J.*, **290**, 665–8

14.   Hames, T.K., Condon, B.R., Fleming, J.S., Phillips, G., Holdstock, G., Smith, C.L., Howlett, P.J. and Ackery, D. (1984). A comparison between the use of shadow shield whole body counter and uncollimated gamma camera in the assessment of 7 day retention of SeHCAT. *Br. J. Radiol.*, **57**, 581–4

15.   Ludgate, S.M. and Merrick, M.V. 91985). The pathogenesis of post-irradiation chronic diarrhoea: Measurement of SeHCAT and B12 absorption for differential diagnosis determines treatment. *Clin. Radiol.*, **36**, 275–8

16.   Merrick, M.V. (1986). The clinical value of the ^{75}SeHCAT retention test. In New radioisotope tests in gastroenterology. In Malaguti, P., Sciarretta, G., Abbati, A. and Funo, A. (eds.) *New Radioisotope Tests in Gastroenterology*, (Milano: pp. 14–19 Masson Italia Editori)

17.   Thayson, E.H., Orholm, M., Arnfred, T. and Podbro, P. (1982). Assessment of ileal function by abdominal counting of the retention of a gamma emitting bile acid analogue. *Gut*, **23**, 862–5

18.   Sciarretta, G., Vicini, G., Fagioli, G., Verri, A., Ginevra, A. and Malaguti, P. (1986). Use of 23-selena-25-homocholyltaurine to detect bile acid malabsorption in patients with ileal dysfunction or diarrhoea. *Gastroenterology*, **91**, 1–9

19.   Hinton, P.J., taylor, D.N., Wyke, R.J. and McIntosh, J.A. (1984). Application of different counting systems in measuring localised retention in the entero-hepatic circulation. *Br. J. Radiol.*, **57**, 799–801

20.   Sciarretta, G., Fagioli, G., Furno, A., Vicini, G., Verri, A. and Malaguti, P. (1986). ^{75}SeHCAT abdominal retention in ileal dysfunction and chronic diarrhoea. In Malaguti, P., Sciarretta, G., Abbati, A. and Furno, A. (eds.) *New Radioisotope Tests in*

Gastroenterology, (Milan: Masson Italia Editori), pp. 22–6.

21. Ferraris, R., Jazrawi, R.P., Bridges, C. and Northfield, T.C. (1986). Use of a γ-labelled bile acid ([75]SeHCAT) as a test of ileal function: Methods of improving accuracy. *Gastroenterology*, **90**, 1129–36

22. Ferraris, R. (1986). [75]SeHCAT gallbladder retention in ileal dysfunction and diarrhoea. In Malaguti, P., Sciarretta, G., Abbati, A. and Furno, A. (eds.) *New Radioisotope Tests in Gastroenterology*, (Milan: Masson Italia Editori), pp. 41–4

23. Schroth, H.J., Berberich, R., Feifel, G., Muller, K.P. and Ecker, K.W. (1985). Tests for the absorption ^{75}Se-labelled homocholic acid conjugated with taurine ([75]SeHCAT). *Eur. J. Nucl. Med.*, **10**, 455–7

24. Jazrawi, R.P., Ferraris, R., Bridges, C. and Northfield, T.C. (1985). Use of a nonabsorbable marker to improve sensitivity of [75]SeHCAT as a test of ileal function. *Gastroenterology*, **88**, 1658 (Abstr.)

25. Jazrawi, R.P., Ferraris, R. and Northfield, T.C. (1986). Daily ileal absorption efficiency for [75]SeHCAT in ileal dysfunction and diarrhoea. In Malaguti, P., Sciarretta, G., Abbati, A. and Furno, A. (eds.) *New Radioisotope Tests in Gastroenterology*, (Milan: Masson Italia Editori), pp. 33–40

26. Fromm, H. and Hofmann, A.F. (1971). Breath test for altered bile acid metabolism. *Lancet*, **2**, 621–5

27. Fromm, H., Thomas, P.J. and Hofmann, A.F. (1973). Sensitivity and specificity of tests of distal ileal function: prospective comparison of bile acid and vitamin B_{12} absorption in ileal resection patients. *Gastroenterology*, **64**, 1077–90

23

Whole Body and Abdominal Retention of [75]SeHCAT

G. Sciarretta, [*]**G. Fagioli,** [*]**A. Furno** [**]**G. Vicini and P. Malaguti**
Gastroenterology Unit; [*]*Department of Nuclear Medicine;* [**]*Department of Health and Medical Physics; Ospedale Maggiore USL 27 Bologna, Italy*

INTRODUCTION

Bile acid malabsorption, (BAM) either idiopathic[1] or resulting from disease or resection of the distal ileum[2,3], is one of the causes of chronic diarrhoea. The diagnosis of structural disease of the ileum is established by radiology and by endoscopy and biopsy. The diagnosis of ileal dysfunction associated with bile acid malabsorption has, however, been based on the Schilling test[4], the ^{14}C-glycocholate breath test[5] and the serum primary bile salt curve following a fat-rich meal[6], none of which is particularly accurate. More specific methods such as measurement of faecal total bile salt excretion[7] or of faecal ^{14}C after the administration of 24-^{14}C-taurocholate[8], are seldom used in clinical practice as they require the collection of faeces.

The demonstration of bile acid malabsorption has been greatly facilitated by the introduction of a gamma-emitting bile acid which can be measured and imaged from outside the abdomen, and is also easily measured in the faeces. This is tauro-23-[^{75}Se]selena-25 homocholic acid (SeHCAT), available from Amersham Radiochemical Centre, England, in 37 kBq (1 μCi) and 370 kBq (10 μCi) capsule form[9,10]. Several European groups have now reported their experience with SeHCAT in various diseases and using different methods of measuring its absorption.

In this chapter we shall discuss the chemical, physical and biological properties of SeHCAT, the measurement of its absorption using whole body counting and abdominal counting.

CHEMICAL, PHYSICAL AND BIOLOGICAL FEATURES OF SeHCAT

In 1973, Fromm *et al.*[4] emphasised that the study of ileal function required a substance that could be absorbed in the ileum, which was not influenced by intraluminal factors, and which behaved like a natural bile acid. SeHCAT possesses all the features of an excellent marker of ileal function.

Abdominal scintigraphy has shown that SeHCAT has an entero-hepatic circulation. It is concentrated in the gallbladder in the fasting state; after a meal it empties from the gallbladder, is distributed down the intestine and then returns to the gallbladder after a varying amount of time (Figure 1). Merrick et al.[10] and Delhez et al.[11] have shown that the absorption and resecretion of SeHCAT closely resembles that of ^{14}C-cholic acid, and that absorption is reduced by resection or by-pass of the distal ileum. Excretion of SeHCAT from the body is biexponential, with a fast initial component including approximately 96% of the activity administered, with a half-life ($t_{1/2}$) of 2.6 ± 0.7 days and a slower component including the remaining 4% of the activity with a half-life of 62 ± 17 days. The latter is the amount distributed uniformly throughout the body and is irrelevant in clinical practise.

SeHCAT is a conjugate of taurine and therefore has a low pKa (pKa = 2), as compared with glycine conjugates (pKa = 4) *and free bile acids (pKa = 6).* It is therefore completely ionised at the pH of intestinal contents and cannot be reabsorbed passively unless it is first deconjugated. The exclusion of the distal ileum abolishes SeHCAT body retention[12] suggesting that it is absorbed specifically in the distal ileum. The efficiency of this absorption is 95–98% at the first pass ileal clearance in normal subjects[13].

The half-life of ^{75}Se itself is 120 days. SeHCAT is stable *in vitro*: less than 5% is deconjugated after 6 months in water solution at room temperature. The linkage between ^{75}Se and the molecule is stable as there are no enzymes capable of cleaving the carbonium–selenium bond. It undergoes little modification during enterohepatic circulation unlike taurocholate which is mostly converted into glycocholate and glycodeoxycholate[9]: about 3% is deconjugated each day in the intestine, compared with 12%/day for taurocholate[14]. This makes SeHCAT specific for ileal absorption even in the presence of small bowel bacterial overgrowth[15].

WHOLE BODY COUNTING TECHNIQUES

The whole body counter (WBC) is capable of measuring very low levels of gamma radioactivity present in the human body. One of the more widely used models for the study of SeHCAT retention is the 'shadow' shield system of Warner and Oliver (1966)[17]. The patient lies in a shielded trough made of lead bricks while the crystal, which is also shielded, is opened to the outside. The detector (or bed) moves longitudinally to record the activity of the whole body. With this system background activity is within acceptable limits.

A 37 kBq (1 μCi) dose of SeHCAT is used for this type of measurement. The patient's background activity, measured before administration, is

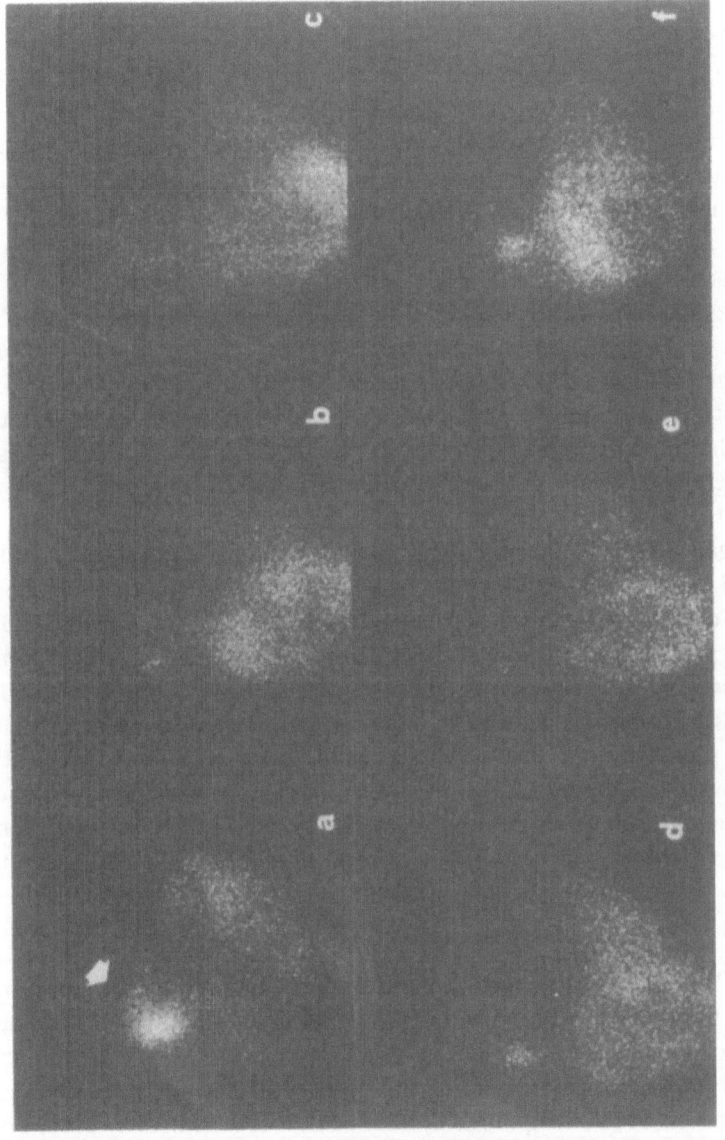

Figure 1 Two enterohepatic cycles of SeHCAT shown by abdominal scintigraphy. The arrow marks the activity in the gallbladder in (a) the fasting state; (b) 30 min after a meal; (c) after 60 min the gallbladder is almost completely emptied; (d) after 75 min the gallbladder is partially refilled; (e) a second emptying of the gallbladder after 120 min; (f) a second refilling after 195 min

subtracted from all subsequent measurements (each taking 6–10 minutes). The next measurement is made 30–60 minutes after administration, and represents the zero time or 100% value; with WBC it is not necessary to wait for the distribution of the SeHCAT to the various compartments. Different investigators then follow different protocols, so that their expressions of absorption also differ.

The first clinical study, conducted by Merrick's group[18], involved 45 patients; the measurements of retention were carried out at both 4 and 7 days after administration and correlated well with the faecal bile salt excretion. A whole body retention <25% on day 4 was considered abnormal, but there was an overlap between results in healthy subjects and in patients. On day 7 retention <12% was considered abnormal and >19% normal; two patients with idiopathic diarrhoea, 1 with ileal resection, one with ileal pathology, two with ileostomy and two with colonic disease lay between these two values[18]. In a later study involving a larger group of subjects, the same authors measured retention on day 7 only, and defined 15% as the lower limit of normal and <8% as definitely abnormal. Patients with diarrhoea of various causes including functional gave results between these two limits[19]. These authors preferred the measurement of retention on day 7 only, thus simplifying the test.

Fagan et al.[20], in a group of 30 subjects, measured retention at 4 and 7 days, and found an overlap between normal controls and patients with ileal disease on day 4, but on day 7 a clear separation between normal controls (10 cases) and patients (20 cases) with a 6% limit value. Scheurlen et al.[21] compared SeHCAT retention, expressed as $t_{1/2}$, with faecal bile salt excretion in 31 subjects with chronic diarrhoea. Measurements were made at 2 and 6 hours, and then daily until day 7. The normal range was taken from Merrick's first study for 18 healthy controls[10], rather than from a personal control group. There is no clinical study comparing the single measurement of retention on day 7 with the calculation of $t_{1/2}$ from repeated daily measurement.

ABDOMINAL RETENTION TESTS

Although WBC allows accurate measurement with only a 1 μCi dose of SeHCAT, the equipment required is not generally available. The gamma-camera technique has been used as an alternative since the first clinical studies. Its use is appropriate because SeHCAT remains effectively confined to the abdomen. A 370 kBq (10 μCi) dose of SeHCAT is usually used. The field of view of the uncollimated gamma-camera (UGC) must include the entire abdomen.

We found it best[22], to keep the crystal 70 cm away from the bed, and to centre a 35% window at 260 keV; the counting time was set at 5 minutes giving an initial count rate of about 6×10^4 cpm and a background count rate around 5×10^3 cpm. The UGC has been compared with the ^{14}C-glycocholate breath test, with the measurement of faecal ^{14}C after ^{14}C-glycocholate[23] and, more importantly, with the WBC technique[24-26]. It has proved valid, in the three WBC comparisons, with positive correlations of $r = 0.98$, 0.96 and 0.96, respectively.

Protocols and expression of results has also varied with this technique in the published reports. Thaysen et al.[23] in an early study of 38 subjects counted at time zero (about 3 hours after administration) and after 5 days. The lower limit or normal was set at 36%, and retention $< 30\%$ considered abnormal, but there were very few healthy controls. In 1986 we reported results of SeHCAT tests using UGC in 66 patients with various intestinal diseases and in 23 healthy controls[22]. We fitted an exponential elimination curve to measurements at time zero and at 1, 3, 5, and 7 days after SeHCAT administration.

The lower limit of normal measured by the gamma-camera was 8% on day 7 and 34% on day 3 from the curve. We used the same method in a study of patients with chronic or recurrent diarrhoea of unknown cause[27].

The slightly better specificity of an exponential curve, based on multiple measurements, does not seem to justify its routine use in the study of patients with diarrhoea; the day 7 retention is shorter and simpler to measure.

COMPARISON OF THE PARAMETERS

Disease Classification

We have analysed our last 100 consecutive tests (carried out over 2 years). We divided the 100 subjects into five groups on clinical grounds:

- healthy subjects with normal bowel habits (13 cases).

- subjects with irregular bowel habits but normal ileum and colon on radiology who had not responded to cholestyramine and who were considered to have irritable bowel syndrome (24 cases).

- subjects with diseases not involving the ileum (duodenal ulcer, gastrectomy, coeliac disease, ulcerative colitis, Crohn's colitis) with normal bowel habit or diarrhoea (22 cases).

- subjects with Crohn's disease, or resection of the distal ileum all but one suffering from chronic diarrhoea (16 cases).

- subjects with chronic or recurrent diarrhoea, with normal bowel

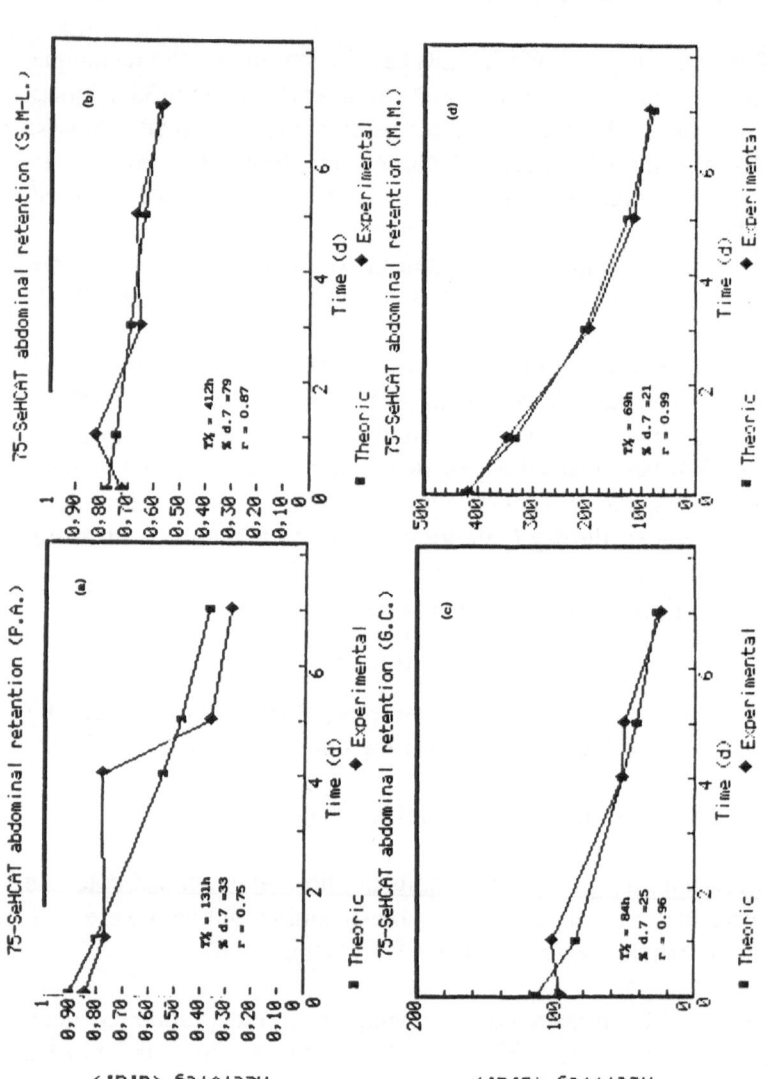

Figure 2 Four curves of SeHCAT abdominal retention with different "*r*" values. (a) shows a curve with a low "*r*" for marked colonic retention; (b) in a coeliac patient with high abdominal retention of SeCAT a wider variability of activity values is possible; (c) a good curve in a normal retention test; (d) a very good curve in a patient suffering from diarrhoea from Crohn's disease of the ileum and colon, with unexpected normal retention test.

radiology, who had responded to cholestyramine and were considered to have probable BAM (25 cases of whom 10 had had a cholecystectomy).

All the subjects in the first three groups had a normal distal ileum and were therefore amalgamated in group 1 (59 cases); the last two groups had structural or functional disorder of the distal ileum and were amalgamated in group 2 (41 cases).

Expression of Results

We used the UGC to measure abdominal retention of SeHCAT at time zero and at 1, 3, 5, and 7 days. We fitted an exponential activity versus time curve (Figure 2), and calculated the half-time $t_{1/2}$ directly from the curve. We also took a direct measurement of percentage retention on day 7. Our lower limit of normal for $t_{1/2}$ was 46 hours, and of retention on day 7 was 8%[22]. There was similar diagnostic accuracy in our population between $t_{1/2}$ and per cent retention on day 7.

SUMMARY

SeHCAT has greatly facilitated the study of ileal function, particularly the absorption of bile salts. The use of the whole body counter, where this is available, is preferable because it allows the most accurate measurement with the lowest dose. The measurement of abdominal retention with an uncollimated gamma camera is more widely available and is valid, but requires a tenfold greater dose. In our experience, confirmed by the last 100 consecutive cases analysed, both the $t_{1/2}$, calculated from a fitted exponential curve, and the percentage retention at day 7 are equally accurate in diagnosis.

REFERENCES

1. Thaysen, E.H. and Pedersen, L. (1976). Idiopathic bile acid catharsis. *Gut*, **17**, 965–70
2. Hofmann, A.F. (1967). The syndrome of ileal disease and broken enterohepatic circulation: cholereic enteropathy. *Gastroenterology*, **52**, 752–7
3. Hofmann, A.F. and Poley, J.R. (1972). Role of bile acid malabsorption in pathogenesis of diarrhoea and steatorrhoea in patients with ileal resection. *Gastroenterology*, **62**, 918–34
4. Fromm, H., Thomas, P.J. and Hofmann, A.F. (1973). Sensitivity and specificity in tests of distal ileal function: prospective comparison of bile acid and vitamin B$_{12}$ absorption in ileal resection patients. *Gastroenterology*, **64**, 1077–90
5. Heaton, K.W. (1977). Disturbances of bile acid metabolism in intestinal disorders. *Clin. Gastroenterol.*, **6**, 69–89
6. Aldini, R., Roda, A., Festi, D., Mazzella, G., Morselli, A.M., Sama, C., Roda, E., Scopinaro, N. and Barbara, L. (1982). Diagnostic value of serum primary bile acids in detecting bile acid malabsorption. *Gut*, **23**, 829–34
7. Sheltawy, M.J. and Losowsky, M.S. (1975). Determination of faecal bile acids by an en-

zymatic method. *Clin. Chim. Acta*, **64**, 127–32

8.   van Blankenstein, M., Hoyset, T., Horschner, P., Frenkel, M. and Wilson, J.H.P. (1977). Faecal bile acid radioactivity, a sensitive and relatively simple test of ileal dysfunction. *Neth. J. Med.*, **20**, 248–52

9.   Boyd, G.S., Merrick, M.V., Monks, R. and Thomas, I.L. (1981). Se-75-labelled bile acid analogues, new radiopharmaceuticals for investigating the enterohepatic circulation. *J. Nucl. Med.*, **22**, 720–5

10. Merrick, M.V., Eastwood, M.A., Anderson, J.R. and Ross, H. McL. (1982). Enterohepatic circulation in man of a gamma-emitting bile-acid conjugate, 23-selena-25-homotaurocholic acid (SeHCAT). *J. Nucl. Med.*, **23**, 126–30

11. Delhez, H., van den Berg, J.W.O., van Blankenstein, M. and Meerwaldt, J.H. (1982). New method for the determination of bile acid turnover using ^{75}Se-homocholic acid taurine. *Eur. J. Nucl. Med.*, **7**, 269–71

12. Merrick, M.V., Boyd, G.S., Eastwood, M.A. and Monks, R. (1982). SeHCAT – a new radiopharmaceutical for evaluating ileal function and the enterohepatic circulation of bile acids. In *Proceedings of the Third World Congress of Nuclear Medicine and Biology*. Vol. III, pp. 2430–33. (Paris: Pergamon Press)

13. Galatola, G., Jazrawi, R.P., Bridges, C., Joseph, A.E. and Northfield, T.C. (1986). First pass ileal clearance of bile acid in man. *Clin. Sci.*, **13**, 71p

14. Ferraris, R., Bridges, C., Jazrawi, R. and Northfield, T.C. (1983). Comparison of different methods of using gamma-labelled bile acid as a test of ileal function. *Clin. Sci.*, **64**, 14p

15. Ludgate, S.M. and Merrick, M.V. (1985). The pathogenesis of post-irradiation chronic diarrhoea: measurement of SeHCAT and B$_{12}$ absorption for differential diagnosis determines treatment. *Clin. Radiol.*, **36**, 275–8

16. Soundy, R.G., Simpson, J.D., Ross, H.McL. and Merrick, M.V. (1982). Absorbed dose to man from the Se-75 labelled conjugated bile salt SeHCAT: concise communication. *J. Nucl. Med.*, **23**, 157–61

17. Warner, G.T. and Oliver, R. (1966). A whole-body counter in clinical measurements utilising the 'shadow-shield' technique. *Phys. Med. Biol.*, **11**, 83–94

18. Nyhlin, H., Merrick, M.V., Eastwood, M.A. and Brydon, W.G. (1983). Evaluation of ileal function using 23-selena-25-homotaurocholate, a gamma-labelled conjugated bile acid. *Gastroenterology*, **84**, 63–8

19. Merrick, M.V., Eastwood, M.A. and Ford, M.J. (1985). Is bile acid malabsorption underdiagnosed? An evaluation of accuracy of diagnosis by measurement of SeHCAT retention. *Br. Med. J.*, **290**, 665–8

20. Fagan, E.A., Chadwick, V.S. and Baird, I. McL. (1983). SeHCAT absorption: a simple test of ileal dysfunction. *Digestion*, **26**, 159–65

21. Scheurlen, C., Kruis, W., Bull, U., Stellaard, F., Lang, P. and Paumgartner, G. (1986). Comparison of ^{75}SeHCAT retention half-life and faecal content of individual bile acids in patients with chronic diarrhoeal disorders. *Digestion*, **35**, 102–8

22. Sciarretta, G., Vicini, G., Fagioli, G., Verri, A., Ginevra, A. and Malaguti, P. (1986). Use of 23-selena-25-homocholyltaurine to detect bile acid malabsorption in patients with ileal dysfunction or diarrhoea. *Gastroenterology*, **91**, 1–9

23. Thaysen, E.H., Orholm, M., Arnfred, T., Carl, J. and Rodbro, P. (1982). Assessment of ileal function by abdominal counting of the retention of a gamma emitting bile acid analogue. *Gut*, **23**, 862–65

24. Freundlieb, O., Szy, D., Balzer, K. and Strotges, M.W. (1983). Comparative study of various methods of measuring bile acid loss using ^{75}SeHCAT. *Nucl. Med.*, **22**, 258–61

25. Hames, T.K., Condon, B.R., Fleming, J.S., Phillips, G., Holdstock, G., Smith, C.L., Howlett, P.J. and Ackery, D.M. (1984). A comparison between the use of a shadow shield whole body counter and an uncollimated gamma camera in the assessment of the seven-day retention of SeHCAT. *Br. J. Radiol.*, **57**, 581–4

26. Holdstock, G., Phillips, G., Hames, T.K., Condon, B.R., Fleming, J.S., Smith, C.L. and

Ackery, D.M. (1985). Potential of SeHCAT retention as an indicator of terminal ileal involvement in inflammatory bowel disease. *Eur. J. Nucl. Med.*, **10**, 528–30

27. Sciarretta, G., Fagioli, G., Furno, A., Vicini, G., Cecchetti, L., Grigolo, B., Verri, A. and Malaguti, P. (1987). [75]SeHCAT test in the detection of bile acid malabsorption in functional diarrhoea and its correlation with small bowel transit. *Gut*, **28**, 970–5

24
Gallbladder Retention of ^{75}SeHCAT

R. Ferraris
Department of Gastroenterology
Ospedale Mauriziano
Torino, Italy
and
Department of Medicine
St. George's Hospital Medical School
London, SW17 0RE, UK

INTRODUCTION

^{75}Se homocholic acid taurine (SeHCAT) is a synthetic gamma labelled bile acid that best fulfils the criteria of a substance suitable for investigating distal ileal function in man[1]. SeHCAT is exclusively absorbed by the active transport site in the terminal ileum[2], since its pK is lower than the physiological intestinal pH and since it is poorly deconjugated by the intestinal bacteria. It is then resecreted in bile.

Early methods of using SeHCAT include faecal excretion and abdominal or whole body retention measurements[3-6]. These methods are inaccurate, since they include as still within the enterohepatic circulation (EHl) unabsorbed SeHCAT that is retained in the colon for an unpredictable period of time before being excreted from the body.

Improved methods have been recently proposed[7] which use a faecal marker, or direct measurement of SeHCAT in the enterohepatic circulation by gallbladder gamma camera scanning. We discuss here the development, validation and clinical performance of the gallbladder retention method.

Development of the Gallbladder Retention Method

SeHCAT, as a gamma emitting bile acid, allows for the first time visualisation of the EHC by external gamma camera scanning over the abdomen[7,11]. Northfield's group in London[7,12] examined sequential gamma camera scans taken at 1 minute intervals for 30–60 minutes following oral ingestion. SeHCAT passed first into the small intestine, but then an area of activity started to appear in the right upper abdomen, indicating intestinal absorption, hepatic secretion and gallbladder storage of SeHCAT. After a subsequent overnight fast, activity concentrated largely over the gallbladder area. Gallbladder activity measured on successive mornings in the fasting state decreased in an exponential manner[2]

We therefore used the gamma camera computer system to delineate the gallbladder as an area of interest separate from the rest of the abdomen, and thus to quantitate daily ileal absorption efficiency for SeHCAT from the rate of its disappearance from the gallbladder area on successive days in the fasting state. We considered that this method would directly reflect SeHCAT retention in the EHC, independently of colonic retention of the isotope, since a constant proportion of the fasting SeHCAT pool[2,9], and of the total bile acid pool[10], lies in the gallbladder on successive mornings and since colonic SeHCAT cannot recycle to the gallbladder because of negligable deconjugation by colonic bacteria.

The SeHCAT was given by mouth at 5.00 p.m., and collimated gamma camera abdominal scans taken over 5–7 successive mornings in the fasting state. The gallbladder counts were calculated following correction for geometry and isotope decay. Our initial method involved 25 μCi of SeHCAT[7], but 10 μCi proved sufficient if $^{51}CrCl_3$ was not used as a colonic marker[15].

SeHCAT half life ($t_{1/2}$) was derived from the slope K of the observed disappearance curve of SeHCAT over the gallbladder area ($t_{1/2} = \ln 2/K$). K represents the fractional turnover rate for SeHCAT in the enterohepatic circulation.

Validation of the Gallbladder Retention Method

We compared the fractional turnover rates of ^{14}C-cholic acid taurine and SeHCAT, both measured using the classical Lindstedt technique (involving subsequent gallbladder bile sampling[16]), with the SeHCAT $t_{1/2}$ using gallbladder scintigraphy in five healthy volunteers. In each subject, $t_{1/2}$ values were similar with each of the three techniques. This indicates that the scintigraphic method does measure the biological $t_{1/2}$ of SeHCAT in the EHC and may provide for the first time a non-invasive method of measuring the fractional turnover rate of bile acid in man[11,14].

Diagnostic Value in Detecting Distal Ileal Disease

SeHCAT whole-body or abdominal retention methods have proved valuable in clinical practice[4,5,15], even though they are less accurate than the gallbladder method for detecting bile acid malabsorption as they do not correct for colonic retention method.

302

Sciarretta *et al.*[15] have, for instance, reported a 94% sensitivity and 100% specificity for their 3–day abdominal retention method in detecting patients with bile acid malabsorption. The high sensitivity they reported may be because 33 out of the 36 patients studied had had an ileal resection – which invariably resulted in a positive test in two other studies[12,16].

In order to define further the diagnostic value of the SeHCAT gallbladder method in detecting terminal ileum disease we are performing a clinical study in Turin. A total of 59 subjects have been studied so far. All of them had radiology of the terminal ileum, a SeHCAT test using the gallbladder method and a 4th day total abdominal retention scan. We used a cut off value for SeHCAT $t_{1/2}$ of 2.3 days to calculate sensitivity and specificity. This value represented our lower limit of normal.

Table 1 Results of SeHCAT $t_{1/2}$ by the gallbladder gamma camera method

Patients	No	$t_{1/2}$ Mean ($\pm$SD)		Altered tests
Ileal resection	8	0.15	(0.2)	8
Ileal Crohn's disease	20	1.65	(1.2)	16
Ulcerative colitis	11	3.7	(1.2)	1
Coeliac disease	4	6.2	(3.1)	0
Controls	16	3.5	(2.0)	1

Table 2 Diagnostic value of the SeHCAT gallbladder (GB) gamma camera method as compared with the total abdominal retention method (4th day) in the same patients

Diagnostic values	GB method	4th day retention
Sensitivity	86%	59%
Specificity	93%	92%
Predictive values:		
Positive	92%	89%
Negative	88%	68%

The disease patients included 8 with ileal resection and 20 with various degrees of Crohn's disease of the terminal ileum. The control patients with normal radiology included 16 with abdominal pain and normal bowel habit, 11 with ulcerative colitis and 4 with untreated coeliac disease.

Preliminary results derived from this study are reported in Tables 1 and 2. Patients with ileal disease tended to have reduced $t_{1/2}$, and patients with colonic disease a normal $t_{1/2}$. Interestingly, patients with coeliac disease had a SeHCAT $t_{1/2}$ higher than normal as expected from their sluggish EHC[17]. An altered SeHCAT $t_{1/2}$ had a 92% probability of indicating disease of the terminal ileum, and a normal SeHCAT $t_{1/2}$ indicated an 88% probability of a normal terminal ileum.

Since these preliminary predictive values are based on an unusual population with a 47% prevalence of terminal ileal disease, they must be applied more generally with caution. There has been no study of the performance of the test in a population more typical of a standard gastroenterological department, where the test is used for diagnosis. A Bayesian approach to this problem would be most helpful. A computer simulation[18] by assuming a 10% prevalence of terminal ileal disease in a standard gastroenterology department suggests that the positive predictive value of SeHCAT test might fall from 92% to 60%.

Clinical Value in Obscure Diarrhoea

The SeHCAT is unlikely to replace radiology as the first test in the detection of terminal ileal disease. It can, however, be best used to detect bile acid malabsorption in patients with diarrhoea and normal terminal ileal radiology[12,15,19,20].

Merrick *et al.*[19] found a positive SeHCAT retention test in 5 out of 42 patients suffering from diarrhoea who were thought to have 'irritable bowel syndrome'. Since the faecal weight was not measured in these patients, the study gives no estimate of the incidence of bile acid malabsorption in patients with confirmed diarrhoea.

We have studied 14 patients with obscure diarrhoea – defined as an increase in faecal wet weight (> 600 g/72 h) and in bowel frequency, with normal colonic and small intestinal radiology, histology and colonoscopy, and no gastrointestinal or systemic condition likely to explain the diarrhoea. The SeHCAT gallbladder $t_{1/2}$ test was reduced in 9 out of the 14 patients indicating bile acid malabsorption. These patients responded to cholestyramine administration with a reduction in faecal wet weight and bowel frequency.

Bile acid malabsorption may be more frequent than generally realised. It may reflect minimal ileal dysfunction, decreased small intestinal transit time or increased bile acid recyling frequency as recently shown[8].

Particular Applications of SeHCAT

The SeHCAT test has been used with success in order to elucidate the mechanism of diarrhoea after cholecystectomy[15], pelvic irradiation[22], excessive alcohol intake[23], or systemic sclerosis[24]. The SeHCAT gallbladder method has been used to evaluate bile acid absorption in patients with a surgically constructed ileal pouch for ileoanal anastomosis[25], most of whom had an abnormal SeHCAT $t_{1/2}$ indicating bile acid malabsorption.

We have used the SeHCAT test to evaluate bile acid absorption in six patients with Crohn's colitis and an intact terminal ileum in radiology. All of them showed a normal SeHCAT $t_{1/2}$ indicating a functioning terminal ileum at least as far as bile acid absorption function is concerned. Others have reported contrasting results[26] and it is clear that bile acid malabsorption is not a constant feature in Crohn's colitis.

SUMMARY

An improved SeHCAT test which is independent of the colonic retention of the isotope has been developed. The SeHCAT disappearance from the gallbladder area over successive mornings in the fasting state by gamma camera measures the biological $t_{1/2}$ of the isotope in the enterohepatic circulation and mirrors the behaviour of the natural bile acid.

SeHCAT $t_{1/2}$ by the gallbladder gamma camera method has a similar specificity but a higher sensitivity than abdominal retention methods in detecting distal ileal diseases. However, caution must be exercised when interpreting the available data on the diagnostic value of SeHCAT. The positive predictive value of the test may be unsatisfactory when the test is being used routinely in a standard gastroenterological department.

The high incidence of altered SeHCAT results in patients with obscure diarrhoea suggests bile acid malabsorption, possibly reflecting minimal ileal dysfunction, increased small intestine transit time or increased bile acid recycling frequency.

REFERENCES

1. Fromm, H., Thomas, P.J. and Hofmann, A.F. (1973). Sensitivity and specificity in tests of distal ileal function: prospective comparison of bile acid and vitamin B_{12} absorption in ileal resection patients. *Gastroenterology*, **64**, 1077–90
2. Ferraris, R., Jazrawi, R. and Northfield, T.C. (1984). Bile acid kinetics using a new gamma labelled bile acid. *Clin Sci*, **66**, 12p
3. Van Blankenstein, M., Van Den Berg, J.W.O., de Groot, R. and Delhez, H. (1981). Radioisotopes in testing ileal function. *Br. J. Radiol.*, **54**, 702
4. Thaysen, E.H., Orholm, M., Arnfred, T., Carl, J. and Rodbro, P. (1982). Assessment of ileal function by abdominal counting of the retention of a gamma emitting bile acid analogue. *Gut*, **23**, 862–5
5. Nyhlin, H., Merrick, M.V., Eastwood, M.A. and Brydon, W.G. (1983). Evaluation of ileal function using 23-selena-25-homotaurocholate, a gamma labelled conjugated bile acid. Initial clinical assessment. *Gastroenterology*, **84**, 63–8
6. Dehlez, H., Van Den Berg, J.W.O., Van Blankenstein, M. and Maarwaldt, J.H. (1982). New method for the determination of bile acid turnover using 75-SeHCAT. *Eur. J. Nucl. Med.*, **7**, 269–71
7. Ferraris, R., Jazrawi, R., Bridges, C. and Northfield, T.C. (1986). Use of a gamma labelled bile acid (75-SeHCAT) as a test of ileal function. Methods of improving accuracy. *Gastroenterology*, **90**, 1129–36
8. Northfield, T.C., Jazrawi, R. and Galatola, G. (1986). Behaviour of the gamma labelled bile acid 75-SeHCAT in the enterohepatic circulation in man. In Malaguti, P. and Sciarretta, G. (eds) *New Radioisotope Tests in Gastroenterology*, pp. 6–11 (Masson Press)
9. Jazrawi, R., Lanzini, A., Britten, A., Meller, S.T. and Northfield, T.C. (1984). Dynamics of gallbladder function and of enterohepatic circulation studies by labelled bile acid.

Clin. Sci., **66**, 10P

10. Jazrawi, R., Kupfer, R.M., Bridges, C., Joseph, A.E. and Northfield, T.C. (1983). Assessment of gallbladder storage function in man. *Clin. Sci.*, **65**, 185–91

11. Jazrawi, R.P., Ferraris, R., Bridges, C. and Northfield, T.C. (1988). Kinetics for the synthetic bile acid [75]SeHCAT in man: Comparison with ^{14}C-taurocholate. *Gastroenterology* (In press)

12. Ferraris, R. (1986). 75-SeHCAT gallbladder retention in ileal dysfunction and diarrhoea. In Malaguti, P. and Sciarretta, G. (eds) *New Radioisotope Tests in Gastroenteroloy*, pp. 41–44 (Masson Press)

13. Lindstedt, S. (1957). The turnover of cholic acid in man. *Acta Physiol. Scand.*, **40**, 1–9

14. Ferraris,, R., Jazrawi, R., Bridges, C. and Northfield, T.C. (1985). Bile acid turnover using SeHCAT. In Barbara, L., Dowling, R.H., Hofmann, A.F., Roda, E. (eds) *Recent Advances in Bile Acid Research*, pp. 81–82. (New York: Raven Press)

15. Sciarretta, G., Vicini, G., Fagioli, G., Verri, A., Ginevra, A. and Malaguti, P. (1986). Use of 23-Selena-25-homocholyl taurine to detect bile acid malabsorption in patients with ileal dysfunction or diarrhoea. *Gastroenterology*, **91**, 1–9

16. Jazrawi, R., Ferraris, R. and Northfield, T.C. (1986). Daily ileal absorption efficiency for 75-SeHCAT in ileal dysfunction and diarrhoea. In Malaguti, P. and Sciarretta, G. (eds) *New Radioisotope Tests in Gastroenterology*, pp. 33–40 (Masson Press)

17. Low-Beer, T.S., Heaton, K.W., Heaton, S.T. and Read, A.E. (1971). Gallbladder inertia and sluggish enterohepatic circulation of bile salts in coeliac disease. *Lancet*, **1**, 991–94

18. Ferraris, R., Colombatti, G., Fiorentini, M.T., Arossa, W. and De La Pierre, M. (1983). Diagnostic value of serum bile acids and routine liver function tests in hepatobiliary diseases; sensitivity, specificity and predictive value. *Dig. Dis. Sci.*, **28**, 129–36

19. Merrick, M.V., Eastwood, M.A. and Ford, M.J. (1985). Is bile acid malabsorption underdiagnosed? An evaluation of accuracy of diagnosis by measurment of SeHCAT retention. *Br. Med. J.*, **290**, 665–8

20. Hardison, W.G. (1986). Technology illuminates a shadowy syndrome. *Gastroenterology*, **91**, 242–9

21. De La Pierre, M., Barlotta, A., Ferraris, R. and Rolfo, P. (1986). ^{14}C-Xylose breath test. In Malaguti, P. and Sciarretta, G. (eds). *New Radioisotope Tests in Gastroenterology*, pp. 62–5 (Masson Press)

22. Merrick, M.V. (1986). The clinical value of the SeHCAT retention test. In Malaguti, P. and Sciarretta, G. (eds) *New Radioisotope Tests in Gastroenterology*, pp. 14–19 (Masson Press)

23. Centi Colella, A., Liberatore, M., Scopinaro, F. and Valentini, G.L. (1986). Changes of 75SeHCAT whole body retention (WBR) induced by alcohol. In Malaguti, P. and Sciarretta, G. (eds) *New Radioisotope Tests in Gastroenterology*, pp. 20–1 (Masson Press)

24. Bagni, B., Pazzi, P., Putinati, S., Feggi, L.M., Prandini, N. and Trotta, F. (1986). Diagnostic value of 75SeHCAT abdominal retention in detecting malabsorption in patients with systemic sclerosis. In Malaguti, P. and Sciarretta, G. (eds) *New Radioisotope Tests in Gastroenterology*, pp. 31–2

25. Fiorentini, M.T., Locatelli, L., Ceccopieri, B., Bertolino, F., Ostellino, O., Barlotta, A., Rolfo, P., Ferraris, R., De La Pierre, M. and Dellepiane, M. (1987). Physiology of ileoanal anastomosis with ileal reservoir for ulcerative colitis and adenomatosis coli. *Dis Colon Rectum*, **30**, 267–72

26. Bracco, E., Argiro, G., Antonacci, P., Castellano, G., Podio, V. and Sategna-Guidetti, C. (1986). Assessment of ileal function by 75SeHCAT retention test. In Malaguti, P. and Sciarretta, G. (eds) *New Radioisotope Tests in Gastroenterology*, pp. 27–8 (Masson Press)

27. Hofmann, A. (1986). Bile acid absorption and malabsorption: state of the art. In Malaguti, P. and Sciarretta, G. (eds) *New Radioisotope Tests in Gastroenterology*, pp. 3–5 (Masson Press)

Index